Biologically Based Methods for Cancer Risk Assessment

NATO ASI Series

Advanced Science Institutes Series

A series presenting the results of activities sponsored by the NATO Science Committee, which aims at the dissemination of advanced scientific and technological knowledge, with a view to strengthening links between scientific communities.

The series is published by an international board of publishers in conjunction with the NATO Scientific Affairs Division

A	Life Sciences	Plenum Publishing Corporation
B	Physics	New York and London
C	Mathematical and Physical Sciences	Kluwer Academic Publishers
		Dordrecht, Boston, and London
D	Behavioral and Social Sciences	
E	Applied Sciences	
F	Computer and Systems Sciences	Springer-Verlag
G	Ecological Sciences	Berlin, Heidelberg, New York, London,
H	Cell Biology	Paris, and Tokyo

Recent Volumes in this Series

Volume 156—Animal Sonar: Processes and Performance
edited by Paul E. Nachtigall and Patrick W. B. Moore

Volume 157—Plasma Membrane Oxidoreductases in Control of Animal and Plant Growth
edited by Frederick L. Crane, D. James Morré, and Hans Löw

Volume 158—Biocompatibility of Co-Cr-Ni Alloys
edited by Hartmut F. Hildebrand and Maxime Champy

Volume 159—Biologically Based Methods for Cancer Risk Assessment
edited by Curtis C. Travis

Volume 160—Early Influences Shaping the Individual
edited by Spyros Doxiadis

Volume 161—Research in Congenital Hypothyroidism
edited by F. Delange, D. A. Fisher, and D. Glinoer

Volume 162—Nematode Identification and Expert System Technology
edited by Renaud Fortuner

Series A: Life Sciences

Biologically Based Methods for Cancer Risk Assessment

Edited by

Curtis C. Travis

Oak Ridge National Laboratory
Oak Ridge, Tennessee

Plenum Press
New York and London
Published in cooperation with NATO Scientific Affairs Division

Proceedings of a NATO Advanced Research Workshop on
Biologically Based Methods for Cancer Risk Assessment,
held June 11–16, 1988,
in Corfu, Greece

Library of Congress Cataloging in Publication Data

NATO Advanced Research Workshop on Biologically Based Methods for Cancer
Risk Assessment (1988: Kerkyra, Greece)
    Biologically based methods for cancer risk assessment.

    (NATO ASI series. Series A, Life sciences; vol. 159)
    'Proceedings of a NATO Advanced Research Workshop on Biologically Based
Methods for Cancer Risk Assessment, held June 11–16, 1988, in Corfu, Greece—
T.p. verso.
    "Published in cooperation with NATO Scientific Affairs Division."
    Includes bibliographies and index.
    1. Carcinogenicity testing—Congresses. 2. Health risk assessment—Con-
gresses. I. Travis, C. C. II. North Atlantic Treaty Organization. Scientific Affairs
Division. III. Title. IV. Series: NATO advanced science institutes series. Series A,
Life sciences; v. 159. [DNLM: 1. Carcinogens—congresses. 2. Neoplasms—
chemically induced—congresses. 3. Risk Factors—congresses. QZ 202 N2784b
1988]
RC268.65.N36   1988   616.99′4075   88-35675
ISBN 0-306-43117-3

© 1989 Plenum Press, New York
A Division of Plenum Publishing Corporation
233 Spring Street, New York, N.Y. 10013

Printed in the United States of America

PREFACE

"Biologically Based Methods for Cancer Risk Assessment", an Advanced Research Workshop, (ARW) sponsored by the North Atlantic Treaty Organization (NATO) was held in Corfu, Greece in June, 1989. The intent of the workshop was to survey available pharmacokinetic and pharmacodynamic methods in cancer risk assessment and identify methodological gaps and research needs for biologically based methods in cancer risk assessment. Incorporation of such methods represents one of the most challenging areas for risk assessment. The workshop included an international group of invited experts in the field and provided for a dynamic exchange of ideas and accomplishments.

Some of the major topics discussed were:

* Inventory of available pharmacokinetic and pharmacodynamic methods for cancer risk assessment.

* Identification of methodology gaps and research needs in biologically based methods in cancer risk assessment.

* Development of a general framework to guide future cancer risk assessment research.

This book is a compilation of the papers presented at the workshop and is intended to provide guidance for future research to reduce uncertainties in the cancer risk assessment process.

The primary sponsorship of this ARW by NATO and the advice and cooperation of Dr. C. Sinclair of the Scientific affairs Division are gratefully acknowledged. Acknowledgement is also given to the National Science Foundation for its support.

The organization of the ARW and the preparation of this book have required considerable help from many other sources. I owe special gratitude to the co-director, Dr. Vincent Covello, and to the many lecturers and participants who shared their knowledge and expertise to help make the ARW a scientifically stimulating and socially enjoyable workshop and last but not least to my assistant, Mary Oran.

Curtis C. Travis

CONTENTS

INTRODUCTION

BIOLOGICAL BASES FOR CANCER MODELS

INTERSPECIES EXTRAPOLATION OF PHARMACOKINETICS

PROMOTION AS A FACTOR IN CARCINOGENESIS

SCREENING FOR CARCINOGENESIS

CANCER RISK ASSESSMENT

RESEARCH NEEDS FOR BIOLOGICALLY BASED RISK ASSESSMENT

Curtis C. Travis

Office of Risk Analysis
Oak Ridge National Laboratory
Oak Ridge, Tennessee 37831-6109

INTRODUCTION

Because of gaps in our current scientific understanding of the cancer-causing process, human risk assessment for chemicals which have demonstrated carcinogenicity in rodents requires the use of a series of judgmental decisions on numerous unresolved scientific issues. Major assumptions are based on the necessity to extrapolate experimental results (1) across species from mice or rats to humans, (2) from the high-dose regions to which animals are exposed in the laboratory to the low-dose regions to which humans are exposed in the environment, and (3) across routes of administration.

Development of tools and methodologies which can help evaluate the scientific bases of these assumptions will reduce the uncertainties in the risk assessment process. A recent development in the cancer risk area is the advent of biologically based pharmacokinetic and pharmacodynamic models. Pharmacokinetic models relate applied dose to effective dose at target tissue, while pharmacodynamic models relate effective dose with biological effect. We will look at each of these areas in turn.

PHARMACOKINETIC MODELING

Pharmacokinetics is the study of the absorption, distribution, metabolism, and elimination of chemicals in man and animals. Predictive, biologically based pharmacokinetic models provide an effective approach for interpreting empirical data relating to pharmacokinetics (Ramsey and Andersen, 1984; Andersen et al., 1987; Reitz et al., 1987; Travis, 1987; Paustenbach et al., 1988; Reitz et al., 1988;

1

Ward et al., 1988). These models utilize actual physiological parameters of the experimental animals such as breathing rates, blood flow rates, tissue volumes, etc., to describe the metabolic process. These models can often quantitatively relate exposure concentrations (in air, water, or food) to concentrations of parent compound or metabolite in various tissues of the body, allowing prediction of the relationship between applied dose of a chemical and effective dose at the target tissue(s). A chief advantage of the pharmacokinetic model is that by simply using the appropriate physiological, biochemical, and metabolic parameters, the same model can describe the dynamics of chemical transport and metabolism in mice, rats, and humans.

PHARMACODYNAMIC MODELING

Biologically based pharmacodynamic models relate fundamental cellular processes to the epidemiology of cancer in animal and human populations. Several authors have developed pharmacodynamic models based on the assumption that normal cells require two genetic alterations to become cancer cells (Moolgavkar et al., 1980; Moolgavkar et al., 1981; Cohen et al., 1983; Ellwein and Cohen, 1986; Moolgavkar, 1986; Thorslund et al. 1987; Ellwein and Cohen, 1988). These genetic alterations are rare and result from a mutation, translocation, or other event on a specific gene. (It is estimated that the background rate of such genetic events in Fischer rat liver is about 1 per 10 million cell divisions.) A cell which has undergone a single genetic alteration is termed initiated. An initiated cell is not malignant, nor will it necessarily progress to malignancy. Initiated cells expand through clonal proliferation to form islands (foci) of initiated cells. When one of these initiated cells undergoes a second genetic alteration, a cancer cell is formed. The vast majority of initiated cells never undergo a second genetic alteration to become cancerous.

This process is most clearly seen in rat liver (Scherer and Emmelot, 1976). Initiated cells are arranged in foci of hepatocytes displaying alterations in phenotype which can be identified by histochemical staining. Initiated cells have higher rates of proliferation than normal hepatocytes. (In control Fischer rats, initiated cells can proliferate at up to 80 times faster than normal hepatocytes). Consider the case of the carcinogen diethylnitrosamine (DEN). A single dose of DEN to rats produces a reproducible number of foci in the liver (each island representing one originally initiated cell). Figure 1 shows the number of foci in rat liver as a function of time after induction by a single dose of 10 mg DEN/kg in rats partially hepatectomized 24 hours previously. The partial hepatectomy is performed to induce cellular proliferation so that all initiated cells will be clonally expanded into visible foci. The number of foci remains constant from the sixth week after induction. Figure 2 presents the dose-response curve for island induction. There is a direct proportionality between the number of foci induced and dose of DEN. These data indicate a consistency and predictability in the early stages of the cancer process. Ongoing research in the pharmacodynamic area is attempting to quantitatively relate the age-specific incidence of initiated cells in rat liver to the age-specific incidence of hepatocellular carcinomas. It is hoped that insights gained from experience with liver carcinogenesis will enable identification of the proper experimental research necessary to understand pharmacodynamics and assist in producing more realistic estimates of risk associated with exposure to environmental carcinogens.

SPECIFIC RESEARCH NEEDS

Biologically based pharmacokinetic and pharmacodynamic models provide the means to develop a defensible methodology to evaluate the low-dose risk of chemical carcinogens. However, several methodological gaps and research needs must be filled before these models can be fully implemented into the risk assessment process. The workshop identified several high priority research needs.

PHARMACOKINETICS

1. PHARMACOKINETIC MODEL DEVELOPMENT. Evaluate the effect of model structure on model output; perform uncertainty and sensitivity analysis to identify most important model parameters; develop user-friendly models to encourage wider participation in modeling efforts.

2. REFERENCE PHARMACOKINETIC PARAMETERS. Develop a standarized list of mouse, rat and human physiological parameters (breathing rates, blood flow rates, tissue volumes, etc.) for use in pharmacokinetic modeling.

3. IN VIVO METABOLISM IN ANIMALS. Perform laboratory experiments to identify metabolic pathways and yields for chemicals of interest. These data would be the basis for development of pharmacokinetic models for specific chemicals; study pharmacokinetics of binary mixtures.

4. IN VITRO/IN VIVO EXTRAPOLATION OF METABOLIC PARAMETERS. Determine in vitro metabolic rates in animal and human tissues for specific compounds; predict human metabolic rates from in vitro/in vivo relationships; validate the use of in vitro/in vivo extrapolations.

5. PHARMACOKINETICS AT LOW EXPOSURES. Current use of pharmacokinetic models for low-dose extrapolation assumes tissue/blood partition coefficients remain constant over

the entire range of exposure levels. Recent evidence for benzene indicates that this is not true. Experimental research is needed to explore this area.

6. ROUTE-TO-ROUTE EXTRAPOLATIONS. Determine the effect of route of administration on dose to target tissue.

7. NONCARCINOGENIC ENDPOINTS. Determine the relationship between dose to target tissue and such noncarcinogenic endpoints as neurotoxicity and systemic toxicity.

PHARMACODYNAMICS

1. MATHEMATICAL MODELS OF PHARMACODYNAMICS. Evaluate the effect of model structure on model output.

2. PHARMACODYNAMIC PARAMETERS. In vivo determination of relevant pharmacodynamic parameters; cell numbers, mitotic rates of normal and initiated cells under different dosing conditions; age-dependent incidence of foci, foci volumes, tumors.

3. MOLECULAR BIOLOGY - DOSE/ADDUCTS RELATIONSHIPS, ONCOGENES ETC. Determine relationship between applied dose, adducts, and probability of initiation and transformation.

4. MODELING OF BACKGROUND LIVER TUMORS IN MICE AND RATS. Apply pharmacodynamic models to data on background foci and liver tumors in mice and rats. Determine background mitotic rates and probability of initiation and transformation; make comparisons between strains and species.

5. MODELING PHARMACODYNAMICS OF KNOWN CARCINOGENS. Apply pharmacodynamic models to data on such known carcinogens as DEN, DMN, Dioxin, etc. Determine effect of pulse and continuous doses on mitotic rates and probability of initiation and transformation.

6. PHARMACODYNAMIC PARAMETERS OF A PROMOTER. Develop necessary in vivo data to relate applied dose, dose to target tissue, mitotic rates of normal and initiated cells, and appearance of tumors in animal bioassays for a promoter. Such data would allow for the first totally biologically based risk assessment for a promoter.

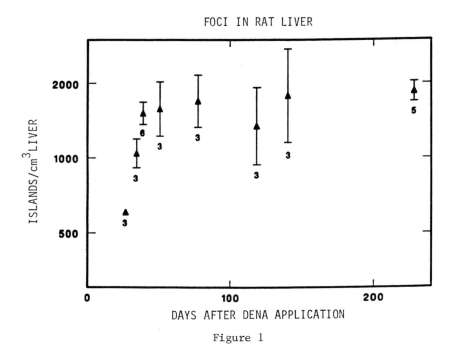

Figure 1

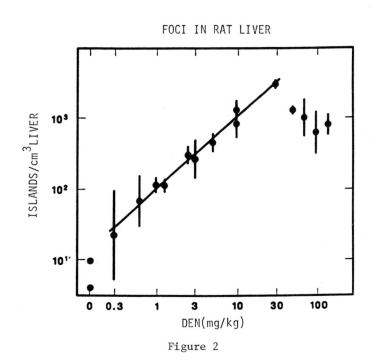

Figure 2

ACKNOWLEDGEMENTS

The primary sponsorship of this ARW by the North Atlantic Treaty Organization, and the advice and cooperation of Dr. C. Sinclair of the Scientific Affairs Division, are gratefully acknowledged. Acknowledgement is also made of support provided by the National Science Foundation.

The organization of the ARW and the preparation of this book have required considerable help from many other sources. I owe my special gratitude to the co-director, Dr. Vincent Covello and to the many lecturers and participants who shared their knowledge and expertise to help make the ARW a scientifically stimulating and socially enjoyable meeting.

REFERENCES

Andersen, M.E., H.J. Clewell, III, M.L. Gargas, F.A. Smith, and R.H. Reitz. (1987). Physiologically based pharmacokinetics and the risk assessment process for methylene chloride. Toxicol. Appl. Pharmacol. 87: 185-205.

Cohen, S.M., R.E. Greenfield, and L.B. Ellwein. (1983). Multistage carcinogenesis in the urinary bladder. Environ. Health Perspectives 49: 202-215.

Ellwein, L.B., and S.M. Cohen. (1986). Modeling of cellular dynamics in carcinogenesis risk assessment. Eppley Institute for Research on Cancer, University of Nebraska. (Unpublished manuscript).

Ellwein, L.B. and S.M. Cohen. (1988). Cellular dynamics model of experimental bladder cancer: Analysis of the effect of sodium saccharin in the rat. Risk Analysis 8: 215-222.

Moolgavkar, S.H., N.E. Day, and R.G. Stevens. (1980). Two-stage model for carcinogenesis: Epidemiology of breast cancer in females. J. National Cancer Institute 65 (3): 559-569.

Moolgavkar, S.H. and A.G. Knudson, Jr. (1981). Mutation and cancer: A model for human carcinogenesis. J. Natl. Cancer Inst. 66: 1037-1052.

Moolgavkar, S.H. (1986). Carcinogenesis modeling: From molecular biology to epidemiology. Ann. Rev. Public Health 7: 151-169.

Moolgavkar, S.H., A. Dewanji and D.J. Venzen. (1988). A stochastic two-stage model for cancer risk assessment I: The hazard function and the probability of tumor. Risk Analysis in press).

Paustenbach, D.J., M.E. Andersen, H.J. Clewell, III, and M.L. Gargas. (1988). A physiologically based pharmacokinetic model for inhaled carbon tetrachloride. <u>Toxicol. Appl. Pharmacol</u>. (in press).

Ramsey, J.C., and M.E. Andersen. (1984). A physiologically based description of the inhalation pharmacokinetics of styrene in rats and humans. <u>Toxicol. Appl. Pharmacol</u>. 73: 159-175.

Reitz, R. H., R.J. Nolan, and A.M. Schumann. (1987). Organohalides. In <u>Proceedings of the National Academy of Science Workshop on Pharmacokinetics</u>, Safe Drinking Water Committee, Subcommittee on Pharmacokinetics, Board on Environmental Studies and Toxicology, National Research Council.

Reitz, R.H., J.N. McDougal, M.W. Himmelstein, R.J. Nolan and A.M. Schumann. (1988). Physiologically-based pharmacokinetic modeling with methylchloroform: implications for interspecies, high dose/low dose and dose route extrapolations. <u>Toxicol. Appl. Pharmacol</u>. (in press).

Scherer, E., and P. Emmelot. (1976). Kinetics of induction and growth of enzyme-deficient islands involved in hepatocarcinogenesis. <u>Cancer Res</u>. 36: 2544-2554.

Thorslund, T.W., C.C. Brown and G. Charnley. (1987). Biologically motivated cancer risk models. <u>Risk Analysis</u> 7: 109-119.

Travis, C.C. (1987). Interspecies and Dose-Route Extrapolations. In <u>Proceedings of the National Academy of Science Workshop on Pharmacokinetics</u>, Safe Drinking Water Committee, Subcommittee on Pharmacokinetics, Board on Environmental Studies and Toxicology, National Research Council.

Ward, R.C., C.C. Travis, D.M. Hetrick, M.W. Andersen, and M.L. Gargas. (1988). Pharmacokinetics of tetrachloroethylene. <u>Toxicol. Appl. Pharmacol</u>. 93: 108-117.

MULTISTAGE MODELS FOR CANCER RISK ASSESSMENT

Suresh H. Moolgavkar

Fred Hutchinson Cancer Research Center
1124 Columbia Street
Seattle, Washington 98104

INTRODUCTION

A biologically realistic quantitative model of carcinogenesis is one component of a scientific approach to cancer risk assessment. The parameters of such a model should have clear interpretation in biological terms and, if their dependence on dose of environmental agent can be measured or inferred, then the model can be used for low-dose and inter-species extrapolation of cancer risk.

In the past inter-species extrapolation has often been based on scaling by body weight or by body surface area. Low-dose extrapolation has been based on the fitting of statistical models to the observed data followed by extrapolation to low doses using the estimated parameters. More recently, a biologically-based model, the Armitage-Doll multistage model (Armitage and Doll, 1954), has been widely used for low-dose extrapolation. The choice of model is rather critical in quantitative cancer risk assessment: while many different models may describe a given set of data adequately, the implications of these models for low-dose extrapolation may be quite different. Thus, it is clear that biologically-based models are to be preferred to statistical descriptions of dose-response. Unfortunately, the Armitage-Doll multistage model has some deficiencies, the most serious of which is that it does not take explicit account of tissue growth and differentiation, which are known to be important in carcinogenesis. Further, current statistical implementation of the model is seriously flawed (Moolgavkar and Dewanji, 1988).

The purpose of my talk is to present a model for carcinogenesis that takes explicit account of recent biological advances in cancer research, and to discuss, in a general way, the implications of this model for environmental carcinogenesis and risk assessment. The model has been shown to be consistent with data from cancer epidemiology and animal experiments in a recent series of papers (e.g., Moolgavkar and Knudson, 1981; Moolgavkar, 1986; Ellwein and Cohen, 1988). Travis and Ellwein (this volume) discuss in some detail experimental hepatocarcinogenesis and bladder carcinogenesis, respectively, within the framework of the model. Wilson (this volume) discusses some implications of the model for quantitative cancer risk assessment.

The process of model building inevitably entails simplification and the making of choices. The model-builder must decide which features of the biological process must be incorporated into the model and which features can be safely ignored. In our current state of knowledge regarding the process of carcinogenesis I believe that the model I shall present here is the most parsimonious model consistent with the facts.

ONCOGENES, ANTIONCOGENES, AND A CANCER MODEL

The basic biological hypothesis underlying the model is that the final common pathway to malignancy is the inappropriate activation of a normally occurring gene belonging to a class of genes called oncogenes. This class of genes was discovered by work on the acutely transforming retroviruses, such as the Rous Sarcoma Virus. Evidence from human epidemiology has implicated another class of genes, the antioncogenes, in human carcinogenesis. Many human cancers occur in two distinct forms, a sporadic form occurring in the general population, and a form that clusters in families, and in which, on pedigree analysis, predisposition to tumor appears to be inherited in an autosomal dominant fashion. Examples are two childhood tumors, retinoblastoma and Wilms' tumor, and an adult tumor, carcinoma of the colon. The gene locus for retinoblastoma is known to be on the long arm of chromosome 13 (band 13q14), tightly linked to the locus for the enzyme esterase D; the gene locus for Wilms' tumor is on the short arm of chromosome 11 (band 11p13), close to the locus for β-globin. Cytogenetic analysis reveals that in many instances of hereditary retinoblastoma and Wilms' tumor, the respective genes are deleted. Thus, in contrast to oncogenes, it is the inappropriate inactivation of these genes that leads to malignancy. Knudson (1985) has coined the term antioncogenes for this class of genes.

A study of the hereditary neoplasms reveals two further facts. First, inheritance of an inactive antioncogene is not sufficient for malignant transformation. In affected individuals, every cell in the target tissue carries the inactivated oncogene; however, only a few of the cells go on to develop malignancy, indicating that at least one other event is necessary for transformation. Second, inheritance of an inactivated antioncogene is the strongest known risk factor for cancer in humans. For example, in non-gene carriers the lifetime risk of retinoblastoma is approximately 1 in 30,000. In contrast, the gene carrier develops three to four tumors on average. Thus, inheritance of the defective gene increases the risk some 100,000-fold (at the level of the target cell, the retinoblast). Similarly, it can be computed that inheritance of the gene for polyposis coli increases the risk for colon cancer some 5,000-fold at age 45.

In 1973, Comings postulated the existence of a genetic regulatory schema involving the oncogenes and antioncogenes (Comings called these regulator genes), the disruption of which would lead to malignancy. Specifically, Comings postulated that all cells contain (tissue-specific) genes capable of coding for transforming factors that can release the cell from normal growth constraints. These oncogenes are expressed during histogenesis and tissue renewal; their expression is controlled by a diploid pair of antioncogenes (regulator genes). Malignant transformation of a cell occurs when the oncogenes are inappropriately turned on and this, in turn, occurs with inactivation of the appropriate (diploid) pair of antioncogenes. This model neatly extends the model proposed by Knudson in 1971 to account for the enormous risk imposed by inheritance of the genes for retinoblastoma and Wilms' tumor. Knudson postulated that two mutations were required for malignant transformation in these cancers, and that the first of these mutations could be either germinal (in the autosomal dominant form of the cancer) or somatic (in the sporadic form of the cancer), whereas the second mutation was always somatic. Thus, according to this model individuals with the gene for retinoblastoma or Wilms' tumor are born with all the cells of the target tissue in the intermediate stage, and only one more mutation is required for malignant transformation. This accounts for the greatly increased risk. Further, the most attractive biological hypothesis is that the two mutations involved in malignant transformation occur at the same locus on homologous chromosomes. Comings' model identified the retinoblastoma and Wilms' tumor genes with genes regulating oncogene function. Recent work in molecular biology leaves little doubt that the salient features of Knudson's model for retinoblastoma and Wilms' tumor are correct (see, e.g., Cavanee et al., 1983; Koufos et al., 1984). However, the normal function of the genes involved is not yet known, and experimental evidence in support of the Comings' model has not yet been obtained.

Knudson and his colleagues showed that a two-mutation model was consistent with the age-specific incidence curves of retinoblastoma and Wilms' tumor (Knudson, 1971; Knudson, Hethcote and Brown, 1975; Hethcote and Knudson, 1978). Later, Moolgavkar and his colleagues showed in a series of papers that, providing the kinetics of tissue growth and differentiation were taken into account, a two-mutation model was consistent with the epidemiology of many human tumors and provided a convenient conceptual framework for interpreting experimental data including the data on initiation-promotion (Moolgavkar and Venzon, 1979; Moolgavkar and Knudson, 1981; Moolgavkar, 1986; Moolgavkar, Dewanji and Venzon, 1988; Dewanji, Venzon and Moolgavkar, 1988).

To recapitulate then, according to the model malignant transformation is due to mutations at each of two homologous antioncogene loci. The first of these mutations is inherited by individuals carrying a dominant cancer gene. These mutations release the oncogenes from normal cellular control and thus lead to cancer. There is evidence, however, that oncogene activation may be brought about directly by, for example, chromosomal translocation as occurs in some leukemias and lymphomas, or by direct mutation of an oncogene that releases it from cellular control. Even in such situations, however, at least two rate-limiting events appear to be necessary for malignant transformation.

The detailed description of a mathematical model that views carcino-genesis as the result of two rare, rate-limiting and (at the level of the cell) heritable events and which incorporates tissue growth and differenti-ation has been presented in previous papers. Figure 1 presents the salient features of the model.

In order to study "dose-response", certain quantities must be derived from the model. For regulatory purposes, the response is often measured in terms of the proportion of animals that develop a particular cancer during a specified period of time. Thus response is measured in terms of the probability of developing a tumor during a specified period of time. In human epidemiology on the other hand, attention is often focussed on the age-specific incidence rate, the appropriate statistical analogue of which is not probability but hazard. The hazard is a measure of the rate at which tumors occur in a previously tumor-free animal. The hazard function completely determines the probability as a function of time, and vice versa, the hazard as a function of time is completely determined by the probability as a function of time. However, it is certainly not true that linearity as a function of dose in one measure of response implies linearity in the other. Further, linearity (as a function of dose) of response at one specified time does not imply linearity at any other time. Thus, for example, if the probability of tumor is found

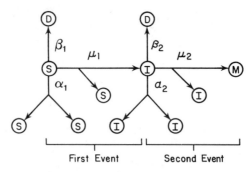

First Event   Second Event

Fig. 1. Two-stage model for carcinogenesis (from Moolgavkar and Knudson, 1981). S = normal stem cell; I = intermediate cell; D = dead or differentiated cell; M = malignant cell. α_1 = rate (per cell per year) of cell division of normal cells; β_2 = rate (per cell per year) of death or differentiation of normal cells; μ_1 = rate (per cell per year) of division into one normal and one intermediate cell. α_2, β_2 and μ_2 are defined similarly. Note that the mutation rate per cell division for normal and intermediate cells is given by $\mu_1/(\alpha_1 + \mu_1)$ and $\mu_2/(\alpha_2 + \mu_2)$, respectively. The rate is to be thought of as the _effective_ mutation rate, i.e., it takes into account host defences such as immune surveillance that may destroy the malignant cell.

to be a linear function of dose one year after exposure, then this certainly does not imply that the probability of tumor will be a linear function of dose a year and a half after exposure.

The hazard function (and thus the probability of tumor) for the model in Figure 1 has been derived in previous papers. The hazard function depends on the mutation rates and on the rates of cell division and differentiation. These, in turn, can be made functions of dose of environmental agents and thus dose-response can be studied within the framework of the model. This is discussed in the next section.

In human populations, the probability of any specific cancer is small, and when the probability of tumor is small, there is a simple approximation to the hazard function predicted by the model. Specifically, the age-specific incidence at age t years per 100,000 individuals per year is given to a good approximation by I(t) × 100,000, where

$$I(t) = \mu_1 \mu_2 \int_0^t X(s) \exp[(\alpha_2 - \beta_2)(t - s)] ds \quad , \tag{1}$$

and X(s) is the (expected) number of susceptible cells at age s in the tissue of interest. This expression is seen to depend on the product of the mutation rates and on the difference $(\alpha_2 - \beta_2)$ so that μ_1, μ_2, α_2 and β_2 are not _individually_ identifiable. The quantity X(s) depends upon $(\alpha_1 - \beta_1)$. For details see the recent paper by Moolgavkar et al.

(1988). Note also that the shape of the age-specific incidence curve is determined by the kinetics of tissue growth and differentiation (as represented by the function X(s) and $\alpha_2 - \beta_2$), whereas the mutation rates determine the overall rates in the population. This simple expression for the hazard function appears to give a good description of the age-specific incidence curves of all human tumors.

In animal experiments, often the probability of tumor is quite large, and the simple approximation given above may no longer be valid. The approximation then overestimates the actual hazard function. For details see Moolgavkar et al. (1988).

ENVIRONMENTAL CARCINOGENESIS, INITIATION AND PROMOTION

According to the model, genetic and environmental factors may influence cancer risk by affecting the mutation rates or the kinetics of growth and differentiation or both. For a discussion of genetic conditions predisposing to cancer within the framework of the model, the reader is referred to some recent papers (Moolgavkar and Knudson, 1981; Knudson and Moolgavkar, 1986).

Recall that in the mathematical formulation of the model, the mutation rates μ_1 and μ_2 are measured per unit time. These mutation rates could be increased by an environmental agent in one of two ways: (1) by direct action on the DNA or (2) by increasing the rate of cell division α_1 or α_2. For any increase in the rate of cell division must result in an increase in the mutation rate per unit time in order that the mutation rate per cell division remain constant.

Any agent that increases the cell division rates α_1 or α_2 or decreases the rates of differentiation β_1 or β_2 will cause an increase in the number of susceptible cells and thus increase the probability of cancer. In particular, any agent that acts on the intermediate stage to increase $\alpha_2 - \beta_2$ will be very effective in increasing the probability of cancer because such an agent will cause an increase in the number of cells that have already sustained the first mutation on the pathway to cancer. In addition, as noted above, any agents that increase α_1 (or α_2) will also increase μ_1 (or μ_2).

The phenomena of initiation and promotion have natural interpretation within the framework of the two-mutation model. There appears to be general consensus that initiators are mutagens and that initiation involves mutation at a specific genetic locus. Thus, within the context of the model, an initiator is any agent that increases the mutation rates μ_1 and μ_2. If the tissue is exposed to an initiator briefly, then the main effect will be to increase the number of cells that have sustained the first mutation, i.e., to increase the pool of intermediate cells by direct mutation of normal cells. Since the number of intermediate cells at any time is small, the probability that one of these will sustain the second mutation and become malignant is vanishingly small. However, with prolonged application of initiator there is a non-negligible probability that one of the cells will sustain both mutations and become malignant. Thus, with prolonged application an initiator is a "complete carcinogen", i.e., the model does not allow for the concept of a 'pure' initiator, unless some agents can preferentially elevate the first mutation rate μ_1 without affecting μ_2. This is biologically plausible only if the nature of the second mutation is quite different from the first. For example, the second mutation may be a deletion of a segment of a chromosome, whereas the first may be a point mutation.

13

The mechanism of promotion is not well understood, and there is some evidence that the process may be further divisible into stages. However, it seems fairly clear that the main effect of promotion is the clonal expansion of initiated cells (Yuspa, 1984). Within the context of the model then a promoter increases α_2 or decreases β_2, or both. In effect, a promoter increases $(\alpha_2 - \beta_2)$ thus increasing the number of intermediate cells and the probability that one of them will sustain the second mutation and become malignant. Examples of visible clones of intermediate cells are provided by the enzyme altered foci in hepatocarcinogenesis experiments and papillomas in skin painting experiments. Putative intermediate lesions in human carcinogenesis are discussed in Moolgavkar and Knudson (1981). In addition, of course, a promoter that increases α_2 will also increase μ_2 as discussed above.

The view initiation-promotion presented above leads to three predictions.

(1) Provided that a metabolically active form of initiator is used, prolonged application should lead to the appearance of malignant tumors (unless the nature of the two mutational events is different). To the best of my knowledge, the existence of a pure initiator has never been convincingly demonstrated.

(2) If it is true that initiation-promotion simply sets the stage for the second genomic event leading to malignancy, then an initiation-promotion-initiation regimen should lead to many more malignant tumors than initiation-promotion alone, which should lead mainly to premalignant lesions (clones of intermediate cells). The initiation-promotion-initiation protocol was suggested on the basis of the model by Moolgavkar and Knudson in 1981. The prediction that this protocol would increase the yield of malignant tumors has recently been verified in mouse skin (Hennings et al., 1983) and in rat liver (Scherer et al., 1984).

(3) If a specific cancer is due to homozygosity at a genomic locus, then any agent that facilitates mitotic recombination should increase the probability of that cancer by increasing μ_2 without increasing μ_1. Indeed, molecular biological techniques (RFLP analysis) have clearly demonstrated that mitotic recombination plays an important role in bringing about homozygosity in retinoblastoma. It is also interesting to note that a recessive condition in humans, Bloom's syndrome, in which there is increased risk of a variety of cancers, is characterized by increased sister chromatid and homologous chromosomal exchanges.

In one experimental system, the liver, enzyme-altered foci, which probably are intermediate lesions, have been carefully studied quantitatively. Thus, information is available on the number and size of such foci under different experimental protocols. In order to analyze these data Dewanji, Venzon and Moolgavkar (1988) derived the corresponding mathematical expressions from the two-mutation model presented here. A study of these mathematical expressions leads to a number of interesting predictions which I would like to briefly discuss.

First, the mean number (expectation) of intermediate cells at time t, denoted by E(t), is given by the expression

$$E(t) = \mu_1 \int_0^t X(s) \; \exp[(\alpha_2 - \beta_2)(t-s)]ds \qquad , \qquad (2)$$

where, for convenience μ_1 is treated as a constant (independent of time), and the other symbols are as in expression (1). By comparing with expression (1) one notes immediately that the approximate hazard function I(t) is simply E(t) multiplied by the second mutation rate μ_2. This result is intuitively appealing. However, while I(t) is only an approximation to the hazard rate, E(t) is the exact expectation. Although I(t) depends only on the product $\mu_1\mu_2$ and on the difference $\alpha_2 - \beta_2$, the exact hazard function (and thus the exact expression for probability of tumor) depends on each of the parameters μ_1, μ_2, α_2 and β_2 individually (see Moolgavkar, Dewanji and Venzon, 1988). In addition the mean number and mean size of intermediate clones depends on μ_1, α_2 and β_2 (Dewanji, Venzon and Moolgavkar, 1988), although the mean number of intermediate cells depends only on μ_1 and $\alpha_2 - \beta_2$ as can be seen in expression (2). Some consequences of these facts are illustrated below.

First, an immediate mathematical consequence of the fact that inter-mediate cells are executing a birth-death process is that there is a non-zero probability that clones of intermediate cells will become extinct, i.e., die out even when β_2, the death rate is smaller than α_2, the birth rate (Figure 2). In fact the probability that an intermediate cell and all its progeny will ultimately die out is given by the ratio β_2/α_2, when $\beta_2 < \alpha_2$. Thus, for example, consider various values of α_2 and β_2 with $\alpha_2 - \beta_2 = 0.2$ a constant. When $\alpha_2 = 0.2$ and $\beta_2 = 0$, the probability that an intermediate cell just produced by mutation and all its daughters will die out is 0; with $\alpha_2 = 0.5$ and $\beta_2 = 0.3$ this probability is 0.6; with $\alpha_2 = 1.0$ and $\beta_2 = 0.8$ this probability is 0.8. In all these examples the mean (expected) number of intermediate cells is the same because this quantity depends only on $\alpha_2 - \beta_2$. One deduces immediately from these facts that, with identical $\alpha_2 - \beta_2$, a high birth rate α_2 leads to a small number of large clones, whereas a low birth rate leads to a large number of small clones (Figure 3). In the examples given above, values of $\alpha_2 = 0.8$ and $\beta_2 = 0.6$ will lead to a smaller mean number of intermediate clones than values of $\alpha_2 = 0.5$, $\beta_2 = 0.3$, but the mean size of the former clones will be larger.

Finally let me recall that the approximate hazard function (and thus the approximate probability of malignant tumor) depends only on the difference $\alpha_2 - \beta_2$. This approximation, however, is poor when probability of malignant tumor is high as in experimental situations. One must then use the exact expressions for the hazard and the probability, and these expressions depend upon α_2 and β_2 individually. Figure 4 shows the behaviour of these exact expressions for $\alpha_2 - \beta_2 = 0.2$ and various values of the pair α_2, β_2. One can see immediately that, whereas the behaviour of the hazards is complicated, at any given time a higher α_2 implies a higher probability of tumor.

To summarize, suppose $\alpha_2 - \beta_2$ is constant (in our examples it is 0.2). Then a high value of α_2 implies a smaller number of larger intermediate clones and a higher probability of malignant tumor when compared to a small value of α_2.

The above facts are simply mathematical consequences of the model. Are there examples of agents that keep $\alpha_2 - \beta_2$ more or less constant but have differential effects on α_2? Recent work by Schwarz et al. (1984, also see this volume) is interesting in this regard. They treated separate groups of female Wistar rats with the hepatocarcinogens 4-dimethylamino-azobenzene (4-DAB) and N-nitrosodiethanolamine (NDEOL), respectively, and studied the effects of these carcinogens on enzyme altered foci and malignant tumors in the liver. To quote from their 1984 abstract, "Treat-ment of rats with either carcinogen alone resulted in similar pattern of increases in the volumetric fraction of liver occupied by ATPase-deficient foci. A differential behaviour, however, was observed with respect to islet size. NDEOL produced large numbers of small foci whereas with 4-DAB

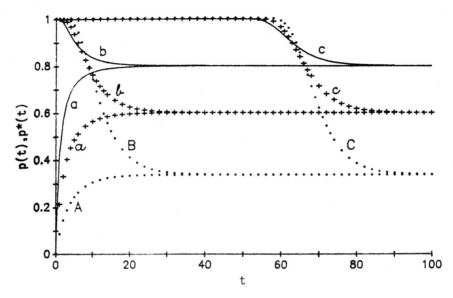

Fig. 2. (From Dewanji, Venzon and Moolgavkar, 1988). Probability of
extinction (p(t)) and non-detection (p*(t)) of premalignant
clones for different values of α_2 and β_2 plotted against time
since appearance of the first cell of the clone. In all plots
$\alpha_2 - \beta_2 = 0.2$; but the values of α_2 and β_2 are individually varied.
The dotted line represents $\alpha_2 = 0.3$ ($\beta_2 = 0.1$); the "+" line
represents $\alpha_2 = 0.5$ ($\beta_2 = 0.3$); the solid line represents $\alpha_2 = 1.0$
($\beta_2 = 0.8$). For each value of α_2, there are three curves. The
curves labelled A, a, α represent the probability of extinction
as a function of time; the curves labelled B, b, ℓ represent
the probability that the clone will be nondetectable when the
threshold size is 10 cells, i.e., the probability that the
clone will never exceed 10 cells in size; the curves labelled
C, c, c represent the probability that the clone will be nondetectable when the threshold size is 10^6 cells.

only few foci were obtained which grew rapidly in the presence of carcinogen." Thus these investigators found that whereas the total number of
intermediate cells were approximately the same with the two treatment
regimens, 4-DAB caused a small number of large foci and NDEOL caused a
large number of small foci. Within the context of the model, the most
parsimonious explanation of this fact is that both carcinogens affect the
kinetics of growth of intermediate cells in such a way that $(\alpha_2 - \beta_2)$ is
similar under both treatments, but α_2 is larger with 4-DAB treatment than
with NDEOL treatment. Further, as discussed above, a consequence of this
is that at any time the probability of malignant tumor is higher (equiva-
lently, the median time to tumor development is lower) with 4-DAB treatment
than with NDEOL treatment (see Figure 4). The findings of Schwarz et al.
confirm this prediction.

CONCLUDING REMARKS

In this paper I have presented a simple model for the process of
carcinogenesis and discussed its implications for environmental carcinogenesis. This model appears to be consistent with much of the experimental

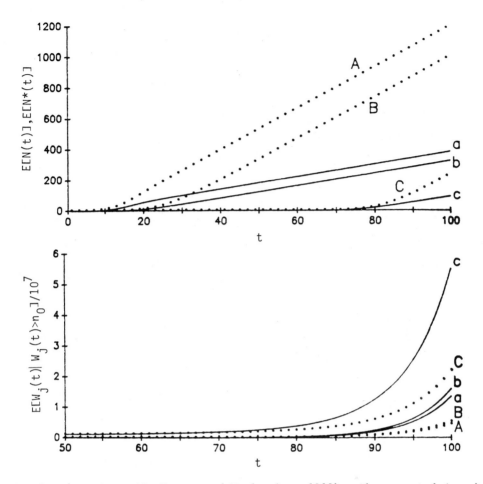

Fig. 3. (From Dewanji, Venzon and Moolgavkar, 1988). The expected (mean) number of non-extinct ($E[N(t)]$) and detectable premalignant clones and their expected (mean) size ($E[W_j(t)|W_j(t) > n_0]$) plotted against time. For all plots, $\mu_1 = 10^{-6}$, $X(s)$ is modelled by a Makeham distribution, the value of $\alpha_2 - \beta_2 = 0.2$ as in Figure 2. The solid line presents $\alpha_2 = 1.0$ ($\beta_2 = 0.8$); the dotted line represents $\alpha_2 = 0.3$ ($\beta_2 = 0.1$). In the upper panel, curves A and a represent the mean number of non-extinct clones; curves B and b represent the mean number of clones with more than 10 cells; curves C and c represent the mean number of clones with more than 10^6 cells. Note that the mean number of clones is smaller with $\alpha_2 = 1.0$ than with $\alpha_2 = 0.3$. In the lower panel curves A and a represent the average size of non-extinct clones; curves B and b represent the average size of clones that are larger than a threshold size of 10 cells; curves C and c represent the average size of clones that are larger than a threshold size of 10^6 cells. Note that the average size of the clones is larger with $\alpha_2 = 1.0$ than with $\alpha_2 = 0.3$.

and epidemiologic data. One of the main purposes of the model is to focus attention on the sorts of data that are needed for rational risk assessment. Not too surprisingly, what is needed is quantitative information on fundamental biological questions. How does the number of stem cells of

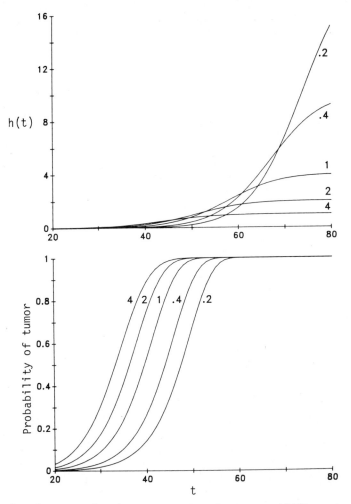

Fig. 4. (From Moolgavkar, Dewanji and Venzon, 1988). The hazard function $h(t)$ and the probability of malignant tumor plotted against time. For all plots $\mu_1 = 10^{-6}$; $X(s)$ is modelled by the Makeham distribution; $\alpha_2 - \beta_2 = 0.2$. The values of α_2 are varied and the curves are labelled by the values of α_2 used. The mutation rate per cell division $\mu_2/(\alpha_2 + \mu_2) = $ constant $= 5 \times 10^{-6}$ for all α_2. Note that the probability of tumor increases with increasing value of α_2; the median time to tumor (time at which probability = 0.5) decreases with increasing α_2. Thus, with $\alpha_2 = 4$, the median time is approximately 32.5 time units; with $\alpha_2 = 0.2$ the median time is approximately 47.5 time units.

a tissue evolve with age? What are the rates of stem cell division and differentiation? What are the locus specific mutation rates? The same questions could be asked about initiated cells. It is clear that a solution to the problem of quantitative risk assessment is not at hand. However, I believe that a beginning has been made in addressing some of the questions raised above, at least in one experimental system, the rat liver.

The discussion of initiation-promotion illustrates the power of simple mathematical analysis. For example, a population of cells undergoing cell division and death may show large fluctuations in total size. Thus, one would expect to see enzyme altered foci of different types in the rat liver. Some foci may appear to be growing, others may appear to be regressing with a large number of dead cells. Although there may be a qualitative biological difference between these two types of foci, one certainly cannot infer that a biological difference must exist. Further, the example of 4-DAB and NDEOL discussed in the previous section has simple interpretation in terms of the growth kinetics of intermediate cells, which is more appealing than previous interpretations of similar experiments in terms of Druckrey's formula.

REFERENCES

Armitage, P., and Doll, R., 1954, The age distribution of cancer and a multistage theory of carcinogenesis, Brit. J. Cancer, 8:1-12.

Cavenee, W. K., Dryja, T. P., Phillips, R. A., Benedict, W. F., Godbout, R., Gallie, B. L., Murphree, A. L., Strong, L. C., and White, R. L., 1983, Expression of recessive alleles by chromosomal mechanisms in retinoblastoma, Nature, 305:779-784.

Comings, D. E., 1973, A general theory of carcinogenesis, Proc. Natl. Acad. Sci. U.S.A., 70:3324-3328.

Dewanji, A., Venzon, D. J., and Moolgavkar, S. H., 1988, A stochastic two-stage model for cancer risk assessment II: The number and size of premalignant clones, Risk Analysis, in press.

Ellwein, L. B., and Cohen, S. M., 1988, A cellular dynamics model of experimental bladder cancer: Analysis of the effect of sodium saccharin in the rat, Risk Analysis, in press.

Hennings, H., Shores, R., Wenk, M. L., Spangler, E. F., Tarone, R., and Yuspa, S. H., 1983, Malignant conversion of mouse skin tumours is increases by tumour initiators and unaffected by tumour promoters, Nature, 304:67-69.

Hethcote, H. W., and Knudson, A. G., 1978, Model for the incidence of embryonal cancers: Application to retinoblastoma, Proc. Natl. Acad. Sci. U.S.A., 75:2453-2457.

Knudson, A. G., 1971, Mutation and cancer: Statistical study of retinoblastoma, Proc. Natl. Acad. Sci. U.S.A., 68:820-823.

Knudson, A. G., 1985, Hereditary cancer, oncogenes, and antioncogenes, Cancer Res., 45:1437-1443.

Knudson, A. G., and Moolgavkar, S. H., 1986, Inherited influences on susceptibility to radiation carcinogenesis, in: "Radiation Carcinogenesis," A. C. Upton, ed., Elsevier, North Holland.

Knudson, A. G., Jr., Hethcote, H. W., and Brown, B. W., 1975, Mutation and childhood cancer: A probabilistic model for the incidence of retinoblastoma, Proc. Natl. Acad. Sci. U.S.A., 72:5116-5120.

Koufos, A., Hansen, M. F., Lampkin, B. C., Workman, M. L., Copeland, N. G., Jenkins, N. A., and Cavenee, W. K., 1984, Loss of alleles at loci on human chromosome 11 during genesis of Wilm's tumour, Nature, 309:170-172.

Moolgavkar, S. H., 1986, Carcinogenesis modeling: From molecular biology to epidemiology, Ann. Rev. Publ. Health, 7:151-169.

Moolgavkar, S. H., and Dewanji, A., 1988, Biologically-based models for cancer risk assessment: A cautionary note, Risk Analysis, 8:5-6.

Moolgavkar, S. H., and Knudson, A. G., Jr., 1981, Mutation and cancer: A model for human carcinogenesis, J. Natl. Cancer Inst., 66:1037-1052.

Moolgavkar, S. H., and Venzon, D. J., 1979, Two-event models for carcinogenesis: Incidence curves for childhood and adult tumors, Math. Biosci., 47:55-77.

Moolgavkar, S. H., Dewanji, A., and Venzon, D. J., 1988, A stochastic two-stage model for cancer risk assessment I: The hazard function and the probability of tumor, Risk Analysis, in press.

Scherer, E., Feringa, A. W., and Emmelot, P., 1984, Initiation-promotion-initiation, Induction of neoplastic foci within islands of precancerous liver cells in the rat, in: "Models, Mechanisms and Etiology of Tumour Promotion," M. Börzsönyi, N. E. Day, K. Lapis, and H. Yamasaki, eds., IARC Scientific Publication No. 56, Lyon.

Schwarz, M., Pearson, D., Port, R., and Kunz, W., 1984, Promoting effect of 4-dimethylaminoazobenzene on enzyme altered foci induced in rat liver by N-nitrosodiethanolamine, Carcinogenesis, 5:725-730.

Yuspa, S. H., 1984, Mechanisms of initiation and promotion in mouse epidermis, in: "Models, Mechanisms and Etiology of Tumour Promotion," M. Börzsönyi, N. E. Day, K. Lapis, and H. Yamasaki, eds., IARC Scientific Publications No. 56, Lyon.

UNDERSTANDING MULTI-STAGE CARCINOGENESIS AT
THE MOLECULAR LEVEL: NOTES ON RECENT PROGRESS

M. Hollstein and H. Yamasaki

International Agency for Research on Cancer
150 cours Albert Thomas
69372 Lyon cedex 08, France

SUMMARY

While it is convenient to separate cancer stages into initiation and
promotion phases, and to classify chemicals based on whether they have
initiation or promoting activity, it is difficult to find mechanistic
definitions that are internally consistent. A transforming point mutation
in c-ras is experimentally inducible by an initiator, yet may occur either
early or late in the development of cancer. Tumor promoters are considered
non-genotoxic, yet TPA does affect the genome and can cause structural
alterations in DNA. A further complication is that inducible cellular
pathways can modulate DNA damage qualitatively and quantitatively. Basic
research on the molecular biology of gene mutation, amplification, rearrangement, and transcription control in simple organisms that lend
themselves to experimental manipulation, coupled with direct analysis of
human tumors for genetic and other molecular changes will be useful in
refining models of the critical steps in human cancer and the mechanisms by
which they come about. Recent work on characterization of oncogenes, on
gene transcription regulation, and on signal transduction pathways already
has advanced our understanding considerably.

INTRODUCTION

Certain observations on cancer have permitted some fundamental
assumptions about the process. One basic concept that usually goes
undisputed is that malignant growth is the consequence of several steps,
one compelling reason for thinking this being that tumor incidence in the
human population increases exponentially with age. This immediately poses
several questions: What are the steps? How can we distinguish them? What is
the sequence of events? It seems that some consensus has been reached
regarding the answers. Carcinogenesis can be divided into at least two
stages, initiation and promotion, and the biological activity of chemicals
that affect cancer incidence are often separated into two categories, each
characterized by certain properties (Table 1). The characteristics
attributed to initiators and promoters should harmonize with what is
currently known about biochemical mechanisms underlying carcinogenesis;
otherwise, some remodeling of classical concepts would be necessary. In
view of recent advances in understanding the molecular biology of growth
control, a refinement of models of carcinogenesis may be appropriate.

Table 1. Properties typically associated with initiating and promoting
activity

Exposure to a chemical with initiating activity	Exposure to a chemical with promoting activity
-causes an early, rare change in an individual cell	-affects entire cell populations, but especially initiated cells
-is genotoxic, e.g., mutagenic	-is non-genotoxic, e.g., DNA not chemically modified
-elicits an irreversible effect	-the effect is reversible
-a single exposure is sufficient	-Multiple exposures are required
Example: NMU	Example: TPA

As summarized in Table 1 and reviewed by Pitot, 1986, results from
decades of study on carcinogenesis were the basis for formulating the
hypothesis that a chemical with initiating activity affects DNA, whereas
the cell membrane is the target of tumor promoting agents. Until recently,
however, neither target genes in the nucleus nor target molecules in the
membrane had been identified. In the last several years advances in the
field of molecular biology have brought about the identification of
critical genes, such as cellular oncogenes (Bishop, 1987), involved in
cancer. In addition, the discovery that protein kinase C is the cellular
receptor of phorbol ester tumor promoters provided a new dimension to
research on promotion since this kinase turned out to be a pivotal
component of a major signal transduction pathway (Nishizuka, 1984). Due to
this finding, and to the identification of phorbol ester responsive
enhancer elements in DNA that increase transcription of specific genes, it
became possible to discuss the molecular links between initiation (gene
damage) and promotion (molecular alterations at the membrane leading to
alterations in gene expression). The notes assembled below do not review
this vast area of research activity. Instead, we have selected a few
examples to illustrate how recently acquired knowledge may bear upon
classical models of multistage carcinogenesis.

INITIATION

If an initiator (carcinogen) causes an irreversible, heritable
structural change in the DNA of a cell that eventually gives rise to a
neoplasm (Pitot, 1986), then we would expect all cells of the tumor to have
this alteration. The notorious instability of genetic material in tumor
cells has added to the inherent difficulty of locating and identifying
relevant changes (mutations) in 3 million kilobases of DNA. The fortuitous
transduction by oncogenic retroviruses of mammalian genes (slightly
altered) has provided us with a first indication about where to look
(reviewed in Bishop, 1987). The human homologues of viral oncogenic DNA,
proto-oncogenes, can transform fibroblasts in culture if these genes have
abnormalities in their structure, expression, or both. This led to the
discovery of some of the other potentially oncogenic sequences in mammalian
DNA not known so far to have been 'cloned' for us by a virus (Marshall,
1985). The question is, then, do we find activated oncogenes in human
tumors and what structural change has rendered them (abnormal)
transforming? Indeed proto-oncogenes with lesions that unleash their
transforming capacities have been identified in human tumors (Table 2).

Specific c-ras Mutations as an Initiating Step in Chemically-Induced Animal Tumors

The most commonly cited example of activated oncogenes in human tumors is the ras gene family (Barbacid, 1987). The c-ras genes can be activated by a single point mutation in any one of a few specific critical codons of the DNA sequences, causing a structural and functional change in the protein product. These point mutations have been detected in a variety of human tumors with a frequency ranging from 0 to 50%, apparently depending in large part on the tumor type (Bos, 1988).

At first glance, this is quite satisfying, because this finding might be predicted by the model of multistage carcinogenesis for cancers resulting from exposure to a mutagenic carcinogen. The reasoning, applied to an initiating dose of NMU, for example, would be as follows: 0-alkylation of guanine residues will cause base mispairing with thymine, and following DNA replication will result in G to A point mutations scattered (though probably non-randomly) throughout the genome and appearing, albeit rarely, in a critical gene controlling cell growth. Fortuitously, the mutation might be positioned in the genome such that the gene product now functions abnormally, providing this mutated cell with the potential for destabilized, disordered growth. Upon further changes, the cell and its descendants give rise to a neoplasm, and eventually cancer. Examination of the tumor DNA will be expected to reveal the precise critical mutation in the growth control gene that occurred in the NMU-initiated cell that eventually gave rise to the tumor.

Experimental studies have substantiated this model: rats exposed to a single dose of NMU develop mammary tumors almost all of which show the presence of an activated H-ras allele (Zarbl et al., 1985). Activation in all cases (61 tumors) is due to an identical base pair substitution (G to A, codon 12). Numerous studies have shown that a single base change in codon 12 of ras genes confers transforming growth properties to the protein product; for example, microinjection of the p21^{H-ras} protein with a substitution of the 12th amino acid residue transforms fibroblasts in vitro (Stacey and Kong, 1984). Thus, it appears that in experiments with NMU-induced animal tumors we have the classic example of an initiation event: a single exposure to a genotoxic chemical causes an early, rare, irreversible and heritable genetic change, a point mutation (G to A) in a gene (H-ras) affecting the growth behavior of cells.

c-ras Mutations in Late Stages of Tumor Development

In human studies, there are data that argue both for and against the notion that an activating ras mutation is typically an early event in human cancers, but it is clear that it can occur relatively late in the course of the disease. On the one hand, in 5/6 human colon cancers with ras mutations the identical base pair change was also present in the adenomatous tissue surrounding the carcinoma (Bos et al., 1987), yet in four cases of acute myeloid leukemia in which N-ras mutations were detected at first presentation of the disease, the mutations were absent in relapse DNA, suggesting that the abnormal pre-malignant cells do not have the mutation and that the N-ras mutations detected at first presentation were not initiation events but rather arose during later steps in the evolution of the disease (Farr et al., 1988). Others (Hirai et al., 1987) have suggested that activating point mutations in N-ras may be related to the transition to leukemic disease in patients with myelodysplastic syndrome. Ras mutation, then, though corresponding to a biochemical event that bears all the hallmarks of initiation (Table 1) can be either an early, intermediate, or late step in cancer depending on as yet undefined parameters, such as the type of tumor, the nature of exposure, if any, to a mutagen, the histological cell type, or other factors. To the wisdom that cancer is many diseases and is usually the result of many deleterious steps we can add the caveat that there is more than one route, as well as more than one possible sequence of events that can lead to a given malignancy.

Resolution of the question: "early or late?", or "what comes first?" is not simple for technical reasons, so it is tempting to rely on animal experimental models to shed light on the matter. The mouse skin initiation/promotion studies, in which tumors are produced from exposure to DMBA followed by repeated applications of TPA, seem promising since the tumors arise first as papillomas, many of which regress, but some of which develop into carcinomas. Balmain and co-workers (Quintanilla et al., 1986) showed that both papillomas (17/19) and carcinomas (12/13) had activated ras alleles and the base pair change (A to T, codon 61, H-ras) is specific and characteristic of the initiator, which supports the model that the mutation occurs early in the evolution of the tumors. We have used a different exposure protocol in which a single administration of DMBA in utero, at doses which do not induce carcinomas, is followed by repeated applications of TPA post-partum. In our experiment only half the papillomas we tested (6/12) showed the presence of the ras mutation, whereas all carcinomas (9/9) were positive for the oncogene activation (Yamasaki et al., 1987). It may be that papillomas without ras mutations are those induced by TPA and destined to regress, but it is also feasible that ras activation can occur "spontaneously" at later stages and contributes to evolution of the neoplasm toward malignancy. We now have found occasional papillomas in mice treated only with TPA that also have the H-ras A to T codon 61 mutation attributed in the initiation promotion studies to the specific binding of DMBA to adenine and subsequent transversion by mispairing of A to T (unpublished results).

Animal Experiments as Models for the Study of Molecular Mechanisms of Multistep Carcinogenesis

In using animal data to interpret or predict the human situation, one is confronted with the usual dilemma regarding possible artifacts due to the high doses necessary to produce tumors in a small group of animals. As alluded to in a recent symposium on theories of carcinogenesis (Mole, 1988), when discussing biochemical mechanisms of action of a compound, can information on frequent biochemical events occurring at high doses necessarily tell us anything about the nature of rare events at low doses? It may be unwise to assume that the nature of a DNA lesion, and the mechanism that governs its occurrence will be the same at high and low doses. This reflection is not an argument in favor of assuming the existence of thresholds in carcinogenesis, rather it is a warning that in some cases the mechanisms we define from animal experiments may prove to be misleading indicators of the cellular events giving rise to human cancers. Although there is no practical alternative that can substitute for the standard high-dose animal cancer test, we can temper our inferences from animal test results with what we do actually find in the human situation. The fact that we can now look at human tumor DNA and ask about the nature of specific and relevant genetic alterations that occurred is quite valuable and should be exploited fully as a corroboration (or not) of hypotheses on mechanisms we have generated from animal tests.

Table 2. Examples of oncogene structural alterations found in human tumor
          DNA

Gene	DNA modification	A cancer in which this change is often seen*
c-ras	Point mutation	Carcinoma of the colon
c-abl	Translocation	Chronic myelogenous leukemia
c-myc	Translocation	Burkitt's lymphoma
L-myc	Amplification	Small cell carcinoma of the lung
N-myc	Amplification	Neuroblastoma
c-erb B	Amplification	Squamous cell carcinoma of the esophagus
c-erb B2	Amplification	Carcinoma of the breast

*Frequency varies depending on the example, e.g., nearly one-half of human
colon tumors tested so far carry an activating (transforming) point
mutation in the K-ras gene, all cases of Burkitt's lymphoma show
translocation of the c-myc gene, and about 10% of esophageal tumors
(Hollstein et al., 1988) have amplified (10x or more) c-erbB sequences.
(Table 2 has been adapted and modified from Bishop, 1987).

Various Inducible Enzyme Pathways May Affect the Nature or Extent of DNA Damage by Initiators

    Examples of global cellular programs induced by biochemical stress have
been described in some detail particularly in lower organisms. A universal
reaction to elevated temperatures, the "heat shock response" occurs in all
prokaryotic and eukaryotic organisms studied (reviewed by Lindquist, 1986);
cells rapidly produce a set of conserved proteins whose function is presumably in part to reduce biochemical damage to macromolecules from heat (one
effect of temperature rise is an increase in DNA damage by depurination).
In bacteria, there is also the example of the SOS response (Echols, 1981),
the induction of a set of genes in response to mutagen-induced DNA damage
which results in error-prone DNA repair, vastly increasing the number of
mutations over what would be seen if the mutagen were allowed to react with
a cell in which this machinery is defective. It is not unlikely that
mammalian cells have processes analogous to this. Inducible enzymes that
fundamentally alter the ultimate genetic consequences of initial DNA base
damage may also be imagined.

    Many oncogenes can be rendered transforming by a genetic alteration
that greatly increases expression of the normal gene product; gene
rearrangement and amplification may be more frequent mechanisms of inducing
genes than point mutations in transcription enhancer or silencer sequences,
for example. At present, it appears that the prevailing mechanism by which
a mammalian oncogene (other than ras) becomes activated in human tumors
involves major re-positioning of large stretches of DNA (Table 2); translocation and amplification of DNA presumably require the complicity of
cellular enzymes such as recombination proteins, some of which may be
induced by exposure to carcinogens (Echols, 1981). Also, there is experimental evidence emerging which supports the long-held suspicion that
transposition of repeated DNA elements occurs in mammalian cells (as it
does in lower eukaryotes) and can be stimulated by a DNA damaging agent
(Lin et al., 1988). Transposition, which has been proposed as a critical
step in the development of some human cancers (Cairns, 1981), can be a very
effective means of generating mutations, and here certain rules regarding
induction of point mutations by initiators may prove to be of no use. The

frequency of transposition in bacteria can be orders of magnitude higher in stationary cells than in dividing cells, and a major fraction of the cell population can experience a particular transposition event.

We may imagine that the induction of certain biochemical pathways will change the kinetics of mutation in conjunction with changing the type of mutation that prevails. If there are quantum leaps in mutation rates, calculations of mutation frequencies in risk estimation would have to be re-considered. There are some striking examples of very high mutation frequencies under certain circumstances. For example, exposure of the multicellular alga volvox to UV light at a certain stage of development can increase the mutation rate at the RegA locus by approximately four orders of magnitude (Kirk et al., 1987). The chemical mutagens bleomycin and 4HAQO are also quite effective. It seems that during a specific developmental stage this gene is exquisitely hypermutable, and this is most likely due to UV-induced malfunctioning of recombinational events involved in genetic rearrangement during development.

Usefulness of Lower Organisms in Studying Mechanisms of Genetic Damage

These observations may be the tip of the iceberg foiling simple models of mutation. Experiments on genetic changes in lower organisms probably will continue to uncover interesting phenomena previously hidden from our sight or inaccessible because appropriate techniques in molecular biology were not yet developed[1]. Typically, simple organisms are used for such studies, but the findings promise to be relevant to mammalian cells given the remarkable phylogenetic conservation in the blueprint for mechanisms of certain fundamental cellular processes. It has been appreciated for some time that genetic material in all organisms is essentially the same chemically and this has been very useful in using easily manipulatable organisms such as bacteria to identify mutagenic carcinogens. In the light of recent experiments, we may now be tempted to add: so is the machinery similar that governs gene function. In the last year, we have learned that a yeast transcription factor will perform properly in a mammalian cell (Webster et al., 1988), and that the human c-fos proto-oncogene product can be fused to the lexA repressor of bacteria to stimulate transcription in yeast (Lech et al., 1988). These and other "mix and match" examples imply that mechanisms of gene regulation are similar across species in overall design as well as molecular detail; understanding gene regulation is proving to be of critical importance in cancer research (see below).

PROMOTION

Tumor promoters affect cells in a plethora of ways, but two constant features seem to be the reversible and non-genotoxic nature of the impact: when the promoter is removed, the stimulus is thereby also removed, the cell returns to its original phenotype, and the exposure has been thought to leave no imprint in the form of measurable DNA damage in the genetic material. The distinct separation sought between the molecular mechanism of an initiator such as a mutagenic carcinogen, and a promoter, such as TPA,

---

[1]One encouraging development is the use of the polymerase chain reaction (PCR) to detect single mutations in the genome (Saiki et al., 1985). This technique is so sensitive that DNA from a single human hair is sufficient material for the analysis (Higuchi, 1988). Detection of point mutations in a single cell is feasible and would allow direct measurement of the frequency of a specific mutation in an exposed cell population.

would thus be achieved. Animal skin painting experiments with TPA have long been cited as a clear example of these truths: tumors do not appear unless the compound is applied often and frequently, and the compound does not bind to DNA or generate base adducts.

Effects of the Tumor Promoter TPA on Genomic Function (Example: Trancription Enhancement)

In recent years, great strides have been made in understanding the molecular biology of TPA effects on the mammalian cell. We now know that TPA binds to and activates protein kinase C, an enzyme that functions in a pathway transmitting growth signals from the cell surface to the nucleus (see M. Castagna, this volume). Rat fibroblasts that are genetically manipulated to produce a vast excess of the kinase acquire some of the phenotypic characteristics of transformed cells, and these cells form tumors when injected into nude mice (Housey et al., 1988). The cellular TPA receptor thus seems to have the properties of an oncogene and is gaining a reputation as such. TPA induces the transcription of many cellular genes some of which are proto-oncogenes (Hollstein and Yamasaki, 1987), and it is known that overabundance of normal protein products of mammalian proto-oncogenes can transform cells. At the molecular level, it has been shown that the cellular oncogene fos, whose expression is abruptly stimulated in quiescent fibroblasts when TPA is added, has a specific short DNA sequence in the upstream enhancer that is required for TPA induction of c-fos transcription (Verma and Sassone-Corsi, 1987).

Effects of TPA on Genomic Structure (Example: Amplification)

In spite of this remarkable molecular detail on the biological effects of TPA, we are still hard put to explain why a certain number of exposures to TPA at a certain frequency is necessary to elicit tumors in the mouse skin experiments. One proposal has been that this tumor promoter causes clonal expansion of initiated cells, so it might be argued that trans-cription stimulation of proto-oncogenes involved in cell division, and preferential priming of the growth machinery in initiated cells will generate a larger population of altered cells in which a second rare genetic event can occur, either spontaneously or as a consequence of exposure to a genotoxic chemical. Additional interpretations may be worth considering, however. It is feasible that the second genetic event can also be the direct consequence of TPA exposure. By repeated transcription stimulus of a TPA-responsive gene, the promoter effect may become fixed in the genome, such that TPA is no longer required for enhanced transcription. One of the genetic alterations that will result in overabundance of a gene product is increase in gene copy number. Both tumor promoters (Barsoum and Varshavsky, 1983; Varshavsky, 1981) and carcinogens (Kleinberger et al., 1986) induce amplification of the dihydrofolate reductase gene in mammalian cells exposed to methotrexate.

The number of oncogenes that can be activated to transforming sequences by this genetic alteration, and the frequency with which c-onc amplifica-tion is found in human tumors are worthy of some reflection (see Table 2). Knowing what internal and external factors induce specific gene amplifica-tion may prove to be as important as identifying what environ- mental compounds cause point mutations in the environment. While the overlap in chemicals that produce these two types of genetic change may be consider-able, the gamut of end-points among the commonly used short-term tests would best be expanded to include amplification as well as other endpoints (see discussion by Ramel, 1988).

DISCUSSION

If gene amplification is important in human cancers, as seems to be the case, and if both genotoxic initiators and "non-genotoxic" promoters can induce this genetic change, there will be exposure situations for which the initiator-promoter model as outlined in Table 1 will not be applicable. The distinction between geno-toxic and non-genotoxic becomes at this point increasingly fuzzy. Though a critical step in some cancers may be a genetic change inducible by chemicals as biochemically different as electrophilic mutagens and phorbol ester promoters, we may regain some footing with the classic paradigms (Table 1), should the pathway by which each class of compound generates amplified sequences turn out to be different. We offer one speculative proposal for the mechanism by which overexpression from a exposure to TPA might lead to gene amplification. The model is prompted by studies reporting an identity between mammalian transcription factors and viral replication proteins (Santoro et al., 1988; Rossi et al., 1988), as well as the experiments on the developmentally regulated amplification of the Drosophila chorion gene locating an upstream control element essential for both transcription and amplification (Orr-Weaver et al., 1986). The model also makes use of the observation that exposure of mammalian cells to TPA stimulates DNA binding activity of the transcription factor Ap1 (Chiu et al., 1987). We propose that specific transcription factors become activated by promoter-stimulated protein kinases, thus greatly increasing transcription protein occupancy of enhancer sequences. If this occurs repeatedly and at inopportune moments in the cell cycle, the presence of the bound transcription factor may facilitate unscheduled replication of adjacent sequences. When promoter exposure is discontinued, a transforming excess of gene product is ensured by the high gene copy number.

It would be exciting should discoveries from basic research in molecular biology put certain principles regarding mechanisms of carcinogenesis to the test. In a recent study with transgenic mice (Muller et al., 1988) even the fundamental concept that multiple steps are required in cancer is challenged, though no generality can be expected to hold always. In any case, the rapid accumulation of knowledge on oncogenes, growth factors, signal transduction and so on, should provide a clearer picture of carcinogenesis and its various stages. This will probably influence the bases of cancer risk assessment, a major theme of this symposium.

ACKNOWLEDGEMENTS

We thank Dr J. Hall and Dr B. Sylla for helpful comments, and Mrs C. Fuchez for secretarial assistance.

REFERENCES (Citations in the text generally provide only one recent illustration or discussion of the point considered).

Barbacid, M. 1987, ras genes. Ann. Rev. Biochem., 56:779.
Barsoum, J., and Varshavsky, A., 1983, Mitogenic hormones and tumor promoters greatly increase the incidence of colony-forming cells bearing amplified dihydrofolate reductase genes. Proc. Natl. Acad. Sci. USA, 80:5330.
Bishop, I.M., 1987, The molecular genetics of cancer, Science, 235:305.

Bos, J.L., 1988, The ras gene family and human carcinogenesis. Mutat. Res., 195:255.

Bos, J.L., Fearon, E.R., Hamilton, S.R., Verlaan-de Vries, M., van Boom, J.H., van der Ebm A.J., and Vogelstein, B., 1987, Prevalence of ras gene mutations in human colorectal cancers. Nature, 327:293.

Cairns, J., 1981, The origin of human cancers. Nature, 289:353.

Chiu, R., Imagawa, M., Imbra, R.J., Bockoven, J.R., and Karin, M., 1987, Multiple cis- and trans-acting elements mediate the transcriptional response to phorbol esters. Nature, 329:648.

Echols, J., 1981, SOS functions, cancer and inducible evolution. Cell, 25:1.

Farr, C.J., Saiki, R.K., Erlich, H.A., McCormick, F., and Marshall, C.J., 1988, Analysis of RAS gene mutations in acute myeloid leukemia by polymerase chain reaction and oligonucleotide probes. Proc. Natl. Acad. Sci. USA, 85:1629.

Higuchi, R., von Beroldingen, C., Sensabaugh, G., Erlich, H., 1988, DNA typing from single hairs. Nature, 332:543.

Hirai, H., Kobayashi, Y., Mano, H., Hagiwara, K., Maru, Y., Omine, M., Mizoguchi, H., Nishida, J., Takaku, F., 1987, A point mutation at codon 13 of the N-ras oncogene in myelodysplastic syndrome, Nature, 327:430.

Hollstein, M., Smits, A.M., Galiana, C., Yamasaki, H., Bos, J.L., Mandard, A., Partensky, C., and Montesano, R., 1988, Amplification of epidermal growth factor receptor gene but no evidence of ras mutations in primary human esophageal cancers. Cancer Res., (in press).

Hollstein, M., and Yamasaki, H., 1987, Tumor promoter-mediated modulation of cell differentiation and communication: the phorbol ester-oncogene connection, in: Tumor Cell Differentiation, J. Aarbakke, P.K. Chiang, and H. P. Koeffler, eds, The Humana Press, Clifton, New Jersey, pp. 317-339.

Housey, G.M., Johnson, M.D., Hsiao, W.L., O'Brien, C.A., Murphy, J.P., Kirschmeier,, P., and Weinstein, I.B., 1988, Overproduction of protein kinase C causes disordered growth control in rat fibroblasts. Cell, 52:343.

Kirk, D.L., Baran, G.J., Harper, J.F., Huskey, R.J., Huson, K.S., and Zagris, N., 1987, Stage-specific hypermutability of the regA locus of volvox, a gene regulating the germ-soma dichotomy, Cell, 48:11.

Kleinberger, T., Etkin, S., and Lavi, S., 1986, Carcinogen-mediated methotrexate resistance and dihydrofolate reductase amplification in Chinese hamster cells. Molec. Cell. Biol., 6:1958.

Lech, K., Anderson, K., and Brent, R., 1988, DNA-bound fos proteins activate transcription in yeast, Cell, 52:179.

Lin, C.S., Goldthwait, D.A., and Samois, D., 1988, Identification of alu transposition in human lung carcinoma cells. Cell, 54:: 153.

Lindquist, S., 1986, The heat-shock response, Ann. Rev. Biochem., 55:1151.

Marshall, C., 1985, Human oncogenes, in: RNA Tumor Viruses, Cold Spring Harbor Laboratory, Cold Spring Harbor, New York.

Mole, R.H., 1988, Radiation-induced acute myeloid leukaemia: an unusually valuable experimental model for testing basic assumptions about the process of carcinogenesis, in: Theories of Carcinogenesis, O.H. Iversen, ed., Hemisphere publishing Co., Washington, D.C., pp. 133-141.

Muller, W.J., Sinn, E.,, Pattengate, P.K., Wallace, R., and Leder, P., 1988, Single-step induction of mammary adenocarcinoma in transgenic mice bearing the activated c-neu oncogene. Cell, 54:105.

Nishizuka, Y., 1984, The role of protein kinase C in cell surface signal transduction and tumour promotion, Nature, 306:693.

Orr-Weaver, T.L., and Spradling, A.C., 1986, Drosophila chorion gene amplification requires an upstream region regulating s18 transcription. Molec. Cell Biol., 6:4624.

Pitot, H.C., 1986, Fundamentals of Oncology, Marcel Dekker, New York.

Quintanilla, M., Brown, K., Ramsden, M., and Balmain, A., 1986, Carcinogen-specific mutation and amplification of Ha-ras during mouse skin carcinogenesis. Nature, 322:78.

Ramel, C., 1988, Short-term testing - are we looking at wrong endpoints? Mutat. Res., 205:13.

Rossi, P., Karsenty, G., Roberts, A.B., Roche, N.S.,, Sporn, M.B., and de Crombrugghe, B., 1988, A nuclear factor 1 binding site mediates the transcriptional activation of a type 1 collagen promoter by transforming growth factor-b. Cell, 52:405.

Saiki, R., Sharf, S., Faloona, F., Mulis, K., Horn, G., Ehrlich, H.A., and Arnheim, N., 1985, Enzymatic amplification of b-globin genomic sequences and restriction site analysis for diagnosis of sickle cell anemia. Science, 230:1350.

Santoro, C., Mermod, N., Andrews, P.C., and Tjian, R., 1988, A family of human CCAAT-box-binding proteins active in transcription and DNA replication: cloning and expression of multiple cDNAs. Nature, 334:218.

Stacey, D.W., and Kung, H.F., 1984, Transformation of NIH 3T3 cells by microinjection of Ha-ras p21 protein. Nature, 310:508.

Varshavsky, A., 1981, Phorbol ester dramatically increases incidence of methotrexate-resistant mouse cells: possible mechanisms and relevance to tumor promotion. Cell, 25:561.

Verma, I.M., and Sassone-Corsi, P., 1987, Proto-oncogene fos: complex but versatile regulation. Cell, 51:513.

Webster, N., Jin, J.R., Green, S., Hollis, M., and Chambon, P., 1988, The yeast UASG is a transcriptional enhancer in human HeLa cells in the presence of the GAL4 trans-activator. Cell, 52:169.

Yamasaki, H., Hollstein, M., Martel, N., Cabral, J.R.P., Galendo, D., and Tomatis, L., 1987, Transplacental induction of a specific mutation in fetal Ha-ras and its critical role in post-natal carcinogenesis. Int. J. Cancer, 40:818.

Zarbl, H., Sukumar, S., Arthur, A.V., Martin-Zanka, D., and Barbacid, M., 1985, Direct mutagenesis of Ha-ras-1 oncogenes by N-nitroso-N-methylurea during initiation of mammary carcinogenesis in rats. Nature, 315:382.

THE USE OF ENZYME-ALTERED FOCI FOR RISK ASSESSMENT OF

HEPATOCARCINOGENS

M. Schwarz, D. Pearson, A. Buchmann and W. Kunz

Institut of Biochemistry
German Cancer Research Center
Im Neuenheimer Feld 280, 6900 Heidelberg (F.R.G.)

INTRODUCTION

Chemically-induced hepatocarcinogenesis is characterized by the sequential appearance of phenotypically altered cell populations which can
be identified by changes in the expression of a variety of markers such
as canalicular adenosine triphosphatase (ATPase), γ-glutamyl transpeptidase, glucose-6-phosphatase and others (for review see Peraino et
al., 1983). There is increasing evidence to suggest that at least some
of these early enzyme-altered foci are precursor lesions which are
causally related to the malignant transformation. This is substantiated
by the sequential appearance of enzyme-altered foci and liver tumors and
by the observation that neoplastic nodules and hepatocellular carcinoma
show enzyme-patterns similar to those seen in preneoplastic foci (Friedrich-Freksa et al., 1969; Goldfarb and Pugh, 1981; Bannasch et al., 1986).
Moreover, strong quantitative relationships between the total volume of
enzyme-altered tissue in liver and the subsequent development of liver
tumors have been established (Emmelot and Scherer, 1980; Kunz et al.,
1983, 1985). Enzyme-altered foci are monoclonal in origin (Rabes
et al., 1982; Williams et al., 1983) and show a growth advantage over
the surrounding normal hepatocytes (Rabes et al., 1979). The analysis
of multiple marker enzymes within individual foci points towards a
marked heterogeneity of phenotypes which is also reflected by differences in the proliferation rates of the foci (Buchmann et al., 1987;
Peraino et al., 1984). The analysis of number and size of enzyme
altered foci in liver can yield quantitative data on the effects of
hepatocarcinogens at low, relevant dose levels. Moreover, these data
inherit information on mechanistic aspects of carcinogenesis which
may be of importance for the improvement of risk assessment of
carcinogens and tumor promoting agents in liver.

INITIATING AND PROMOTING ACTIVITY OF HEPATOCARCINOGENS

Carcinogens are agents that produce cancer in their target organ
when administered at sufficiently high doses. In contrast, tumor promotors, almost by definition, do not induce tumors when given alone but
enhance the neoplastic response when administered following an initiating carcinogen. There is evidence to assume that carcinogens may
possess in addition to their tumor-initiating activity the potential

31

to enhance the carcinogenic process by acting on stages subsequent to initiation. In analogy to the initiation-promotion model this latter activity of the carcinogen will be referred to as "promoting" activity, or, since both initiating and promoting activities are combined within one and the same molecule as "intrinsic promoting" activity.

The azodye 4-dimethylaminoazobenzene (4-DAB, also known as butter yellow) and the nitrosamine N-nitrosodiethanolamine (NDEOL) were chosen as model carcinogens to investigate possible differences in their initiating and "intrinsic promoting" activities. 4-DAB has already been used in the 1950th by Druckrey to study quantitatively the effect of continuous and discontinuous carcinogen exposure (Druckrey, 1967). In his pioneering studies he could demonstrate a quantitative relationship between daily exposure level of rats to 4-DAB and the median induction times (t_{50}) of liver tumors that developed in these animals. T_{50}-values were thereby defined as those time-points when 50 % of animals of a given treatment group had died from the particular tumor. With 4-DAB the product of daily carcinogen dose and t_{50} was constant over almost all treatment groups. This relationship yields a straight line in a log-log plot as is shown in Figure 1. This is also true for NDEOL as for all other carcinogens tested sofar. The slope of the regression lines, however, are characteristically different between 4-DAB and NDEOL (see Figure 1).

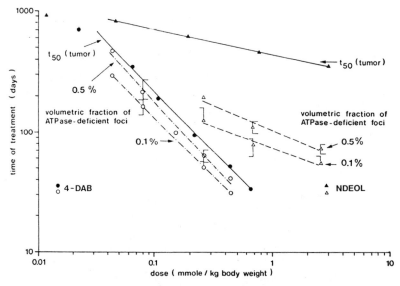

Fig. 1.   Dose-time relationships for the induction of liver tumors and defined volumetric fractions of ATPase-deficient foci in liver. Liver tumor data are taken from the literature (4-DAB; Druckrey, 1969; NDEOL, Preussmann et al., 1982). For the analysis of preneoplastic response female Wistar rats were treated continuously with different doses of 4-dimethylaminoazobenzene and N-nitrosodiethanolamine. Rats were sacrificed sequentially and the time periods to reach 0.1 % and 0.5 % enzyme-altered tissue in liver were determined for each dose group by regression analysis of time-dependent increases in the volumetric fraction of ATPase-deficient foci.

Doubling the daily exposure level of 4-DAB will cut the median tumor induction time into half. An approximately 50-fold increase in daily dose, however, is necessary with NDEOL to obtain the same effect. The relationship between carcinogen exposure level d and tumor induction time t_{50} can be described as $d \times t_{50}^n$ = constant, where the socalled "time reinforcing factor n" has a numerical value of approximately 1 for 4-DAB and approximately 5 for NDEOL (Druckrey, 1967; Preussmann et al., 1982).

It can be assumed that the velocity of the carcinogenic process is predominantly governed by the transition probabilities between subsequent stages and the kinetics of cell birth and death of intermediate cell populations (Moolgavkar 1983, 1986; see also this volume). Each transition can occur spontaneously at a low probability. Initiating agents will increase the probability of the transition from a normal cell to an initiated cell (and from initiated to tumor cells). Tumor promotors will increase the growth rate of intermediate cell populations and might also affect the transition rates between stages subsequent to initiation (Kunz et al., 1983, 1985). They might also slow down cell death of intermediate cell populations (see Schulte-Hermann, this issue). If one assumes that carcinogens like 4-DAB would, in a dose-related manner, initiate the carcinogenic process and in addition to this show an enhancing activity on subsequent stages, we would expect very short tumor induction times at high dose levels and a rapid loss in efficiency with a decrease in dose. On the contrary, if a compound like NDEOL would only initiate, but not possess "intrinsic promoting" activity even at high doses, the velocity of the carcinogenic process would be predominantly governed by the probability of spontaneously occuring changes and would be much less influenced by changes in carcinogen dose.

QUANTITATIVE ANALYSIS OF ENZYME-ALTERED FOCI

Quantitative analyses of early enzyme-altered foci in liver of rats treated continuously with either carcinogen yielded several lines of evidence which favour this hypothesis. Enzyme-altered foci were quantitated by means of a computer-assisted system; stained tissue sections were projected onto a digitizer screen and the focal transections and the outlines of the tissue sections were scored manually with a cursor. The number of foci in the three-dimensional space, their size distribution and the volumetric fraction occupying the liver were calculated on the basis of stereological methods (for review see Campbell et al., 1986).

In a first experiment rats were treated continuously with different doses of 4-DAB or NDEOL and killed sequentially after start of treatment. The increase in the volumetric fraction in liver occupied by ATPase-deficient foci as a function of time of treatment was quantitated and the time points where 0.1 and 0.5 % volumetric fraction were reached in liver were calculated from the regression lines for each dose group. These time points were plotted against dose in a double logarithmic net. The slopes of these regression lines were found to be very similar to the ones observed with respect to tumor induction and characteristically different for 4-DAB and NDEOL (see Figure 1). Moreover, there were striking differences between NDEOL and 4-DAB in the time periods between the appearance of early enzyme-altered foci and the later manifestation of liver tumors. This time interval was short for 4-DAB but much longer for NDEOL. The analysis of size class distribution of the enzyme-altered foci pointed towards a growth-stimulating activity of 4-DAB at the high doses. This was substantiated by thymidine-pulse-labeling experiments which demonstrated a very high frequency of labeled hepatocytes in liver foci of continuously 4-DAB treated rats indicating ongoing DNA synthesis in these cells. In contrast, foci generated in rats by continuous NDEOL exposure seemed to lack such proliferative response even at very high carcinogen dose levels. A direct comparison can be taken from data shown in Figure 2.

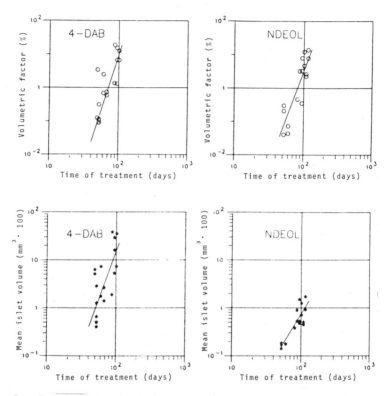

Fig. 2. Increase in the volumetric fraction of ATPase-deficient foci (upper part) and the mean volume of foci (lower part) as a function of time of treatment with 4-dimethylamino-azobenzene and N-nitrosodiethanolamine. 4-DAB was given in the diet (0.06 %) and NDEOL was administered via the drinking water (2000 ppm). Each point represents the value from one animal (taken from Schwarz et al., 1984).

At concentrations of 0.06 % in diet (4-DAB) and 2000 ppm in the drinking water (NDEOL) the volumetric fraction in liver occupied by ATPase-deficient foci (or the total number of enzyme-altered cells per unit liver) increased almost identically for either carcinogen (upper two graphs). With respect to this parameter these dose levels of NDEOL and 4-DAB were therefore equipotent. However, with NDEOL the increase in the volumetric islet fraction was mainly mediated by an increase in islet number whereas with 4-DAB the increase was predomi- nantly due to an enhancement of individual islet size. Thus, the mean islet volume calculated from data on the volumetric fraction in liver divided by islet number - was always smaller for NDEOL-induced foci and only about 1/10th of that generated by 4-DAB at a treatment period of 100 days. From these data we conclude that NDEOL has comparatively strong initiating potencies leading to the formation of many preneo- plastic foci but does not possess the activity to stimulate these foci to grow. In contrast, 4-DAB demonstrates weak initiating activity but exhibits at high dose levels a strong potency to stimulate the growth of enzyme-altered foci.

The volumetric fraction occupied by enzyme-altered tissue in liver is the integral of the number of foci and their size. Therefore, this value gives a direct estimate on the number of enzyme-altered cells per liver. At the two selected doses of 4-DAB and NDEOL shown in Figure 2 the number of enzyme-altered cells in liver increased almost identically. However, the time intervals between a defined preneoplastic response (0.1 or 0.5 % ATPase-deficient tissue in liver) and the appearance of liver tumors (50 % liver tumor-lethality) were markedly different for these dose levels of 4-DAB and NDEOL. Therefore, the proliferation rate of individual foci rather than the total number of enzyme-altered cells seems to be of importance for the transition to malignant cell populations.

Time-related increase in foci volume is an indirect measure of foci growth. As was expected, mean foci volumes determined at defined end-points differed considerably between various carcinogens but were less affected by carcinogen dose.

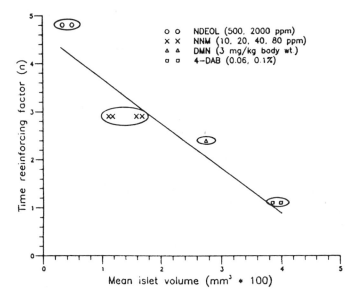

Fig. 3. Relation between mean volume of ATPase-deficient foci and time reinforcing factor n for tumor induction. ATPase-deficient foci were induced by continuous treatment of rats with various doses of the indicated carcinogens. Rats were killed sequentially and the time-dependent increases in number and volumetric fraction of ATPase-deficient foci in liver were determined by means of stereological procedures. Mean foci diameters at an arbitrarily chosen end-point of 1 % of liver being occupied by enzyme-altered tissue were calculated from these data. Data on time reinforcing factors n for tumor induction were taken from the literature.

Data shown in Figure 3 stem from experiments with continuous exposure of rats to different doses of NDEOL, 4-DAB, N-nitrosodimethylamine (DMN) and N-nitrosomorpholine (NNM). Mean volumes of ATPase-deficient foci were calculated on the basis of data describing the time-dependent increases in the volumetric tissue fraction and the number of foci per unit liver. As is demonstrated in Figure 3 there seems to exist a relation between mean foci volumes and time-reinforcing factors n determined in long-term tumor studies with the same hepatocarcinogens (Preussmann et al., 1982; Druckrey, 1967; Peto et al., 1984; Kunz et al., 1983). We conclude that the various carcinogens possess to a differing degrees the potency to stimulate growth of enzyme-altered foci, an effect which is inversely related to the numerical value of their time-reinforcing factor for tumor induction.

GROWTH PROPERTIES AND PHENOTYPE OF FOCI

The differences in the growth rate of enzyme-altered foci are reflected by a marked heterogenicity of foci phenotypes. The relationship between foci phenotype and proliferation kinetics was studied in detail using diethylnitrosamine (DEN) as a model carcinogen. Discrimination into different phenotypes was performed on the basis of serial liver sections stained enzyme- and immunohistochemically for a variety of different marker enzymes such as ATPase, γ-glutamyltranspeptidase (γ-GT), epoxide hydrolase (EH) and various cytochrome P-450 (cyt. P-450) isozymes. This study which has been reported elsewhere (Buchmann et al., 1987) demonstrated that those liver lesions which were characterized by decreased levels of three or four cyt. P-450 isozymes possessed a clear growth advantage over lesions with no or only one cyt. P-450 isozyme being altered. This result is in accordance with similar observations on other enzyme changes (Pugh and Goldfarb, 1978; Peraino et al., 1984; Estadella et al., 1984) and indicates that the proliferation behaviour of different lesions is correlated with their phenotypic complexity level. Similar findings were obtained in experiments with 4-DAB and NDEOL (Table 1).

As demonstrated in Table 1 the frequency of lesions with characteristically different phenotypes varied considerably between 4-DAB and NDEOL. With NDEOL the number of foci showing ATPase-deficiency without additional changes in any of the other markers was higher, whereas the number of lesions showing concomitant alterations in 2, 3 or all markers investigated was considerably lower than with 4-DAB. This phenotype distribution is characteristic for the slow proliferation rate of the majority of foci generated by NDEOL. In contrast, continuous administration of 4-DAB led to a comparatively high number of lesions showing changes in ATPase, γ-GT and all four cyt. P-450 isozymes, a phenotype which has been demonstrated in the experiments with DEN (see above) to be characteristic for rapidly growing lesions.

CONCLUSIONS

There is strong evidence to suggest that enzyme-altered foci in liver represent precursor lesions for tumors in this organ. Quantitative and qualitative analyses of early preneoplastic lesions can add significant information to our understanding of the mechanistic principles by which carcinogens and promoting agents enhance the carcinogenic process. Quantitative analyses of foci number and growth kinetics can be used to obtain precise data on effects of carcinogens at low dose levels and to discriminate between initiating and promoting activities. This is of importance for the improvement of models presently used for extrapolating animal carcinogenicity data into concentration ranges relevant to humans. Qualitative analyses of enzyme markers demonstrate a heterogeneity of foci phenotypes which reflects differences in their growth rates. The data indicate that not the total number of enzyme-altered cells per liver but rather the proliferation rate of individual lesions is of major importance for the additional transition(s) to malignant cell populations.

Table 1. Phenotypes of liver foci generated by continuous
treatment of rats with 4-DAB (0.06 %) or NDEOL
(2000 ppm). Serial liver sections from 4 rats
per treatment group were stained for the different
enzymes indicated in the table. – Phenotypes were
analyzed following computer-assisted 3-dimensional
reconstruction of the serial sections in a total
number of 41 (4-DAB) and 42 (NDEOL) foci which were
identified by ATPase-deficiency in the first and
last section of the series. Since the number of
permutations with 7 markers is extremely high,
the frequency of some selected phenotypes is given
only.

Phenotype	4-DAB	NDEOL
total number of ATPase-deficient foci	41	42
ATPase only	1	5
*ATPase + γ-GT	33	17
*ATPase + γ-GT + EH	14	4
*ATPase + γ-GT + 4 cyt. P-450 isozymes	12	2

*Lesions of these phenotypes show at least the indicated enzyme
alterations irrespective of additional marker changes.
Individual foci may therefore be scored in more than one of
these phenotype classes. Moreover, some lesions cannot be
classified into any of the indicated phenotypes. As a result
the sum of foci of the selected phenotypes does not equal the
total number of foci analyzed.

REFERENCES

1. Bannasch, P., Enzmann, H., and Zerban, H., 1986, Preneoplastic lesions as indicators of the carcinogenic risk caused by chemicals, in "Cancer Risks; strategies for elimination", P. Bannasch (ed.) Springer Verlag 47–64.

2. Buchmann, A., Schwarz, M., Schmitt, R., Wolf, C.R., Oesch, F., and Kunz, W., 1987, Development of cytochrome P-450 altered preneoplastic and neoplastic lesions during nitrosamine-induced hepatocarcinogenesis in the rat, Cancer Res., 47:2911–2918.

3. Campbell, H.A., Yuan-Ding Xu, Hanigan, M.H., and Pitot, H.C., 1986, Application of quantitative stereology to the evaluation of phenotypically heterogenous enzyme-altered foci in the rat liver, J. Natl. Cancer Inst., 76:751–767.

4. Druckrey, H., 1967, Quantitative aspects in chemical carcinogenesis, U.I.C.C. Monographs, 7:60–78.

5. Emmelot, P. and Scherer, E., 1980, The first relevant cell stages in rat liver carcinogenesis: a quantitative approach, Biochim. Biophys. Acta, 605:247–304.

6. Estadella, M.D., Pujol, M.J., and Domingo, J., 1984, Enzyme pattern and growth rate of liver preneoplastic clones during carcinogenesis by diethylnitrosamine, Oncology 41:276–279.

7. Friedrich-Freksa, H., Gössner, W., and Börner, P., 1969, Histochemische Untersuchungen der Cancerogenese in der Rattenleber nach Dauergabe von Diäthylnitrosamin, Z. Krebsforsch. 72:226–239.

8. Goldfarb, S. and Pugh, T.D., 1981, Enzyme histochemical phenotypes in primary hepatocellular carcinomas, Cancer Res., 41:2092–2095.

9. Kunz, H.W., Tennekes, H.A., Port, R.E., Schwarz, M., Lorke, D., and Schaude, G., 1983, Quantitative aspects of chemical carcinogenesis and tumor promotion in liver, Environ. Health Perspect., 50:113–122.

10. Kunz, H.W., Schwarz, M., Tennekes, H.A., Port, R., and Appel, K.E., 1985, Mechanism and dose-time response characteristics of carcinogenic and tumor promoting xenobiotics in liver, in "Tumorpromotoren, Erkennung, Wirkungsmechanismen und Bedeutung", K.E. Appel and A.G. Hildebrandt (eds), MMV Medizin Verlag München, BGA-Schriften 6, pp. 76–94.

11. Moolgavkar, S.H., 1983, Model of human carcinogenesis: action of environmental agents, Environm. Health Perspect., 50:285–291.

12. Moolgavkar, S.H., 1986, Carcinogenesis modeling: From Molecular Biology to Epidemioly, Ann. Rev. Public Health, 7:151–169.

13. Peraino, C., Richards, W.L., and Stevens, F.J., 1983, Multistage Hepatocarcinogenesis, in:"Mechanisms of Tumor Promotion", Vol. 1, T.J. Slaga (ed.), CRC Press, Inc., Boca Raton, Florida.

14. Peraino, C., Staffeldt, E.F., Carnes, B.Y., Ludemann, V.A., Blomquist, J.A., and Vesselinovictch, S.D., 1984, Characterisation of histochemically detectable altered hepatocyte foci and their relationship to hepatic tumorigenesis in rats treated once with diethylnitrosamine or benzo(a)pyrene one day after birth, Cancer Res., 44:3340–3347.

15. Peto, R., Gray, R., Brastom, P., and Grasso, P., 1984, Nitrosamine carcinogenesis in 5120 rodents: chronic administration of sixteen different concentrations of NDEA, NDMA, NPYR, and NPIP, in the water of 4440 inbred rats, with parallel studies on NDEA alone of the effect of age of starting (3, 6 or 20 weeks) and the species (rats, mice, hamsters), IARC Monography Series, 57:627–665.

16. Preussmann, R., Habs, M., Habs, H., and Schmähl, D., 1982, Carcinogenicity of N-nitrosodiethanolamine in rats at five different dose levels, Cancer Res., 42:5167–5171.

17. Pugh, T.D. and Goldfarb, S., 1978, Quantitative histochemical and autoradiographic studies of hepatocarcinogenesis in rats fed 2-actylaminofluorene followed by phenobarbital, Cancer Res., 38:4450-4457.
18. Rabes, H.M. and Szymkowiak, R., 1979, Cell kinetics of hepatocytes during the preneoplastic period of diethylnitrosamine-induced liver carcinogenesis, Cancer Res., 39:1298-1304.
19. Rabes, H.M., B§cher, T., Hartmann, A., Linke, I., and D§nnwald, M., 1982, Clonal growth of carcinogen-induced enzyme deficient pre-neoplastic cell population in mouse liver, Cancer Res., 42:3220-3227.
20. Schwarz, M., Pearson, D., Port, R., and Kunz, W., 1984, Promoting effect of 4-dimethylaminoazobenzene on enzyme altered foci induced in rat liver by N-nitrosodiethanolamine, Carcinogenesis, 5:725-730.
21. Williams, E.D., Wareham, K.A., and Howell, S., 1983, Direct evidence for the single cell origin of mouse liver cell tumours, Br. J. Cancer, 47:723-726.

This paper is dedicated to Prof. Dr. Rolf Preussmann on the occasion of his 60th birthday.

PATHOGENIC INTERRELATIONSHIP OF FOCAL LESIONS, NODULES, ADENOMAS AND

CARCINOMAS IN THE MULTISTAGE EVOLUTION OF AZASERINE-INDUCED RAT PANCREAS

CARCINOGENESIS

E. Scherer[1], J. Bax and R.A. Woutersen[2]

Division of Chemical Carcinogenesis, The Netherlands Cancer
Institute (Antoni van Leeuwenhoekhuis), 121 Plesmanlaan
1066 CX Amsterdam, The Netherlands

[1] To whom correspondence should be addressed
[2] Department of Biological Toxicology, TNO-CIVO Toxicology and Nutrition
Institute, P.O. Box 360, 3700 AJ Zeist, The Netherlands

INTRODUCTION

It is widely accepted now that cancer develops in a cellular
multistage proces in which cell populations of increasing neoplastic
potential develop in a stochastic (and probably clonal) way from less
neoplastic precursor cell populations. The increasing malignancy of
tumors in time (progression, Foulds [1969]) has since long been explained
in this way, but recent results from *i.a.* rat hepatocarcinogenesis
(Scherer [1987]) and mouse skin carcinogenesis (Hennings and Yuspa
[1985]) indicate that a similar stochastic process operates in the
development of the tumor from initiated cell clones and intermediate
neoplastic cell populations (promotion).

For the purpose of risk assessment and regulatory decisions it is of
paramount importance to know the relationship between precancerous cell
populations and the ultimate formation of tumors. This knowledge can also
help to identify initiating carcinogens and promoting or anticarcinogenic
factors by short term experiments.

In the present communication we present a careful analysis of the
histo- and cytological properties of azaserine-induced focal lesions in
exocrine rat pancreas carcinogenesis. Particular attention was paid to
topological relationships between focal lesions, especially to lesions
within lesions, indicating the development of more advanced focal cell
populations - including carcinoma-in-situ and carcinoma - within lesions
of already changed acinar tissue (foci, nodules or adenomas).

This approach led to the recognition of various focus-in-focus
patterns (FIF), and enabled us to establish the often slight differences
between cell populations related to each other in a precursor-product
relationship. This allowed the distinction of the acidophilic acinar
foci, nodules and adenomas on basis of cyto- and histologic/histochemical
properties, and on the FIF interrelationships observed, rather than on

size. Strong evidence was obtained that exocrine pancreatic cancer of the rat develops from the azaserine-induced acidophilic foci via several acidophilic and later eventially basophilic intermediate cell populations. Occasionally carcinoma exhibiting a ductal pattern with the involvement of stroma - similar to human pancreatic adenocarcinoma - was found as part of acidophilic acinar pancreatic carcinoma. As acidophilic pancreatic lesions similar to those of the rat were observed in human pancreatic autopsy material (Longnecker et al., [1980]) and in cancer specimens (preliminary studies) a sequence as derived for the rat could well apply to man.

MATERIALS AND METHODS

Hematoxylin and eosin (H&E) stained rat pancreas sections were obtained from a study into the modulating effect of ethanol and coffee on dietary fat promoted pancreatic carcinogenesis (Woutersen et al., submitted).

One hundred and sixty male weanling SPF albino Wistar rats (Cpb:WU; Wistar random) were obtained from the TNO Central Institute for the Breeding of Laboratory Animals, Zeist, The Netherlands. They were kept on softwood bedding in macrolon cages, five animals per cage, under standard laboratory conditions. All rats were given a single i.p. injection of 30 mg L-azaserine/kg body wt. (Calbiochem-Behring Corp., La Jolla, CA; dissolved freshly in 0.9 % NaCl solution) at 19 days of age, and allocated to 4 different groups by a computer randomization procedure. Each group consisted of 40 rats which were maintained on: (A) a low fat (LF) control diet (5% corn oil); (B) a high fat (HF) diet (25% corn oil); (C) a HF diet in combination with coffee (instead of drinking water); and (D) a HF diet in combination with ethanol (10% in drinking water). The diets were compounded from natural feed ingredients and stored at - 20 °C until needed. They contained equal amounts of protein, minerals, trace elements and vitamins per unit energy. The percentage composition of the diets is summarized in a previous paper (Woutersen et al., [1986]).

General condition and behaviour of the animals were checked daily. Terminal autopsy was 15 months after the injection with azaserine. The animals were anesthesized by ether, exsanguinated by cannulating the abdominal aorta, autopsied and then examined for gross pathological changes. The entire pancreas, liver, lungs, kidneys and all gross lesions from each animal were excised, and fixed in 10% buffered formalin. The pancreas and liver were weighed before fixation. The paraffin-embedded pancreata were step sectioned at 5 μm, and stained with H&E. From selected animals fresh pancreas samples were also quickly frozen for the preparation of ATPase-stained cryostat sections (Bax et al., [1986]).

RESULTS

In agreement with earlier reports (Bax et al., [1986], Longnecker et al., [1974,1975], Roebuck et al., [1984]) various phenotypically different populations of foci and nodules were observed in the pancreata of azaserine-treated rats. 15 Months after treatment, in many animals - especially of the high fat groups - virtually 100% of the pancreatic tissue consisted of altered acinar cells, mainly present as acidophilic nodules and adenomas. Remnants of normal acini were often confined to little areas compressed between the nodular/adenoma populations.

Acidophilic focal lesions

Early focal lesions of altered acinar cells are difficult to recognize in H&E stained sections as long as they are small. These lesions can, however, easily be evaluated in cryostat sections stained for ATPase activity (Bax *et al.*, [1986]). Cytologically these lesions (fig. 2) are characterized by slightly increased size of the individual acini, pronounced acidophilic staining of the apical part of the acinar cells and decreased area as well as basophilic staining intensity of basal cytoplasm. The nuclei are of about the same size as those of normal acinar tissue (Fig. 1).

Cytologically very similar to the above foci are lesions which reach nodular dimensions (> 1mm, fig. 3). The main difference as compared to the foci (fig. 2) is in the decreased size of the acinar cells. Due to the resulting closer package of the nuclei and the generally larger size of the acini these lesions are easily recognized in H&E stained sections. Individual acini are separated - as in normal or focal pancreas - by connective tissue. The nuclear diameter is similar to that of normal acinar cells. As compared with the foci the ATPase staining intensity was increased.

Acidophilic lesions of adenoma size (>3mm) were observed in two different forms, exhibiting both a still closer nuclear package than in the nodular lesions; they either retained the acinar differentiation (fig. 4), or lost it together with even smaller cell size and cellular and nuclear pleomorphism (fig. 5). The former type of adenoma was the most prominent one in this series of slides. A characteristic of this type is a considerable reduction in connective tissue separating the acini in normal, focal and nodular tissue. This reduction in connective tissue might be due to the high mitotic activity of acinar cells seen in these adenomas. ATPase staining was very strong in these lesions.

The latter type of lesion was frequently associated which a thin capsule. Together with the pronounced pleomorphism this indicates carcinoma-in-situ. ATPase staining was strong, but less intense than in the former lesions.

Basophilic focal lesions

Early basophilic focal lesions induced by azaserine are characterized by the lack of acidophilic cytoplasmic staining and by huge acini composed of large cells comprising large nuclei (fig. 6).

Basophilic nodules and adenomas were generally observed in close association, or within, acidophilic nodules or adenomas (figs. 7-9; see below). They were characterized by either a broadened area of basal basophilic cytoplasm, or by diffuse basophilic staining all over the acinus. The cytoplasm exhibited pronounced or decreased acidophilia. As in acidophilic nodules and adenomas, the relative size of the acinar cells is decreased, leading to a smaller internuclear distance. Nuclei were either of the same size as in the acidophilic foci, or enlarged.

After ATPase staining the basophilic cell populations were not or only slightly stained (fig. 9). This sharply contrasts with the strong ATPase staining of the adjacent acidophilic cell populations.

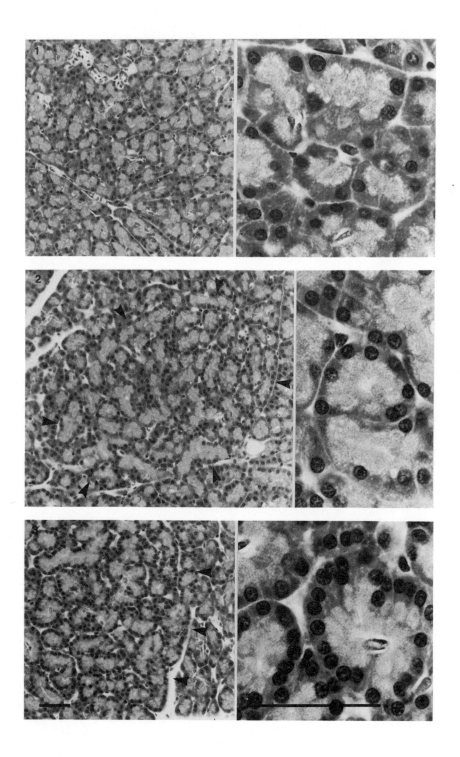

44

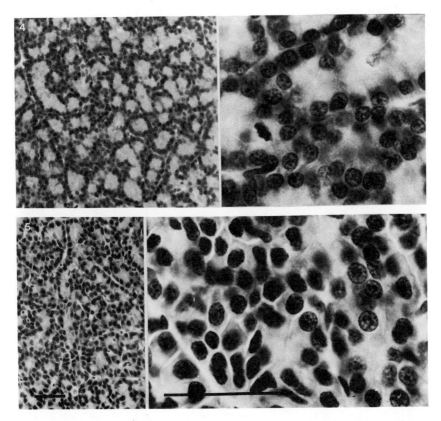

Figure 1. Unaltered part of pancreas of a rat treated once with azaserine at age 19 days, and fed a low fat (5%) diet for 15 months. Left: overview, right: individual acini. H&E; Bar 50μm.

Figure 2. The central circumscribed focus of altered acinar cells (arrows in the left panel, surrounded by normal acinar tissue) is characterized by increased size of individual acini and decreased intensity and area of cytoplasmic basophilia (right panel). Same pancreas as fig. 1; H&E; Bar 50 μm.

Figure 3. The acini of the circumscribed acidophilic nodule (arrows in the left panel, 1.5 mm in diameter) are characterized by decreased size of the acinar cells resulting in a smaller internuclear distance (right panel). Same pancreas as fig. 1; H&E; Bar 50 μm.

Figure 4. Part of a circumscribed acidophilic adenoma (left panel, 4 mm in diameter). Note (right panel) the lack of separation of individual acinar structures by connective tissue. The cytoplasmic basophilia is further decreased. From a rat fed a high fat (25%) diet; H&E; Bar 50 μm.

Figure 5. Part of a less well differentiated acidophilic adenoma or carcinoma-in-situ (left panel, 3 mm in diameter). Note (right panel) the small cell size, the considerable loss of acinar differentiation, and the nuclear pleomorphism. Same pancreas as fig. 4; H&E; Bar 50 μm.

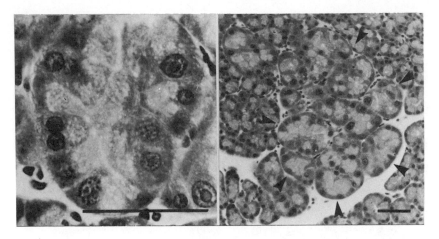

Figure 6. Circumscribed primary basophilic focus (left panel, arrows) surrounded by normal acinar tissue. It consists (right panel) of large cells with large nuclei. The cytoplasm is hardly stained by the acidic dye eosin. Same pancreas as Fig. 1; Bar 50 μm.

Focus-in-focus (FIF) interrelationship between various populations of altered acinar cells.

FIF patterns were first observed in ATPase-stained sections between basophilic cell populations (ATPase deficient) and acidophilic nodule or adenoma tissue surrounding them (strongly ATPase positive, fig. 9). Such patterns are also easy to find in H&E-stained sections (figs. 7, 8), provided the surrounding cell population is large enough to be recognized, *i.e.* consists of more than only a thin rim of cells.

Much less prominent are FIF patterns between acidophilic cell populations. From the careful evaluation of thousands of foci, nodules and adenomas we conclude, however, that a FIF histogenesis is indicated also for more advanced acidophilic lesions, such as the nodules, adenomas and carcinoma-in-situ. A typical example is given in figure 10 of a small population resembling cytologically an acidophilic nodule (fig. 3) surrounded by acinar tissue with characteristics of the early focus (fig. 2). The putative step from nodular to adenomatous phenotype is illustrated in figure 11. Since a FIF ethiology is indicated for nodules and adenomas the respective phenotype is not restricted to a certain size group (> 1 mm, and > 3 mm), but holds also for the earlier and thus smaller forms.

Similar FIF patterns have been observed between acidophilic cell populations differing to each other with respect to characteristics such as nuclear shape or diameter, nuclear staining intensity, cytoplasmic acidophilia, degree of pleomorphism or amount of connective tissue between acini.

Carcinoma stages

Carcinoma was generally associated with altered acinar tissue of nodular and/or adenomatous type (fig. 12). Often more than one form of carcinoma was observed in the same tumor, indicating that progression is by similar histogenic processes as the development of nodules and

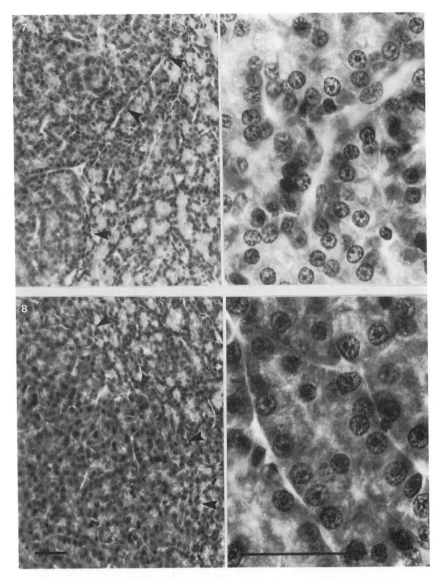

Figure 7. Part of a circumscribed basophilic nodule (left portion of the left panel, arrows) surrounded by (right portion) acidophilic nodule tissue. The basophilic cell population exhibits acinar differentiation (right panel), the cytoplasm containing both acidophilic and basophilic material. H&E; Bar 50 μm.

Figure 8. Part of a basophilic carcinoma-in-situ which is surrounded by acidophilic adenoma tissue (right portion of the left panel). It is characterized (right panel) by acinar differentiation, strong cytoplasmic basophilia and enlarged nuclei. H&E; Bar 50μm.

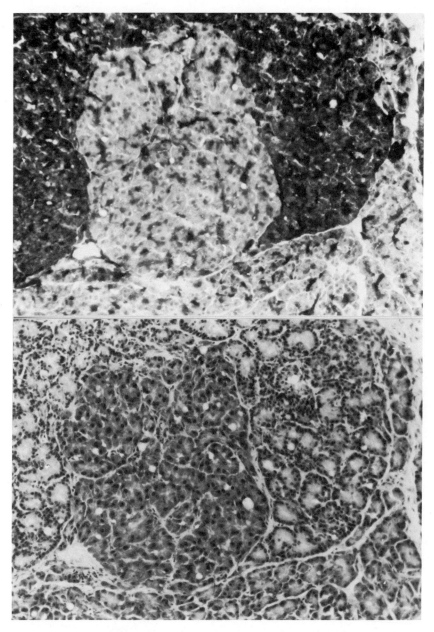

Figure 9. Focus-in-focus: The central ATPase deficient nodule cell population (top panel, ATPase staining) is surrounded by ATPase positive focus/nodule tissue. The nodule cell population is characterized by basophilic cytoplasm (bottom panel, H&E staining). The slightly stained tissue at the bottom edge is normal pancreas. Cryostat section, Bar: 50μm.

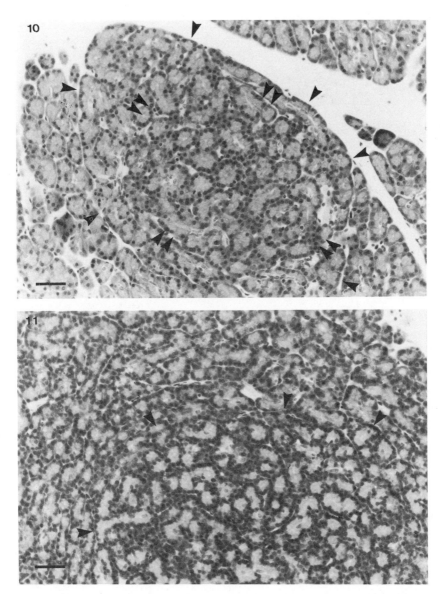

Figure 10. Focus-in-focus: An acidophilic cell population similar to that shown in fig. 3 (nodule, double arrows) is partially surrounded by a cell population as shown in fig. 2 (focus, arrows). The tissue in the corners is normal pancreas. Same pancreas as fig. 1; H&E; Bar 50 μm.

Figure 11. Focus-in-focus: A circumscribed acidophilic cell population (arrows) similar to that shown in fig. 5 (adenoma) is completely surrounded by a nodule cell population as shown in fig. 3. Same pancreas as fig. 4; H&E; Bar 50 μm.

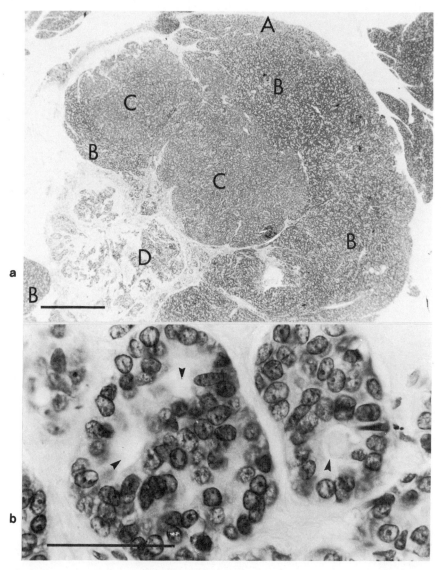

Figure 12. Panel a: Pancreatic carcinoma being composed of various cell populations. Two independent basophilic CIS populations (C) and poorly differentiated carcinoma (D) are surrounded by acidophilic adenoma (B) and acidophilic focus/nodule (A) tissue. Left and right upper corners: normal acinar tissue, lower left corner: adenoma tissue contigous with (B); Bar: 1mm. Panel b: Poorly differentiated carcinoma area (D) with stroma, composed of cells with centroacinar-like nuclei. Some ductal organization (arrows) is present. High fat (25%) group; H&E; Bar: 50μm.

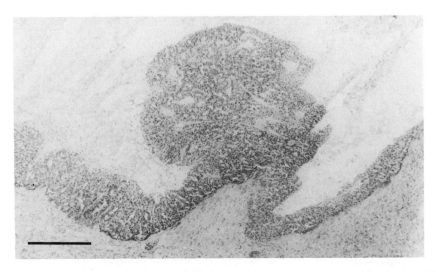

Figure 13. Papillary pancreatic carcinoma. The tumor cells are acidophilic (ATPase reaction is positive) and exhibit some acinar differentiation. High fat (25%) + coffee group; Cryostat section, H&E; Bar: 250 μm.

adenomas, *i.e.* by generation of deviating cells within an already altered cell population followed by selection for the most proliferative variants.

As for nodules/adenomas two main lines could be distinguished on basis of the cytoplasmic staining. The *acidophilic* line led to carcinoma of acinar differentiation (ATPase positive), of either solid or papillary growth pattern with stroma (fig. 13) and to poorly differentiated carcinoma (massive stroma) characterized by rather 'empty', centroacinar-like nuclei and the tendency to form ductal structures (fig. 12B). A rare type of carcinoma developed from an acidophilic acinar carcinoma, and was charcterized by small cells arranged in a multilayered, adenomatous pattern (fig. 14).

The *basophilic* line led to nodular, often encapsulated lesions of some mm in diameter. These basophilic carcinoma-in-situ or microcarcinoma were cytologically similar to the secondary basophilic nodules, and only rarely showed indications of further progression. The trabecular carcinoma (relatively large nuclei, prominent nucleolus, eventually liver characteristics like glycogen and glucose-6-phosphatase) which was occasionally observed, could, however, belong to this series.

CONCLUSIONS

In the present evaluation of azaserine-induced pancreatic carcinogenesis in the rat we observed numerous FIF patterns between distinguishable acidophilic cell populations and between acidophilic and secondary basophilic cell populations. The occurrence of such FIF patterns is in agreement with an ordered evolutionary sequence (chart 1) in which cells of a new phenotype develop after a specific rare event has taken place in cells of already altered populations.

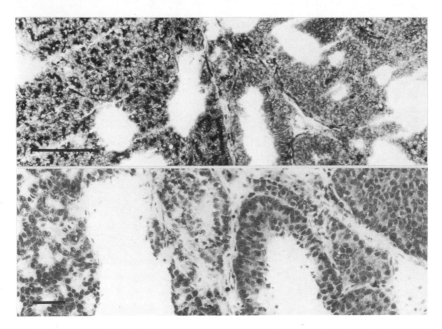

Figure 14. The acidophilic pancreatic carcinoma in the left portion of this field (ATPase positive, especially at the apical site of the acini) contains a poorly differentiated subpopulation (right portion, slightly ATPase positive only) which tends to form adenomatous, multilayered structures. High fat (25%) group; Cryostat sections; Upper half: ATPase; Bar: 250 μm. Lower half: H&E; Bar: 50 μm.

Two main lines of development were indicated which shared the acidophilic acinar focus as a common root: from initiated acinar cells growing out to acidophilic foci, via acidophilic nodules and adenomas (figs. 10,11) to (i) (acidophilic) lesions consisting of small cells, and eventually further to microinvasive and anaplastic carcinomas (Figs. 12-14), and (ii) to secondary basophilic nodules (Figs. 7-9), carcinoma-in-situ and well differentiated acinar carcinoma (Fig. 12A - populations C). While the latter line is characterized by increased cellular/nuclear size, basophilic cytoplasma and retained acinar differentiation of the

carcinoma, the former line shows stepwise decrease of cytoplasmic basophila, of cell size, and later of acidophilic staining intensity. It is characterized in its late stages (carcinoma-in-situ and poorly differentiated carcinoma) by densely packed small cells (Fig. 12B-14), resulting in an overall basophilic appearance.

In contrast to the numerous FIF originating in the acidophilic foci, we have never seen in the present series of slides any FIF relationship originating in the primary basophilic focus. This suggests that the primary basophilic focus/nodule cell population is unrelated to pancreatic carcinogenesis under the present experimental conditions. This lack of progression could result from a lower probability per focus cell to undergo changes, which may be related, as stressed by Rao et al. [1982], to the low proliferative capacity of the basophilic foci as compared to that of the acidophilic foci/nodules/adenomas.

```
                    POORLY DIFFERENTIATED CARCINOMA
                               ∧
                               │    step, proliferation
                               │
               ACIDOPHILIC CIS
                    ∧
                    │    step, proliferation
                    │
            ACIDOPHILIC ADENOMA  -------------
               ∧                              │    step, proliferation
               │    step, proliferation       │
               │                              V
        ACIDOPHILIC NODULE  -----------       V
          ∧                                   │   .
          │    step, proliferation            │  step, proliferation
          │                                   V   .
    ACIDOPHILIC FOCUS    - - - ? - >   BASOPHILIC NODULE
                                              │   .
       ∧                                      │   . step, proliferation
       │    step, proliferation               V V
       │                              BASOPHILIC CIS
  NORMAL ACINAR CELL                          │
       │                                      ?
       │    step, proliferation               V
       V                              TRABECULAR CARCINOMA
  PRIMARY BASOPHILIC
  FOCUS
```

Chart 1. Putative pathogenic interrelationship between focal cell populations in rat pancreas carcinogenesis.

The absence of surrounding putative precursor tissue was also regularly encountered, especially in case of large acidophilic or basophilic nodules or adenomas. This lack can, however, not been taken as evidence that nodules or adenomas do develop without precursor cell populations. It is more likely that the apparently lacking precursor-product relationship is due to the pronounced proliferation of a more advanced cell population overgrowing any slowly proliferating precursor cell population within a short time. In addition, the chance to cut by the section plane through both the nodule and its precursor lesion becomes smaller the larger the nodule is.

From the FIF patterns observed one may conclude that pancreatic cancer of the rat develops through a relatively high number of rare events/steps, about 5 for the endpoint 'poorly differentiated carcinoma' of the acidophilic series (focus->nodule->adenoma->CIS->carcinoma). This deviates from the two-step model as proposed currently - mainly on base of tumor kinetics - for the formation of various human tumors (Moolgavkar, this volume). The number of steps involved in pancreatic carcinogenesis could, however, be lower if not all the observed steps are obligatory, *i.e.* if shorter routes skipping some of the stages are possible. On the other hand, the kinetics of tumor formation reflect only *rate-limiting* steps. If some steps in this process occur with relatively high probability - which seems not so unlikely for later steps seen the large number of intermediate cells at risk and their generally increased proliferation rate - tumors can develop through more than two steps, and nevertheless follow kinetics consistent with a two-step process.

Compared to other experimental models such as rat liver (Scherer, [1987]), the frequency by which FIF were observed was exceptionally high in rat pancreas, and even increased by a diet high in unsaturated fat. Apart from the FIF and nodules harbouring multiple subpopulations, large nodules or adenomas exhibiting no indications for the presence of subclones were observed. This indicates that the probability of clonal progression is specific for each lesion of altered pancreatic cells. The key question is which phenotype - and underlying genotype - is linked to a high progression probability, and thus may be the most relevant precancerous lesion for the formation of pancreatic cancer.

ACKNOWLEDGEMENTS

The skilled technical assistance by A. van Garderen-Hoetmer and C. Schippers-Gillissen, as well as the financial support by Koningin Wilhelmina Fonds (Grant CIVO 84-1) is greatfully acknowledged. We are indepted to Dr. D.S. Longnecker for valuable discussions during his sabbatical leave at TNO-CIVO.

REFERENCES

Bax, J. , Feringa, A. W. , Van Garderen-Hoetmer, A. , Woutersen, R. A. , and Scherer, E. Adenosine triphosphatase, a new marker for the differentiation of putative precancerous foci induced in rat pancreas by azaserine. Carcinogenesis, 7: 457-462, 1986.

Foulds, L. , Neoplastic development, Vol. I, II. London, New York.: Academic Press, 1969.

Hennings, H. , and Yuspa, S. H. Two-stage tumor promotion in mouse skin: An alternative interpretation. J. Natl. Cancer Inst., 74: 735-740, 1985.

Longnecker, D. S. , and Crawford, B. G. Hyperplastic nodules and adenomas of exocrine pancreas in azaserine-treated rats. J. Natl. Cancer Inst., 53: 573-577, 1974.

Longnecker, D. S. , and Curphey, T. J. Adenocarcinoma of the pancreas in azaserine-treated rats. Cancer Res., 35: 2249-2258, 1975.

Longnecker, D. S. , Shinozuka, H. , and Dekker, A. Focal acinar cell dysplasia in human pancreas. Cancer, 45: 534-540, 1980.

Rao, M. S. , Upton, M. P. , Subbarao, V. and Scarpelli, D. G. Two populations of cells with differing proliferative capacities in atypical acinar cell foci induced by 4-hydroxyaminoquinoline-1-oxide in the rat pancreas. Lab. Invest., 46: 527-534, 1982.

Roebuck, B. D. , Baumgartner, K. J. , and Thron, C. D. Characterization of two populations of pancreatic atypical acinar cell foci induced by azaserine in the rat. Lab. Invest., 50: 141-146, 1984.

Scherer, E. Relationship among histochemically distinguishable early lesions in multistep-multistage hepatocarcinogenesis. Arch. Toxicol. Suppl., 10: 81-94, 1987.

Woutersen, R. A. , Van Garderen-Hoetmer, A. , Bax, J. , Feringa, A. W. , and Scherer, E. Modulation of putative preneoplastic foci in exocrine pancreas of rats and hamsters. I. Interaction of dietary fat and ethanol. Carcinogenesis, 7: 1587-1593, 1986.

Woutersen, R. A. , Van Garderen-Hoetmer, A. , Bax, J. , and Scherer, E. Modulation of dietary fat promoted pancreatic carcinogenesis in rats and hamsters by chronic ethanol ingestion. Carcinogenesis, submitted.

Woutersen, R. A. , Van Garderen-Hoetmer, A. , Bax, J. , and Scherer, E. Modulation of dietary fat promoted pancreatic carcinogenesis in rats and hamsters by chronic coffee ingestion. Carcinogenesis, submitted.

PHENOTYPIC CELLULAR CHANGES IN MULTI-

STAGE CARCINOGENESIS

Peter Bannasch

Institut für Experimentelle Pathologie
Deutsches Krebsforschungszentrum
6900 Heidelberg, Federal Republic of Germany

INTRODUCTION

The concept that carcinogenesis is a multistage process comprising initiation, promotion and progression has mainly been inferred from experiments
in which certain operational steps were used to induce tumors of the skin,
liver or other tissues (Pitot, 1988). However, an unequivocal explanation
of initiation, promotion and progression in biological terms has not been
reached by this experimental approach. The more recent discovery of characteristic sequential cellular changes during neoplastic development in different organs, especially in the liver, has opened a new approach for the
distinction of stages of carcinogenesis which can now be defined by biological rather than operational criteria (Bannasch, 1988). In many tissues, preneoplastic foci composed of phenotypically altered cells emerging weeks and
months before benign or malignant tumors appear have been described (Carter,
1984; IARC, 1986). The diagnosis of foci implies that the altered cell populations are perfectly integrated into the normal architecture of the respective tissue and do not show any expansive growth. At the histological level,
preneoplasia may be defined as a phenotypically altered cell population which
has no obvious neoplastic nature but has a high probability of progressing
to a benign or malignant neoplasm (Bannasch, 1986). Frequently, the transition from preneoplastic foci into benign or malignant tumors is associated
with additional changes of the cellular phenotype. A precise knowledge of
the sequence of phenotypic cellular changes during carcinogenesis is not only
a prerequisite for the elucidation of the mechanism of oncogenesis but is also
of increasing importance in the assessment of the carcinogenic risk caused
by chemicals. In the past few years, preneoplastic lesions have been used
with advantage as end points in carcinogenicity testing in a number of laboratories. Sequential cellular changes induced with chemicals in the liver and
kidney of rodents will be presented as examples for modulations of the cellular phenotype during carcinogenesis which may help to unravel a general
principle underlying the phenotypic diversity of preneoplastic and neoplastic
cells, and may improve the evaluation of bioassays for carcinogenicity.

PHENOTYPIC CELLULAR CHANGES IN RENAL CARCINOGENESIS

In rodents, chemical carcinogens may induce nearly all types of kidney
tumors known from human pathology, namely chromophobic, basophilic, clear
cell, acidophilic and oncocytic tumors (Bannasch et al., 1986). The tumors
develop after long lag periods and often appear multicentrically and bilate-

rally. Different parts of the renal tubular system are the site of origin of the cytologically different tumor types which are preceded by characteristic preneoplastic tubular lesions. Thus, chromophobic tubules and tumors originate from the proximal nephron. They store excessive amounts of substances the nature of which is not entirely clear. Sometimes glycosaminoglycans can be demonstrated by staining with alcian blue. Basophilic tubules (often also storing small amounts of glycosaminoglycans) likewise arise from the proximal tubule. They represent prestages of basophilic tumors which share a number of enzymatic aberrations with the basophilic tubules (Tsuda et al., 1986). Clear cell tubules storing glycogen in excess are precursors of clear and acidophilic cell tumors developing from the epithelium of the collecting duct and the connecting tubule (Bannasch et al., 1988). A fourth preneoplastic tubular lesion are oncocytic tubules which give rise to oncocytomas and may rarely contain clear (glycogenotic) cells. Like the clear cells, the oncocytes develop from the epithelium of the collecting duct and the connecting tubule (Nogueira, 1987; Nogueira and Bannasch, 1988). All renal lesions described may be induced by a single dose of N-nitrosomorpholine (NNM), and they frequently appear side by side in the same kidney. The reason for the divergent reactions of the renal epithelia to the primary biochemical alteration produced by the carcinogenic agent has not been clarified, but it seems that the well-known variations in the morphological and functional differentiation of normal epithelia along the nephron may play a crucial role in determining the phenotype of preneoplastic and neoplastic lesions. Ultrastructural and histochemical findings suggest that a disturbance of energy metabolism leading to an excessive storage of polysaccharides (clear and chromophobic cells), to an increased activity of the pentose phosphate pathway (basophilic cells) or to an increase in the activity of mitochondrial enzymes associated with a reduced activity of the pentose phosphate pathway (oncocytes) may be a common denominator of the phenotypic cellular changes observed (Bannasch et al., 1986). The single dose experiments prove that the development of both the preneoplastic and the neoplastic phenotypes initiated by the carcinogen are due to a self-propagating process which does neither need the further action of the carcinogen nor any other exogenous stimulus.

PHENOTYPIC CELLULAR CHANGES IN HEPATOCARCINOGENESIS

A variety of cellular phenotypes have been described in preneoplastic hepatic foci which precede the development of hepatic adenomas (HA) and carcinomas (HCC) induced in rats with chemicals (Bannasch, 1986; Goldsworthy et al., 1986; Moore and Kitagawa, 1986). According to cytoplasmic tinctorial changes the following types of foci may be distinguished (Bannasch, 1986; Weber et al., 1988a): 1) clear cell foci storing glycogen in excess, 2) acidophilic cell foci exhibiting both a proliferation of the smooth endoplasmic reticulum and an excessive storage of glycogen (in glycogenotic foci clear and acidophilic cells often appear together), 3) basophilic cell foci poor in glycogen but rich in homogeneously distributed basophilic material (ribosomes), 4) mixed cell foci composed of cell types 1-3, 5) tigroid cell foci showing a prominent lamellar cytoplasmic basophilia due to abundant stacks of highly ordered rough endoplasmic reticulum, 6) amphophilic cell foci poor in glycogen and staining with both acidophilic and basophilic dyes, and finally 7) intermediate cell foci composed of a more or less uniform population of intermediate cell types. Most of these phenotypically altered foci represent different stages in an ordered sequence of cellular changes leading from the clear and acidophilic cell foci through mixed and basophilic cell foci to HA and HCC (Bannasch, 1968). However, the tigroid cell foci which have been explicitly described in rats after oral application of a single dose of aflatoxin (Bannasch et al., 1985) and after treatment with hexachlorocyclohexanes (Schröter et al., 1987) are apparently characteristic for another cell lineage leading to hepatic tumors. No clearcut prestages for the tigroid cell foci have been identified so far, but we tentatively assume that they might originate from the large X-cells described earlier (Bannasch et al., 1980). In this context it should be mentioned that morphometric studies in extrafocal hepatocytes of NNM-treated rat liver revealed a significant nuclear and cytoplasmic enlargement in many cells, especially in perivenular hepatocytes, persisting up to 40 weeks after the end of treatment (Enzmann and Bannasch, 1987a). Although the foci of altered hepatocytes are apparently the most typical and the most important features of early stages in hepatocarcinogenesis, some participation of the persisting extrafocal changes cannot be ruled out. Like the tigroid cell foci, the amphophilic cell foci are not a regular part of the sequence of cellular changes mentioned above. They appear to be the consequence of a modulation of this sequence stimulated, for instance, by an additional treatment with dehydroepiandrosterone (Weber et al., 1988a and b).

The morphological changes in preneoplastic hepatic foci are regularly associated with a decrease or an increase in the amount and/or activity of various enzymes, particularly enzymes of the carbohydrate and drug metabolism (Friedrich-Freksa et al., 1969; Bannasch et al., 1984; Scherer, 1984; Goldsworthy et al., 1986; Moore and Kitagawa, 1986; Farber and Sarma, 1987; Seelmann-Eggebert et al., 1987; Klimek et al., 1988; Tatematsu et al., 1988a and b). Some of these enzymatic alterations have frequently been used as "negative or positive markers", respectively, for the detection of preneoplastic hepatic foci. Examples for negative markers are the decreased activities of the adenosine triphosphatase and the glucose-6-phosphatase, and for positive markers the increased activities of the γ-glutamyltransferase, the glutathione S-transferase and the glucose-6-phosphate dehydrogenase. It is important to realize, however, that no universal marker for preneoplastic foci is available. In addition to a considerable heterogeneity of the morphological and enzyme histochemical phenotypes of the foci, a remarkable reversion- or progression-linked phenotypic instability has been observed in cells composing the foci under certain experimental conditions (Bannasch, 1986). In spite of this shortcoming, many results suggest that the phenotypic heterogeneity in preneoplastic hepatic foci is to a large extent due to well-controlled patterns of ordered morphological and metabolic changes resulting in HA and HCC (Bannasch et al., 1984). Although adenomas are often the direct precursors of the carcinomas, the latter may also develop from focal lesions without passing an adenomatous intermediate stage.

It has been widely accepted that the preneoplastic hepatic foci originate from single or a few initiated hepatocytes (Rabes, 1983 and 1988) but some earlier results favor the development from larger fields of the liver parenchyma (Bannasch, 1968). On an average, cell proliferation is increased in the foci as compared to the surrounding liver parenchyma (Rabes, 1983 and 1988). However, when the different types of foci are studied separately, remarkable variations are evident. As demonstrated by the incorporation of ^{3}H-thymidine, the early clear or acidophilic glycogen storage foci only show a slightly increased cell proliferation, but a pronounced and steadily rising cell proliferation is linked with the appearance of mixed and basophilic cell populations in foci, HA and HCC (Zerban et al., 1985). Recently, Tatematsu and colleagues (1988a) reported an inverse relationship between the development of glutathione S-transferase positive liver foci and proliferation of the surrounding liver parenchyma in rats.

The importance of taking cell death into account in the analysis of hepatocarcinogenesis has been emphasized in recent years by Columbano and colleagues (1984) and by Bursch and colleagues (1984). Small non-persisting foci of altered hepatocytes which apparently disappear due to cellular necrosis have also been observed in stop experiments with NNM (Enzmann and Bannasch, 1988).

The sequential changes in hepatocellular morphology and proliferation during progression from foci to HA and HCC are often accompanied by additional enzymatic alterations (Bannasch et al., 1984; Buchmann et al., 1985). As to the carbohydrate metabolism enzyme histochemical and microbiochemical studies in rats suggest a gradual shift from glycogen metabolism to alternative metabolic pathways, such as the pentose phosphate pathway and glycolysis. Similar changes in a number of other species, including primates (Ruebner et al., 1976; Vesselinovitch et al., 1985; Limmer et al., 1988), support the hypothesis that the disturbance in glucose metabolism may be causally related to neoplastic transformation of the hepatocytes (Bannasch, 1988). Interestingly, an increase of the central metabolite glucose-6-phosphate has recently been found in preneoplastic glycogenotic liver cell lines (Mayer, 1988) and in early stages of NNM-induced hepatocarcinogenesis in rats (Enzmann et al., 1988). In the latter case, it is not yet clear, however, whether this metabolic alteration is correlated with hepatic preneoplasia or is due to unspecific toxic alterations of hepatocytes.

QUANTITATIVE ASPECTS OF HEPATOCARCINOGENESIS

A close statistical correlation between the total number and size of hepatic foci and the development of hepatic tumors in rodents has been reported by a number of authors (Emmelot and Scherer, 1980; Kunz et al., 1982; Vesselinovitch and Mihailovich, 1983; Goldsworthy and Pitot, 1985; Zerban et al., 1988a and b).

Quantitative stereological studies according to the procedures proposed by Scherer (1981) and by Enzmann and colleagues (1987) in rat liver treated with NNM have shown that in addition to the total number and size of the focal hepatic lesions their cellular composition strongly depends on the dose and duration of the carcinogenic treatment and on the time point of the carcinogenic process investigated (Moore et al., 1982; Enzmann and Bannasch, 1987b; Weber and Bannasch, 1988). After limited (7 weeks) oral administration of NNM (stop model) in a concentration of 120 mg/l drinking water a chronological sequence was observed leading from clear and acidophilic (glycogenotic) foci of early appearance to mixed and basophilic foci occurring at later time points (Moore et al., 1982; Enzmann and Bannasch, 1987b). Eventually HA and HCC developed. The results are in line with the concept that the phenotypically different types of foci essentially reflect different stages in the process of hepatocarcinogenesis.

When the dose-dependence of the preneoplastic lesion phenotype was studied in greater detail, we found that the mean of over-all number of preneoplastic lesions and the incidence of HA and HCC were dose-dependent ranging from 1000 foci/cm^3, 1% HA and no HCC after single oral dose (SD) of NNM (200mg/kg b.w.) to 3200 foci/cm^3, 48% HA and 27% HCC in the group permanently treated with NNM (12mg/kg/d) (Weber and Bannasch, 1988). While in all groups the majority of lesions was of clear cell type, the group treated permanently with NNM showed the highest frequency of acidophilic, mixed and basophilic cell foci. Tigroid cell foci, rarely found under the conditions used, appeared predominantly in the SD-group indicating that low-dose treatment was associated with this type of focal lesion as demonstrated earlier for single dose treatment with aflatoxin (Bannasch et al., 1985). With respect to the other types of focal lesions, all groups showed the same time-dose-dependence in the appearance of the different phenotypes of lesions: first the number of clear cell foci increased to a maximum and started to fall when the number of mixed cell foci began to increase while somewhat later HA and HCC appeared. The speed of this process was dose-dependent and showed its highest value in the group permanently treated with the highest dose of NNM. A considerable part of the lesions in this group was of acidophilic character corresponding to lesions which have frequently also been induced by initiation-promotion-protocols and were thought to have very little probability to proceed to HCC. The quantitative results indicate, however, that the acidophilic foci have also the potential to progress to HA and HCC.

CONCLUSIONS

The phenotypic cellular changes observed in a number of tissues during chemical carcinogenesis permit the dissection of stages of carcinogenesis on biological grounds. Preneoplastic lesions can be identified and studied in detail as to their cytology, biochemistry, molecular biology and proliferation kinetics. It is evident, however, that a distinction of phenotypically different focal lesions is imperative if we are to understand the complex process of carcinogenesis. It is no longer sufficient to group all types of carcinogen-induced alterations in a given tissue with "preneoplastic foci", "adenomas" or "carcinomas". A careful classification of preneoplastic and neoplastic lesions based on phenotypic cellular changes appears to be a prerequisite for successful further studies of the mechanism of multistage carcinogenesis.

ACKNOWLEDGEMENTS

I am indebted to Dr. Heide Zerban for support in the preparation of this manuscript and to Antje Groh for secretarial help. The work outlined in this paper has been supported by the Deutsche Forschungsgemeinschaft.

REFERENCES

Bannasch, P., 1968, The cytoplasm of hepatocytes during carcinogenesis. Light and electron microscopic investigations of the nitrosomorpholine-intoxicated rat liver, Rec. Res. Cancer Res., 19:1.
Bannasch, P., 1986, Preneoplastic lesions as end points in carcinogenicity testing. I. Hepatic preneoplasia and II. Preneoplasia in various non-hepatic tissues, Carcinogenesis, 7:689 and 849.
Bannasch, P., 1988, Phenotypic cellular changes as indicators of stages during neoplastic development, in: "Theories of Carcinogenesis", O.H. Iversen, ed., Hemisphere Publishing Corporation, Washington.
Bannasch, P., Mayer, D., and Hacker, H.J., 1980, Hepatocellular glycogenosis and hepatocarcinogenesis, Biochim. Biophys. Acta, 605:217.
Bannasch, P., Hacker, H.J., Klimek, F., and Mayer, D., 1984, Hepatocellular glycogenosis and related pattern of enzymatic changes during hepatocarcinogenesis, Adv. Enzyme Regul., 22:97.
Bannasch, P., Benner, U., Enzmann, H., and Hacker, H.J., 1985, Tigroid cell foci and neoplastic nodules in the liver of rats treated with a single dose of aflatoxin B_1, Carcinogenesis, 6:1641.
Bannasch, P., Hacker, H.J., Tsuda, H., and Zerban, H., 1986, Aberrant carbohydrate metabolism and metamorphosis during renal carcinogenesis, Adv. Enzyme Regul., 25:279.
Bannasch, P., Nogueira, E., Zerban, H., Beck, K., and Mayer, D., 1988, Sequential phenotypic conversion of renal epithelial cells during neoplastic development, in: "Chemical Carcinogenesis: Models and Mechanisms, F. Feo, ed., Pergamom Press, London, in press.
Buchmann, A., Kuhlmann, W.D., Schwarz, M., Kunz, H.W., Wolf, C.R., Moll, E., Friedberg, T., and Oesch, F., 1985, Regulation and expression of four cytochrome P-450 isoenzymes, NADPH-cytochrome P-450 reductase, the glutathione transferases B and C and microsomal epoxide hydrolase in preneoplastic and neoplastic lesions in rat liver, Carcinogenesis, 6:513.
Bursch, W., Lauer, B., Timmermann-Trosiener, T., Barthel, G., Schuppler, J., and Schulte-Hermann, R., 1984, Controlled cell death (apoptosis) of normal and putative preneoplastic cells in rat liver following withdrawal of tumor promoters, Carcinogenesis, 5:453.

Carter, R.L., 1984, "Precancerous States", Oxford University Press, London, New York, Toronto.

Columbano, A., Ledda-Columbano, G.M., Rao, P.M., Rajalakshmi, S., and Sarma, D.S.R., 1984, Occurrence of cell death (apoptosis) in preneoplastic and neoplastic liver cells: A sequential study, Am. J. Pathol., 116:441.

Emmelot, P., and Scherer, E., 1980, The first relevant cell stage in rat liver carcinogenesis: a quantitative approach, Biochim. Biophys. Acta, 605: 247.

Enzmann, H., and Bannasch, P., 1987a, Morphometric studies of alterations of extrafocal hepatocytes of rat liver treated with N-nitrosomorpholine, Virchows Arch. B Cell Pathol., 53:218.

Enzmann, H., and Bannasch, P., 1987b, Potential significance of phenotypic heterogeneity of focal lesions at different stages in hepatocarcino-genesis, Carcinogenesis, 8:1607.

Enzmann, H., and Bannasch, P., 1988, Non-persisting early foci of altered hepatocytes induced in rats by N-nitrosomorpholine, J. Cancer Res. Clin. Oncol., 114:30.

Enzmann, H., Edler, L., and Bannasch, P., 1987, Simple elementary method for the quantification of focal liver lesions induced by carcinogens, Carcinogenesis, 8:231.

Enzmann, H., Dettler, T., Ohlhauser, D., and Bannasch, P., 1988, Elevation of glucose-6-phosphate in early stages of hepatocarcinogenesis induced in rats by N-nitrosomorpholine, Horm. metabol. Res., 20:128.

Farber, E., and Sarma, D.S.R., 1987, Hepatocarcinogenesis: A dynamic cellular perspective, Lab. Invest., 56:4.

Friedrich-Freksa, H., Papadopulu, G., and Gössner, W., 1969, Histochemische Untersuchungen der Cancerogenese in der Rattenleber nach zeitlich begrenzter Verabfolgung von Diäthylnitrosamin, Z. Krebsforsch., 72:240.

Goldsworthy, T.L., and Pitot, H.C., 1985, The quantitative analysis and stability of histochemical markers of altered hepatic foci in rat liver following initiation by diethylnitrosamine administration and promotion with phenobarbital, Carcinogenesis, 6:1261.

Goldsworthy, T.L., Hanigan, H.M., and Pitot, H.C., 1986, Models of hepato-carcinogenesis in the rat - Contrasts and comparisons, CRC Crit. Rev. Toxicol., 17:61.

IARC, 1986, "Long-term and short-term assays for carcinogens: A critical appraisal", R. Montesano, H. Bartsch, H. Vainio, J. Wilbourn and H. Yamasaki, eds., IARC Scientific Publications, Lyon.

Klimek, F., Moore, M.A., Schneider, E., and Bannasch, P., 1988, Histochemical and microbiochemical demonstration of reduced pyruvate kinase activity in thioacetamide-induced neoplastic nodules of rat liver, Histo-chemistry, in press.

Kunz, W., Schaude, G., Schwarz, M., and Tennekes, H., 1982, Quantitative aspects of drug-mediated tumour promotion in liver and its toxico-logical implications, in: "Carcinogenesis - A Comprehensive Survey", E. Hecker, N.E. Fusenig, W. Kunz, F. Marks and M.W. Thielmann, eds., Raven Press, New York.

Limmer, J., Fleig, W.E., Leupold, D., Bittner, R., Ditschuneit, H., and Beger, H.G., 1988, Hepatocellular carcinoma in type I glycogen storage disease, Hepatology, 8:531.

Mayer, D., 1988, Regulation of carbohydrate metabolism in a glycogen-storing liver cell line, in: "Experimental Hepatocarcinogenesis", M.B. Roberfroid and V. Préat, eds., Plenum Press, New York, London.

Moore, M.A., and Kitagawa, T., 1986, Hepatocarcinogenesis in the rat; the effect of the promoters and carcinogens in vivo and in vitro, Int. Rev. Cytol., 101:125.

Moore, M.A., Mayer, D., and Bannasch, P., 1982, The dose-dependence and sequential appearance of putative preneoplastic populations induced in the rat liver by stop experiments with N-nitrosomorpholine, Car-cinogenesis, 3:1429.

Nogueira, E., 1987, Rat renal carcinogenesis after chronic simultaneous exposure to lead acetate and N-nitrosodiethylamine, Virchows Arch. B Cell Pathol., 53:365.

Nogueira, E., and Bannasch, P., 1988, Cellular origin of rat renal oncocytoma, Lab. Invest., in press.

Pitot, H.C., 1988, Hepatic neoplasia: Chemical induction, in: "The Liver. Biology and Pathobiology", J.M. Arias, W.B. Jakoby, H. Popper, D. Schachter and D.A. Shafritz, eds., Raven Press, New York.

Rabes, H.M., 1983, Development and growth of early preneoplastic lesions induced in the liver by chemical carcinogens, J. Cancer Res. Clin. Oncol., 106:85.

Rabes, H.M., 1988, Cell proliferation and hepatocarcinogenesis, in: "Experimental Hepatocarcinogenesis", M.B. Roberfroid and V. Préat, eds., Plenum Press, New York, London.

Ruebner, B.H., Michas, C., Kanayama, R., and Bannasch, P., 1976, Sequential hepatic histologic and histochemical changes produced by diethylnitrosamine in the Rhesus monkey, J. Natl. Cancer, Inst., 57:1261.

Scherer, E., 1981, Use of a programmable pocket calculator for the quantitation of precancerous foci, Carcinogenesis, 2:805.

Scherer, E., 1984, Neoplastic progression in experimental hepatocarcinogenesis, Biochim. Biophys. Acta, 738:219.

Schröter, C., Parzefall, W., Schröter, H., and Schulte-Hermann, R., 1987, Dose-response studies on the effects of α-, β-, γ-hexachlorocyclohexane on putative preneoplastic foci, monooxygenases and growth in rat liver, Cancer Res., 47:80.

Seelmann-Eggebert, G., Mayer, D., Mecke, D., and Bannasch, P., 1987, Expression and regulation of glycogen phosphorylase in preneoplastic and neoplastic hepatic lesions in rats, Virchows Arch. B Cell Pathol., 53:44.

Tatematsu, M., Aoki, T., Kagawa, M., Mera, Y., and Ito, N., 1988a, Reciprocal relationship between development of glutathione S-transferase positive liver foci and proliferation of surrounding hepatocytes in rats, Carcinogenesis, 9:221.

Tatematsu, M., Mera, Y., Inoue, T., Satoh, K., Sato, K., and Ito, N., 1988b, Stable phenotypic expression of glutathione S-transferase placental type and unstable phenotypic expression of γ-glutamyltransferase in rat liver preneoplastic and neoplastic lesions, Carcinogenesis, 9:215.

Tsuda, H., Hacker, H.J., Katayama, H., Masui, T., Ito, N., and Bannasch, P., 1986, Correlative histochemical studies on preneoplastic and neoplastic lesions in the kidney of rats treated with nitrosamines, Virchows Arch. B. Cell Pathol., 51:385.

Vesselinovitch, S.D., and Mihailovich, N., 1983, Kinetics of diethylnitrosamine hepatocarcinogenesis in the infant mouse, Cancer Res., 43:4253.

Vesselinovitch, S.D., Hacker, H.J., and Bannasch, P., 1985, Histochemical characterization of focal hepatic lesions induced by single diethylnitrosamine treatment in infant mice, Cancer Res., 45:2774.

Weber, E., and Bannasch, P., 1988, Dose-dependence of preneoplastic lesion phenotype in N-nitrosomorpholine-induced hepatocarcinogenesis, Falk-Symposium No. 51, Liver Cell Carcinoma, 43.

Weber, E., Moore, M.A., and Bannasch, P., 1988a, Enzyme histochemical and morphological phenotype of amphophilic foci and amphophilic/tigroid cell adenomas in rat liver after combined treatment with dehydroepiandrosterone and N-nitrosomorpholine, Carcinogenesis, 9:1049.

Weber, E., Moore, M.A., and Bannasch, P., 1988b, Phenotypic modulation of hepatocarcinogenesis and reduction in N-nitrosomorpholine-induced hemangiosarcoma and adrenal lesion development in Sprague-Dawley rats by dehydroepiandrosterone, Carcinogenesis, 9:1191.

Zerban, H., Rabes, H.M., and Bannasch, P., 1985, Kinetics of cell proliferation during hepatocarcinogenesis, Europ. J. Cancer Clin. Oncol., 21:1424.

Zerban, H., Preussmann, R., and Bannasch, P., 1988a, Dose-time-relationship of the development of preneoplastic liver lesions induced in rats with low doses of N-nitrosodiethanolamine, Carcinogenesis, 9:607.

Zerban, H., Preussmann, R., and Bannasch, P., 1988b, Quantitative morphometric comparison between the expression of two different "marker
enzymes" in preneoplastic liver lesions induced in rats with low
doses of N-nitrosodiethanolamine, Cancer Lett., submitted.

INTERSPECIES EXTRAPOLATION

Curtis C. Travis

Office of Risk Analysis
Oak Ridge National Laboratory
Oak Ridge, Tennessee   37831-6109

INTRODUCTION

One of the fundamental problems in the cancer risk assessment area is the extrapolation of observed experimental results between animal species and man. Lacking detailed information on interspecies differences, it is frequently assumed that experimental results can be extrapolated between species when administered dosage is standardized as either mg/kg body weight per day (body weight scaling) or mg/m^2 per day (surface area scaling). Several investigators have argued for the efficacy of one or the other of these procedures (Pinkel, 1958; Freireich et al., 1966; Crouch and Wilson, 1978; Hoel, 1979; Crump and Guess, 1980; Hogan and Hoel, 1982; MRI, 1986; FASEB, 1986; Travis and White, 1988). It is well recognized that neither of these extrapolation procedures will be exactly correct for all compounds and that when species-specific data are available, they should be used in risk assessment. In their absence, body weight or surface area extrapolations are used with the explicit knowledge that they are only approximately correct.

With the advent of biologically based pharmacokinetic models (Gerlowski and Jain, 1983; Ramsey and Andersen, 1984; Andersen et al., 1987; and Ward et al., 1988), it has become possible to provide an accurate description of the pharmacokinetics of the parent compound and metabolites in mice, rats, and humans. These models, thus, provide a tool to quantitatively evaluate the scientific bases for the choice of an interspecies scaling metric.

The purpose of this paper is to use physiologically based pharmacokinetic models to demonstrate that if toxic response is proportional to the area under the curve of the concentration of the toxic moiety in the target tissue, then, regardless of the mechanism of action (direct-acting compound, reactive metabolite, or stable metabolite), the appropriate interspecies scaling law for administered dose is the 3/4 power of body weight (modified surface area scaling).

In cases where pharmacokinetic models exist, it is no longer necessary to extrapolate experimental results on the basis of administered dose. Effective dose to target tissue can be estimated using the pharmacokinetic model, and interspecies extrapolations made on this basis. When the toxic moiety is the parent compound or a stable metabolite, this poses no problem. However, reactive metabolites are often too short-lived to measure directly and the intermediate metabolic rates of reactive metabolites are generally unknown, making tissue dose of a reactive metabolite difficult to predict even with the use of a pharmacokinetic model. To circumvent this problem, total reactive metabolite (TRM) (the integral of the rate of formation of reactive metabolite) has been suggested as a tissue dose surrogate. In a pharmacokinetically based risk assessment for methylene chloride, Andersen et al. (1987) argued that TRM divided by liver weight was the proper measure of dose, while the Environmental Protection Agency (EPA) argued that TRM divided by body weight to the 2/3 power was more appropriate (U.S. EPA, 1987). Thus, the historical debate regarding the proper scaling law (body weight or surface area) for administered dose was transferred to dose to target tissue.

The second purpose of this paper is to use physiologically based pharmacokinetic models to demonstrate that if a pharmacokinetic model is used to estimate dose to target tissue, then the appropriate measure of tissue dosimetry for a reactive metabolite is TRM divided by the 3/4 power of body weight.

PHYSIOLOGICALLY BASED PHARMACOKINETIC MODELS

Physiologically based pharmacokinetic models divide the body into physiologically realistic compartments connected by the arterial and venous blood flow pathways (Gerlowski and Jain, 1983; Ramsey and Andersen, 1984; Andersen et al., 1987; Paustenbach et al., 1988; Ward et al., 1988). The tissue groups generally include: (1) organs such as brain, kidney, and viscera, (2) muscle, (3) fat, and (4) metabolic organs (principally liver). The models use actual physiological parameters such as breathing rates, blood flow rates, blood volumes, and tissue volumes to describe the pharmacokinetic process. These physiological parameters are coupled with chemical specific parameters such as blood/gas partition coefficients, tissue/blood partition coefficients, and metabolic constants to predict the dynamics of a compound's movement through an animal system. An advantage of the physiologically based model is that by simply using the appropriate physiological, biochemical, and metabolic parameters, the same model can be utilized to describe the dynamics of chemical transport and metabolism in any species, including mice, rats, and humans. It is the interspecies scaling of these physiological, metabolic, and biochemical parameters that controls interspecies extrapolation of pharmacokinetics.

SCALING PHYSIOLOGICAL AND METABOLIC PARAMETERS

Many of the physiological and metabolic parameters used in pharmacokinetic modeling are directly correlated to the body weight of the particular organism (Adolph, 1949). These physiological parameters generally vary with body weight according to a power equation expressed as:

$$y = a \, BW^b \qquad\qquad (1)$$

where y is a physiological parameter of interest, and a and b are constants (Adolph, 1949; Schmidt-Nielsen, 1970, 1984; Lindstedt, 1987). If the constant b equals one, the physiological parameter y correlates directly with body weight. If the constant b equals 2/3, the parameter y correlates with surface area. I will briefly review the empirical scaling laws for physiological and metabolic parameters used in pharmacokinetic modeling.

Organ Volumes

Organ volumes tend to scale across species with the first power of body weight (Schmidt-Nielsen, 1984; NRC, 1986). Examples are total blood volume which scales across species with the 1.02 power of body weight (Stahl, 1967) and the mass of the mammalian heart which scales with the 0.98 power of body weight (Prothero, 1979). The liver is an exception scaling with 0.87 power of body weight (Stahl, 1965). Following the National Academy of Sciences (NRC, 1986), I will assume that the appropriate scaling law for volume of tissue group i is:

$$V_i = V_{i\theta}BW^{1.0},$$ (2)

where $V_{i\theta}$ is a species-independent allometric constant.

Cardiac Output

Cardiac output is defined as the volume of blood pumped by each ventricle of the heart per minute. There is considerable evidence that cardiac output is related to metabolic rate (Guyton, 1971) and that metabolic rates across species are related to the 3/4 power of body weight (Kleiber, 1961; Holt et al., 1968; White et al., 1968; Schmidt-Nielsen, 1970). The most commonly assumed scaling law for cardiac output has the form:

$$Q_b = Q_{b\theta}BW^{0.75},$$ (3)

where $Q_{b\theta}$ is a species-independent allometric constant.

The percent of cardiac output distributed to different organs is approximately constant across species (Arms and Travis, 1988). Thus, cardiac output, Q_i, to tissue group i has the form:

$$Q_i = Q_{i\theta}BW^{0.75},$$ (4)

where $Q_{i\theta}$ is a species-independent allometric constant.

Alveolar Ventilation

Ventilation is a cyclic process of circulation and exchange of gases in the lungs that is basic to respiration. Total ventilation or minute volume is defined as the volume of air exhaled per minute. The fraction of minute volume available for gas exchange in the alveolar compartments is termed the alveolar ventilation rate. Minute volume and, hence, alveolar ventilation has been shown to scale across species with the 3/4 power of body weight (Guyton, 1947; Adolph, 1949; Stahl, 1967). The most commonly assumed scaling law for alveolar ventilation rate has the form:

$$Q_{alv} = Q_{alv\theta}BW^{0.75},$$ (5)

where $Q_{alv\theta}$ is a species-independent allometric constant.

Renal Clearance

Clearance is the amount of a substance removed from the blood per unit of time. Renal clearance relates the kidneys' rate of elimination of a given compound to the concentration of the compound in the blood. Adolph (1949) first showed that renal clearance of inulin in four species scaled with body weight to the 3/4 power. Studies by Brody (1945), Edwards (1975), Lindstedt and Calder (1981), Boxenbaum (1982), Schmidt-Nielsen (1984), and Mordenti (1986) support a general scaling law for renal clearance:

$$K_r = K_{r\theta} BW^{0.75} \quad , \quad (6)$$

where $K_{r\theta}$ is a species-independent allometric constant.

Metabolic Parameters

Oxygen consumption rates have been shown to scale across species with the 3/4 power of body weight (Kleiber, 1932; Brody, 1945; Benedict, 1938; McMahon, 1973; Schmidt-Nielsen, 1984; Lindstedt and Calder, 1981; Lindstedt, 1987). There are limited data on interspecies scaling of metabolic enzymatic activity. Cytochrome oxidase has been found to scale with the 3/4 power of body weight (Kunkel et al., 1956; Jansky, 1961; Jansky, 1963). The number of mitochondria in mammalian liver scales with the 0.72 power of body weight (Smith, 1956) and mitochondria densities in 13 species of mammals have been shown to closely parallel maximal rates of oxygen consumption (Mathieu et al., 1981). However, information on interspecies scaling of metabolic parameters is inadequate and further studies are needed. Nevertheless, we assume that the appropriate scaling law for metabolic parameters is:

$$V_{max} = V_{max\theta} BW^{0.75} \quad (7)$$

and

$$K_f = K_{f\theta} BW^{0.75} . \quad (8)$$

The Michaelis-Menten constant, K_m, is generally assumed to be approximately constant across species (NRC, 1987).

Partition Coefficients

Partition coefficients are an expression of a chemical's solubility in tissues. The partition coefficient of a given chemical between two media is defined as the ratio of the equilibrium chemical concentration in the first medium to the chemical concentration in the second medium. The most common measurements are blood/air and tissue/air partition coefficients with tissue/blood derived as the ratio of tissue/air to blood/air. Tissue/air partition coefficients tend to be constant across species (NRC, 1986), while blood/air partition coefficients show some species-dependent variability. As a general rule, however, I will assume that partition coefficients are approximately constant across species (NRC, 1987).

PHYSIOLOGICAL TIME

The presence between species of a biologically variable time scale has been asserted by several authors (Carrel, 1931; Huxley, 1927; Brody, 1945; Hill, 1950; Adolph, 1949; Dedrick, 1973; Boxenbaum, 1982; Mordenti, 1986; Yates and Kugler, 1986). Hill (1950) first suggested that body size served as the regulating mechanism for an internal biological clock, making the rate of all biological events constant across species when compared per unit physiological time. His conclusions are supported by Adolph (1949), Stahl (1967), Gunther and Leon de la Barra (1966), Calder (1968), Dedrick (1973), Lindstedt and Calder (1981), Boxenbaum (1982, 1986), Mordenti (1986), and Lindstedt (1987), who have shown that breath duration, heartbeat duration, longevity, pulse time, breathing rates, and blood flow rates are approximately constant across species when expressed in internal time units. These time units have been termed physiological time (t') and can be defined in terms of chronological time (t) and body weight (BW) as:

$$t' = t/BW^{0.25}. \tag{9}$$

Thus, while chronological time is the same for all species, physiological time is different for each species. The value of this concept is that all species have approximately the same physiological and metabolic rates when measured in the physiological time frame (Dedrick, 1973; Boxenbaum, 1986; Mordenti, 1986, Yates and Kugler, 1986; Lindstedt, 1987).

INTERSPECIES EXTRAPOLATION OF PHARMACOKINETICS

Interspecies extrapolation of toxic effect attempts to find a measure of administered dose (i.e., mg/kg or mg/m^2) which produces the same measure of effect in all species. It is understood that any such extrapolation procedure is only approximately correct and should be used only when species-specific data are unavailable. Historically, it has been assumed that a single extrapolation procedure would work for all chemicals regardless of their mechanism of action. More recently, Andersen (1987) and the National Academy of Sciences (NRC, 1986, 1987) have suggested that interspecies extrapolation rules should depend on the mechanism of action. They distinguish three classes, depending on whether the parent compound, stable metabolite, or reactive metabolite produces the toxic response.

Measure of Effective Dose

I assume that the proper measure of dose to target tissue is the area under the tissue concentration curve (AUC) of the toxic moiety (Andersen, 1987; NRC, 1986, 1987). Thus, the question of interspecies extrapolation of pharmacokinetics reduces to, "Is it possible to choose a measure of administered dose so that AUC of the toxic moiety is the same in all species?" I will investigate this question using the pharmacokinetic equations expressed in physiological time.

Direct Acting Compounds

Direct acting compounds are those which do not require metabolic transformation to be active. As I have stated, I am assuming that the proper measure of dose to target tissue for a direct acting compound is the AUC of the tissue concentration (mg/kg) of the administered compound. For specificity, I will look at AUC of liver concentration. Using a change of variable from chronological time to physiological time,

$$AUC = \int_0^\infty C_1(t)dt \qquad\qquad (10)$$

$$= \frac{1}{V_1} \int_0^\infty A_1(t)dt$$

$$= \frac{1}{V_{1\theta}} \int_0^\infty A_1{}'(t)dt$$

$$= \frac{1}{V_{1\theta}} \int_0^\infty A_1{}'(t')dt' \; BW^{0.25}$$

However, it is shown in Travis et al. (1988) that A'_1 (t') is identical for all species; that is, tissue concentration curves are species-independent when measured in physiological time. Thus, $AUC/BW^{0.25}$ is constant across species when administered dose is normalized by body weight (i.e., mg/kg). Stated in a slightly different fashion, area under the tissue concentration curve of parent compound will be constant across species if administered dose is measured in $mg/kg^{0.75}$. As a computational verification of this statement, the pharmacokinetic model, together with the physiological and metabolic scaling laws (Eqs. 1-8), were used to predict AUC of the concentration of parent compound in livers of mice, rats, and humans for different intravenous administered doses.

Figures 1A-C present the relationship between AUC, $AUC/BW^{0.33}$ and $AUC/BW^{0.25}$ of the parent compound, respectively and intravenously by administered dose (mg/kg). In Figure 1A, area under the human curve (represented by squares) is larger than that for rats (circles), which is larger than that for mice (triangles). Thus, traditional body weight scaling (mg/kg) would underpredict toxic effect of a direct acting compound in humans based on animal data.

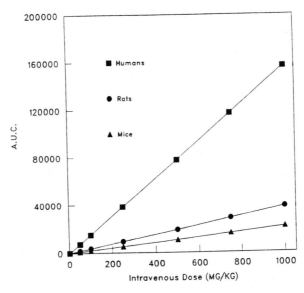

FIGURE 1A

In Figure 1B, the area under the human curve is less than that for rats, which is less than that for mice. Thus, traditional surface area scaling ($mg/kg^{0.67}$) would overpredict toxic effect of a direct acting compound in humans based on animal data. In Figure 1C, the area under the human, rat, and mouse curves are identical. Thus, when a direct acting compound is the toxic moiety, interspecies scaling should be on the basis of $mg/kg^{0.75}$.

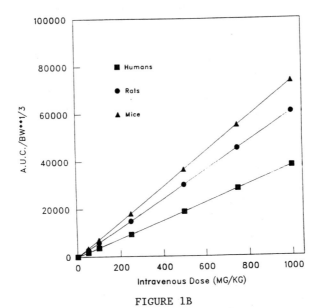

FIGURE 1B

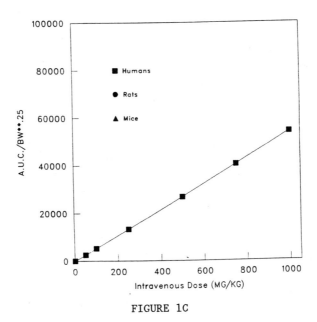

FIGURE 1C

Reactive Metabolite

When the toxic effect is caused by a short-lived by-product of the metabolic process which interacts with the cellular constituents, the toxic moiety of concern is a reactive metabolite. In what follows, I assume that the reactive metabolite is metabolically degraded. I am assuming that the proper measure of dose to target tissue for a reactive metabolite is the area under the tissue concentration (mg/kg) curve (AURMC). For specificity, I will again look at AURMC of liver concentration. Using a change of variable from chronological time to physiological time,

$$AURMC = \int_0^\infty C_{rml}(t)dt \qquad (11)$$

$$= \frac{1}{V_1} \int_0^\infty A_{rml}(t)dt$$

$$= \frac{1}{V_{1\theta}} \int_0^\infty A'_{rml}(t)dt$$

$$= \frac{1}{V_{1\theta}} \int_0^\infty A'_{rml}(t')dt' \ BW^{0.25}$$

It is shown in Travis et al. (1988) that $A'_{rml}(t')$ is identical for all species; that is, tissue concentration curves are species-independent when measured in physiological time. Thus $AURMC/BW^{0.25}$ is constant across species when administered dose is normalized by body weight (i.e., mg/kg). Therefore, area under the tissue concentration curve of a reactive metabolite will be constant across species if administered dose is measured in $mg/kg^{0.75}$.

Andersen (1987) and the National Academy of Sciences (NRC, 1986, 1987) state that body weight is the proper scaling law for reactive metabolites. Rather than using AURMC as a surrogate of tissue exposure to a reactive metabolite, they used the integral of the rate of formation of the reactive metabolite divided by tissue volume. Interspecies comparisons using this dose surrogate assume that the degradation rate of the reactive metabolite is approximately constant across various species (Andersen, 1987). However, in the case of a reactive metabolite which is metabolically degraded, these rate constants (1/hr) will scale with $BW^{-0.25}$ (Boxenbaum, 1982, 1986; Mordenti, 1986; Lindstedt, 1987).

Figures 2A-C present the AUC of the concentration of reactive metabolite in livers of mice, rats, and humans following an intravenous administered dose (mg/kg). These curves were generated using the pharmacokinetic model, together with the physiological and metabolic scaling laws (1-8). Figures 2A and 2B demonstrate that traditional body weight scaling (mg/kg) underpredicts toxic effect of a reactive metabolite in humans based on animal data, while traditional surface area scaling ($mg/kg^{0.67}$) overpredicts toxic effect. In Figure 2C, the area under the human, rat, and mouse curves are identical. This figure presents a computational verification of the fact that when a reactive metabolite which is metabolically degraded is the toxic moiety, interspecies scaling should be on the basis of $mg/kg^{0.75}$.

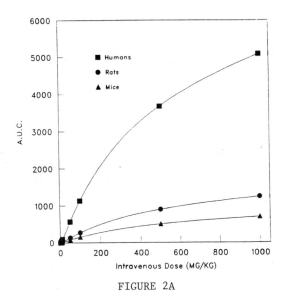

FIGURE 2A

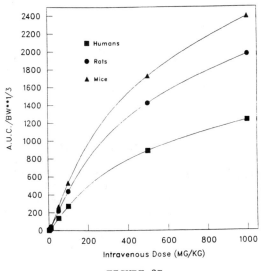

FIGURE 2B

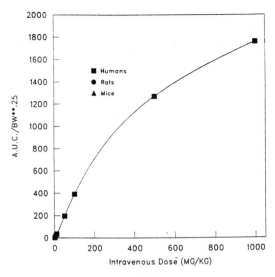

FIGURE 2C

Stable Metabolite

A stable metabolite is one which does not undergo further metabolite transformation. As I have stated, I am assuming that the proper measure of dose to target tissue for a stable metabolite is the area under the tissue concentration (mg/kg) curve (AUSMC). For specificity, I will again look at AUSMC of liver concentration. Again, using a change of variable from chronological time to physiological time,

$$
\begin{aligned}
\text{AUSMC} &= \int_0^\infty C_{sml}(t)dt \\
&= \frac{1}{V_l} \int_0^\infty A_{sml}(t)dt \\
&= \frac{1}{V_{l\theta}} \int_0^\infty A'_{sml}(t)dt \\
&= \frac{1}{V_{l\theta}} \int_0^\infty A'_{sml}(t')dt' \ BW^{0.25}
\end{aligned}
\tag{12}
$$

It is shown in Travis et al. (1988) that $A'_{sml}(t')$ is identical for all species; that is, tissue concentration curves are species-independent when measured in physiological time. Thus $\text{AUSMC}/BW^{0.25}$ is constant across species when administered dose is normalized by body weight (i.e., mg/kg). Therefore, area under the tissue concentration curve of a stable metabolite will be constant across species if administered dose is measured in $mg/kg^{0.75}$.

Figures 3A-C present the AUC of the concentration of stable metabolite in livers of mice, rats, and humans following an intravenous administered dose (mg/kg). In Figure 3A, area under the human curve (represented by squares) is larger than that for rats (circles), which is larger than that for mice (triangles). Thus, traditional body weight scaling (mg/kg) would underpredict toxic effect of a stable metabolite in humans based on animal data. In Figure 3B, the area under the human curve is less than that for rats, which is less than that for mice. Thus, traditional surface area scaling (mg/kg$^{0.67}$) would overpredict toxic effect of a stable metabolite in humans based on animal data. In Figure 3C, the area under the human, rat, and mouse curves are identical. Thus, when a stable metabolite is the toxic moiety, interspecies scaling should be on the basis of mg/kg$^{0.75}$.

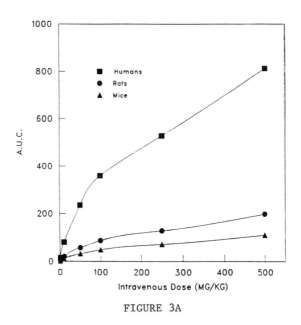

FIGURE 3A

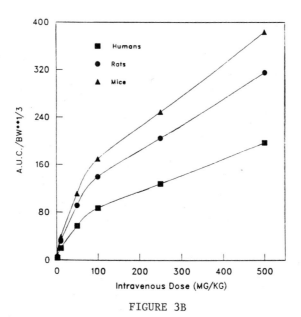

FIGURE 3B

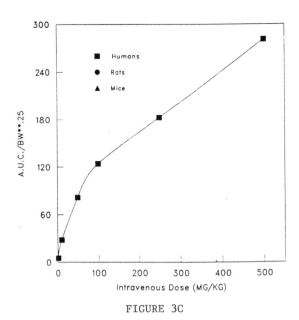

FIGURE 3C

TISSUE DOSIMETRY OF A REACTIVE METABOLITE

I will now address the question of the proper metric for tissue dosimetry when metabolized dose to target tissue is estimated using a pharmacokinetic model (Travis, 1988). I will treat the case of a reactive metabolite, which I again assume is metabolically degraded. Stable metabolites can be handled in a similar fashion. I assume that the proper measure of dose to target tissue for a reactive metabolite is the area under the liver concentration (mg/kg) curve (AURMC). Using a change of variable from chronological time to physiological time, I have shown that $AURMC/BW^{0.25}$ is constant across species when administered dose is normalized by body weight (mg/kg). That is, AURMC will be constant across species if administered dose is measured in $mg/kg^{0.75}$.

This answers the question of how to extrapolate toxic effect due to a reactive metabolite across species on the basis of administered dose. However, when one uses pharmacokinetic models in risk analysis, one is interested in extrapolating toxic effect across species on the basis of dose to target tissue, and as I have already stated, I assume that the proper measure of dose to target tissue is the AURMC (Andersen, 1987; NRC, 1986, 1987).

In the case of methylene chloride, however, rather than using AURMC as a measure of dose, Andersen et al. (1987) and the EPA (U.S. EPA, 1987) used the integral of the rate of formation in the liver of the reactive metabolite. That is, they used TRM produced in the liver. Andersen et al. (1987) argued that TRM divided by liver weight was the proper measure of dose, while the EPA argued that TRM divided by $BW^{0.66}$ was more appropriate. To resolve this issue, I must determine how TRM is related to AURMC. However,

$$TRM = \int_0^\infty \frac{dA_{rml}(t)dt}{dt} = \int_0^\infty \frac{dA'_{rml}(t')dt'BW.}{dt'} \qquad (13)$$

Since $A'_{rml}(t')$ is identical for all species, TRM/BW is constant across species. Thus, TRM = k_1 BW, while AURMC = k_2 $BW^{0.25}$. Consequently,

$$AURMC = (k_1 k_2) \, TRM/BW^{0.75} \qquad (14)$$

and shows that TRM divided by body weight to the 0.75 power is proportional to AURMC. Consequently, the proper measure of tissue dosimetry (for interspecies extrapolation) of a reactive metabolite which is metabolically degraded is TRM divided by body weight to the 0.75 power.

CONCLUSIONS

A long standing problem in toxicology is the extrapolation of observed experimental results between animal species and man. It has historically been assumed that experimental results can be extrapolated between species if administered dose is standardized in one of two metrics: mg/kg body weight/day (body weight scaling) or mg/m^2/day (surface area scaling). More recently, Andersen (1987) and the National Academy of Sciences (NRC, 1986, 1987) point out that scaling should depend on the kinetic behavior of the toxic moiety and its mechanism of toxicity. They suggest that if carcinogenic response is proportional to the area under the curve of the concentration of the toxic moiety in the target tissue, then the appropriate scaling laws for cancer risk assessment interspecies extrapolations are 0.7 power of body weight for direct acting compounds and stable metabolites, and body weight scaling for reactive metabolites.

With the advent of biologically based pharmacokinetic models, it has become possible to present a scientifically defensible justification for the choice of an interspecies scaling metric. It has been established that biologically based pharmacokinetic models provide an accurate description of the pharmacokinetics of parent compound and metabolites in mice, rats, and humans (Ramsey and Andersen, 1984; NRC, 1986; Andersen et al., 1987; Paustenbach, 1988; Ward et al., 1988). Thus, pharmacokinetic models provide a tool to quantitatively evaluate the scientific bases for interspecies extrapolation of experimental results.

The parameters controlling pharmacokinetics in a given species are physiological (breathing rates, blood flow rates, blood volumes, tissue volumes, etc.), biochemical (partition coefficients), and metabolic. It is the extrapolation of these parameters across species that controls interspecies extrapolation of pharmacokinetics. It has long been established that tissue volumes tend to extrapolate across species with the first power of body weight (Schmidt-Nielsen, 1984; NRC, 1986; Lindstedt, 1987), biological times extrapolate with the 1/4 power of body weight (Adolph, 1949; Stahl, 1967; Gunther and La Barra, 1966; Calder, 1968; Dedrick, 1973; Lindstedt and Calder, 1981; Boxenbaum, 1982, 1986; Mordenti, 1986; Lindstedt, 1987), and volume rates (i.e., volume divided by time such as clearance rates, cardiac output, alveolar ventilation, etc.) vary to the 3/4 power of body weight (Guyton, 1947; Adolph, 1949; Kleiber, 1961; Stahl, 1967; Lindstedt and Calder, 1981; Boxenbaum, 1982; Schmidt-Nielsen, 1984; Mordenti, 1986; Lindstedt, 1987). These allometric relationships, together with physiologically based pharmacokinetic models, provide the basis for the derivation of scientifically defensible interspecies scaling laws.

In the present report, I have demonstrated that if toxic response is proportional to the area under the curve of the concentration of the toxic moiety in the target tissue, then regardless of the mechanism of action (direct-acting compound, reactive metabolite, or stable metabolite), the appropriate interspecies scaling law for administered dose is the 3/4 power of body weight (modified surface area scaling).

Currently available biologically based pharmacokinetic models make it possible to accurately estimate dose to target tissue, eliminating the need to extrapolate experimental results on the basis of administered dose. The question arises however as to the proper measure of tissue dosimetry for a reactive metabolite (Andersen et al., 1987; U.S. EPA, 1987). In the present report, I have also demonstrated that if toxic response is proportional to the area under the curve of the concentration of the toxic moiety in the target tissue, then the appropriate measure of tissue dosimetry for a reactive metabolite which is metabolically degraded is TRM divided by the 3/4 power of body weight.

ACKNOWLEDGMENTS

Research sponsored by the National Science Foundation and the U.S. Environmental Protection Agency under Interagency Agreements applicable under Martin Marietta Energy Systems, Inc. Contract No. DE-AC05840R21400.

REFERENCES

Adolph, E. F. (1949). Quantitative relations in the physiological constitutions of mammals, Science 109: 579-585.

Andersen, M. E. (1987). Tissue Dosimetry in Risk Assessment, or What's the Problem Here Anyway? in: Drinking Water and Health, Volume 8, Pharmacokinetics in Risk Assessment. National Academy Press, Washington, DC.

Andersen, M. E., Clewell, H. J. III, Gargas, M. L., Smith, F. A., and Reitz, R. H. (1987). Physiologically based pharmacokinetics and the risks assessment process for methylene chloride, Toxicol. Appl. Pharmacol. 87: 185-205.

Arms, A. D., and Travis, C. C. (1988). Reference Physiological Parameters In Pharmacokinetic Modeling. US Environmental Protection Agency, Washington, DC. EPA/600/6-88/004.

Benedict, F. G. (1938). Vital Energetics: A Study in Comparative Bacal Metabolism. Washington, DC, Carnegie Institute of Washington

Boxenbaum, H. (1986). Time concepts in physics, biology, and pharmacokinetics, J. Pharmaceutical Sci. 75 (11): 1053-62.

Boxenbaum, H. (1982). Interspecies scaling, allometry, physiological time, and the ground plan of pharmacokinetics, J. Pharmacokinet. Biopharm. 10: 201-227.

Brody, S. (1945). Bioenergetics and Growth: With Special Reference to the Efficiency Complex in Domestic Animals. Reinhold, New York. (reprinted 1964. Darien, CT: Hafner).

Calder, W. A. (1968). Respiration and heart rates of birds at rest. Condor 70: 358-365.

Carrell, A. (1931). Physiological time, Science 74: 618-621.

Crouch, E., and Wilson R. (1978). Interspecies Comparison of Carcinogenic Potency, Journal of Toxicology and Environmental Health 5: 1095-1118.

Crump, K. S. and Guess H. A. (1980). Drinking Water and Cancer: Review of Recent Findings and Assessment of Risks. Science Research Systems Inc., Ruston, Louisiana, CBQ Contract No. EQ10AC018.

Dedrick, R. L. (1973). Animal scale-up, J. Pharmacokinetics and Biopharmaceutics 1 (5): 435-461.

Edwards, N. A. (1975). Scaling of renal functions in mammals, Comp. Biochem. Physiol. 52A: 63-66.

Federation of American Societies for Experimental Biology (FASEB) (July, 1986). Biological Bases for Interspecies Extrapolation of Carcinogenicity Data, (Eds. Thomas Hill, Ralph Wands, and Richard Leukroth, Jr.) Prepared for the FDA by Life Sciences Research Office of the FASEB.

Freireich, E. J., Gehan, E. A., Rall, D. P., Schmidt, L. H. and Skipper, H. E. (1966). Quantitative comparison of toxicity of anticancer agents in mouse, rat, hamster, dog, monkey and man, Cancer Chemotherapy Reports 50(4): 219-244.

Gerlowski, L. E. and Jain, R. K., (1983). Physiologically based pharmacokinetic modeling: Principles and applications, J. Pharm. Science., 72: 1103-1126.

Gunther, B. and Leon de la Barra, B. (1966). On the space-time continuum in biology, Acta Physiol. Latinamerica 16: 221-231.

Guyton, A. C. (1947). Measurement of the respiratory volumes of laboratory animals, Amer. J. Physiol. 150: 70-77.

Guyton, A. C. (1971). Textbook of Medical Physiology. 4th Edition. Philadelphia, PA, W. B. Saunders Company.

Hill, A. V. (1950). The dimensions of animals and their muscular dynamics. Proc. Roy. Inst. G.B., 34: 450-471.

Hoel, D. G. (1979). Low-Dose and Species to Species Extrapolation for Chemically Induced Carcinogenesis, in: Banbury Report No. 1: Assesing Chemical Mutagens: The Risks to Humans, ed. V. McElheny. New York: Cold Spring Harbor Laboratory, pp. 135-145.

Hogan, M. and Hoel, D. G. (1982). Extrapolation to man, in: Principles of Toxicology, ed. A. W. Hayes, New York, Raven Press.

Holt, J. P., Rhode, E. A., and Kines, H. (1968). Ventricular volumes and body weight in mammals, Amer. J. Physiol. 215 (3) pp. 704-715.

Huxley, J. S. (1927). On the relation between egg-weight and body-weight in birds, J. Linnean Soc. Zoology 36: 457-466.

Jansky, L. (1961). Total cytochrome oxidase activity and its relation to basal and maximal metabolism, Nature 189: 921-922.

Jansky, L. (1963). Body organ cytochrome oxidase activity in cold-and-warm acclimated rats, Can. J. Biochem. Physiol., 41: 1847-1854.

Kleiber, M. (1932). Body size and metabolism, Hilgardia 6: 315-353.

Kleiber, M. (1961). The Fire of Life. An Introduction to Animal Energetics. New York, Wiley Publications.

Kunkel, H. O., Spalding, J. F., de Franciscis, G. and Futrell, M. F. (1956). Cytochrome oxidase activity and body weight in rats and in three species of large animals, Amer. J. Physiol., 186: 203-206.

Lindstedt, S. L. and Calder, W. A. (1981). Body size and physiological time, and longevity of homeothermic animals, The Quarterly Review of Biology 56: 1-16.

Lindstedt, S. L. (1987) Allometry: Body size constraints in animal design, in: Drinking Water and Health. Pharmacokinetics in Risk Assessment Volume 8. National Academy Press, Washington, DC.

Mathieu, O., Krauer, R., Hoppeler, H., Gehr, P., Lindstedt, S. L., Alexander, R., Taylor, C. R., and Weibel, E. R., (1981). Design of the mammalian respiratory system. VII. Scaling mitochondrial volume in skeletal muscle to body mass, Resp. Physiol., 44: 113-128.

McMahon, T. (1973). Size and shape in biology, Science 179: 1201-1204.

Midwest Research Institute (MRI) (July 31, 1986). Risk Assessment Methodology for Hazardous Waste Management. (Final Report.) Prepared for the US EPA and Council on Environmental Quality.

Mordenti, J. (1986). Man versus beast: pharmacokinetic scaling in mammals, J. Pharmaceutical Science 75 (11): 1028-1040.

National Research Council (NRC) (1987). Drinking Water and Health. Volume 6. National Academy Press, Washington, DC.

National Research Council (NRC) (1986). Drinking Water and Health. Pharmacokinetics in Risk Assessment Volume 8. National Academy Press, Washington, DC.

Paustenbach, D. J., Andersen, M. E., Clewell, H. J. III, Gargas, M. L., (1988). A physiologically based pharmacokinetic model for inhaled carbon tetrachloride in the rat, Toxicol. Appl. Pharmacol. (In press.)

Pinkel, D. (1958). The use of body surface area as a criterion of drug dosage in cancer chemotherapy, Cancer Research 18 (1):853-856.

Prothero O. (1979). Heart weight as a function of body weight in mammals, Growth 43: 139-150.

Ramsey, J. C., and Andersen, M. E. (1984). A physiologically based description of the inhalation pharmacokinetics of styrene in rats and humans, Toxicol. Appl. Pharmacol. 73: 159-175.

Schmidt-Nielsen K. (1970). Energy metabolism, body size and problems of scaling. Fed. Proc. 29: 1524-1532.

Schmidt-Nielson, K. (1984). Scaling: Why is Animal Size So Important? Cambridge: Cambridge University Press.

Smith, R. E. (1956). Quantitative relations between liver mitochondria metabolism and total body weight in mammals, Ann. NY Acad. Sci. 62: 403-422.

Stahl, W. R. (1965). Organ weights in primate and other mammals, Science 150: 1039-1042.

Stahl, W. R. (1967). Scaling of respiratory variables in mammals, J. Appl. Physiology 48: 1052-1059.

Travis, C. C. and White, R. K., (1988). Interspecific scaling of toxicity data, Risk Analysis 8: 119-125.

Travis, C. C., White, R. K., and Ward, R. C. (1988). Interspecies extrapolation of pharmacokinetics, Fundamentals Applied Toxicology (Submitted).

Travis, C. C. (1988). Tissue dosimetry in risk assessment, Risk Analysis (Submitted).

U. S. Environmental Protection Agency (EPA) (1987). Update of the Health Assessment Document and Addendum for Dichloromethane (Methylene Chloride): Pharmacokinetics, Mechanisms of Action, and Epidemiology. EPA/600/8-87/030A.

Ward, R. C., Travis, C. C., Hetrick, D. M., Andersen, M. E., and Gargas, M. L., (1988). Pharmacokinetics of tetrachloroethylene, Toxicol. Appl. Pharmacol. 93: 108-117.

White, L., Haines, H. and Adams, T. (1968). Cardiac output related to body weight in small mammals, Comp. Biochem. Physiol. 27: 559-565.

Yates, F. E. and Kugler, P. N. (1986). Similarity principles and intrinsic geometrics: contrasting approaches to interspecies scaling, J. Pharmaceutical Sci. 75 (11): 1019-1027.

COMPARATIVE CARCINOGENESIS :

IS THERE A THEORETICAL APPROACH TO INTER-SPECIES SIMILARITY ?

P.Tautu

German Cancer Research Centre
Institute of Epidemiology and Biometry
Department of Mathematical Models
D-6900 Heidelberg , INF 280

Abstract.Comparative carcinogenesis should be understood as
the scientific activity dealing with rational analyses and
syntheses of the essential differences and similarities between
experimental and observed carcinogenesis ('the mouse-to-man
problem'). In this area,two extreme positions can be made out:
(1)the 'optimistic' one (frequent among regulatory authorities),
which accepts a direct "extrapolation" of all kinds of xenobiotic effects from strains of small laboratory animals to the
human species, and (2)the 'pessimistic' position,which relies
upon the argument that no animal data has any value for humans
("man is not a big rat").
   The paper puts forward the essential mathematical concepts
involved and shows some of the fallacies observed in biological applications. By comparing the enunciation of the empirical
problem with the suggested dimensional-analytical one,it
appears that a scientific solution cannot be envisaged without
a deep and novel study of the process of carcinogenesis get
rid of current beliefs.

I.INTRODUCTION:THE PROBLEM

   It is an ascertained fact that in all empirical sciences a
propensity exists for discovering some universal invariant but
simple "laws of nature". Yet,since Galileo it has also been

generally accepted that the road to such a discovery is strewed with numerous serious obstacles. One should frequently mention the advice given by C.S.Peirce(1892):

> "Try to verify any law of nature,and you will find
> that the more precise your observations,the more
> certain they will be to show irregular departures
> from the law...Trace their causes back far enough,
> and you will be forced to admit they are always due
> to arbitrary determination,or chance."

The reader is referred to the enlightening paper by T.S.Kuhn, "The Function of Measurement in Modern Physical Science"(1961), and courteously invited to cogitate on his thesis : "To discover quantitative regularity one must normally know what regularity one is seeking and one's instruments must be designed accordingly; even then nature may not yield consistent or generalizable results without a struggle"(see also the 1968 paper by A.Ehrenberg).

The plenary illustration of the above is the attempt to "extrapolate" to man the experimental data of chemical carcinogenesis,with the purpose to find an invariant quantitative relationship between the "carcinogenic dose" for laboratory animals and the dose inducing human neoplasias. It is requested pragmatically to predict the location of the point "man" on the Salmonella-elephant dose-response curve or,if restricted to mammals,on the mouse-elephant curve.

From scientific but mostly from regulatory objectives,the problem of "predictive toxicology" can be formulated as follows:

Empirical instances:(1)there are batteries of in vitro/in vivo tests developed for the identification of a chemical compound as carcinogen; (2)there are dose-effect relationships for many chemical carcinogens,obtained from small laboratory animals.

Empirical Problem 1(P1):Find(predict) the carcinogenic(or safety)doses for humans of a chemical compound evidenced as carcinogenic in animal experiments and/or in vitro tests.

This problem has the following (dreamlike) delineation:

> "Ideally,one would want to develop a smooth mathematical function which would be based upon experimental data and permit extrapolation from a single species of placental mammal to any other species within the same class"(Hart and Fishbein,1985,p.15).

80

One of the purposes of this paper is to discuss the essential
difficulties in finding the way "from the laboratory to Park
Avenue and 59th Street" and to suggest some adjustments to the
present road map. Actually,all cartographers know that on every
blueprint there are a lot of "detours,chuckholes,swamps,quag-
mires,and dead ends"(Schneiderman et al.,1975). It would not
be very complicated to demonstrate that the empirical Problem 1
is not correctly posed and,furthermore to show that also in
carcinogenesis "the road from scientific law to scientific
measurement can rarely be travelled in the reverse direction"
(Kuhn,1961). The certitude in a positive answer to P1 is,for
the time being,a belief in the successful movement in the opposite direction. Yet,the main intention of the present paper
is to consider Problem 1(as such) above all as a biological one,
but in the modern right sense,that is as a theoretical-biologi-
cal problem. It led to the idea of "comparative carcinogenesis".
  Obviously,the first question would be : compared to what ?
If one cannot compare oranges and apples,what can we do in
cancer research with Salmonella,Marion's tortoise and mouse ?
The reader will find in an editorial by F.E.Yates(1979)the brief
description of three approaches to comparative physiology.
An analogous concept in cancer research is "comparative oncology",defined as "that branch of oncology seeking to improve
understanding of neoplasia by identifying the differences and
similarities among neoplasms in man,in other animals,and even
in plants"(Dawe,1973,1983). Thence,"comparative carcinogenesis"
should constitute a primary branch of comparative oncology
consisting not at all of cumulative retention of empirical facts
but mainly of the critical examination of
  -the amount and the weight of experimental data supporting a
solution of P1,
  -the amount and the weight of the so-called "empirical
anomalies" (in reality:the existence and action of antimutagens,
anticarcinogens,etc.),and
  -the number and centrality of the conceptual fallacies (or
falsities) contained in the enunciation of P1 and in the hypotheses behind it.
  To some extent,this satisfies Yates' idea about the comparative investigation which is intended to reduce "our sense of
being engulfed by a flood tide of raw data,and confused by
complexity. Only concepts(theories)can help us." Thus,compara-

tive carcinogenesis could be a special exercise for lateral thinking.

Remarks on the empirical instances of Problem 1. (1).Recent controversy of the value of detection tests(see Ashby,1986) revealed two or three important aspects:

(i)There is no evidence that rodent assays are superior to short-term tests(STTs)in detecting human carcinogens. The sensitivity rank of the usual in vitro tests is as follows:

[short term tests] > [sister chromatid exchange]=

=[mouse lymphoma tests] > [chromosome aberration]=

=[Salmonella/microsome reverse-mutation assay] ;

the tests' specificity is the reciprocal of this ranking(Brockman and DeMarini,1988).

(ii)If mouse carcinogenicity results are measured against rat carcinogenicity results,concordance equals 67%,which is not significantly different from the concordance values shown for the STTs in comparison with rodent results. Only 63% of rat carcinogens are detected correctly by mouse bioassays and only 79% of rat non-carcinogens are correctly identified. "An intelligent rat might be less than satisfied with this results" (Heddle,1988;see also Brusick,1983).

A considerable effort for a correct statistical analysis must be noticed;the reader is referred to the recent papers by H.S. Rosenkranz and F.K.Ennever,L.P.Claxton et al.,S.Parodi et al., published in the special issue(205)of Mutation Res.,"Strategies for the Deployment of Batteries of Short-Term Tests"(1988). The investigation of the relationships between the molecular structure of a chemical compound and its carcinogenic activity (see Ashby,1985;Ashby and Tennant,1988),mostly known as QSAR (extrathermodynamic and connectivity)approach,comes slowly into view(Frierson et al.,1986;Benigni and Giuliani,1987). Recently, Š.Baláž et al.(1988)suggested the direct incorporation of the time of exposure into the relationships between biological and physico-chemical properties of a substance(i.e.QSTAR). The relationships between the molecular structure and the reactivity properties(e.g.,molecular electrostatic potentials)of carcinogens may be used for establishing how the information necessary for recognition and activation of the biological receptors at which a carcinogen acts is encoded in its molecular structure(Weinstein et al.,1981). Actually,the connection between the receptor modifications and the induced biological response is the most loosely defined step in carcinogenesis.

(2).Hesitations about the accuracy and reproducibility of dose-response curves have also been set down:

(i)The intra- and inter-laboratory variability of tumour incidence frequently exceeded what "one would expect to find by chance alone"(Haseman,1983).

(ii)Dose-response curves vary with different classes of xenobiotica(and,also some of these agents may be carcinogenic at one site but anticarcinogenic at another site).

(iii)"Dose" can be defined in different ways and at different steps. See Ehrenberg et al.(1983):their Eq.34 represents the general dose-response function.

II.HOW TO SOLVE IT ?

1.Analysis of conjectures. In order to find a solution to Problem 1, I will adapt some of the recommendations suggested by G.Pólya in his book "How To Solve It.A New Aspect of Mathematical Method"(1945),namely

(I)the analysis of the conjecture(s) underpining the statement of a problem,

(II)the search for a similar problem,

(III)the substitution of problem's terms by their definitions,

(IV)the decomposition and recombination of the elements of the problem.

It appears that for P1 at least two conjectures are essential:

(C1)The unity of biology : Humans and laboratory rodents have many physiologic and biochemical processes in common (Rodricks and Tardiff,1983) and,after all,the human genome is similar to those of the plant and animal kingdoms (Calabrese, 1984). Thus,mouse(Grasso and Crampton,1972) and rat(Oser,1981) are adequate experimental species for human carcinogenesis (see also Ashby,1983).

(C2)The general biological regularity : There exists an appropriate scale on which the parameters of a process can be similarly expressed in different species. This is the approach promoted by F.E.Yates(1979) in comparative physiology : "It is comparison by dimensional analysis,using the similitude theory of physics...What I look for in Comparative Physiology is a demonstration of similarity in the comparison across species, according to a criterion arising out of dimensional analysis."

Conjecture C1 is an empirical general statement which,in fact, has no direct application(like "All men are mortal");its truth or falsity depends upon the truth(or falsity)of other general statements with which it is deductively connected and which do have direct application.

Recent experimental results (Ashby,1986,1988;Tennant et al., 1986,1987;Natarajan and Obe,1986;Clayson,1987,etc.) indicate that carcinogens can be classified according to different criteria,e.g.,species and sex,site of action,chemical structure, etc.(with the mention that no classification is definitive). For instance,one can distinguish carcinogens as being

-uni-species : carcinogens inducing tumours in both species of only one of the two exposed rodent species(mouse and rat);

-uni-sex/species : inducing tumours in only one sex of either species;

-trans-species : inducing tumours in at least one sex of both species;

-trans-sex/species : inducing tumours in both sexes of both species (Tennant et al.,1986).

Also,according to the common criterion of the nature of effects,one distinguishes (1)genotoxic, (2)non-genotoxic(epi-genetic), and (3)misclassified(dubious)carcinogens(Ashby,1986).

Therefore,we have to suppose that there is a group of female rat genotoxic carcinogens distinct from the group of female mouse genotoxic carcinogens and,consequently,that "the human carcinogens so far identified are a special group of carcino-gens"(Shelby et al.,1988). Such a conjecture is far from the certitude of ten years ago that all chemicals that are carcino-genic in rodents are carcinogenic in human populations (see,e.g., Rall,1979;Teichmann and Schramm,1979). The present consensus may be that the trans-species/multi-tissue/genotoxic carcino-gens are of maximum potential hazard to man,while selective/ non-genotoxic carcinogens represent a negligible hazard in iso-lation(Ashby and Purchase,1988). The reader is referred to A.M. Jeffery(1987) for a topical classification of chemical carcino-gens and to G.M.Williams(1987),particularly for the classifica-tion of non-genotoxic carcinogens(neoplasm-promoting/endocrine-modifying/immunosuppressants/cytotoxic/peroxisome-proliferating).

Another consequence affects our scientific language : the word "carcinogen" alone,without any specification,has become imprecise. In the sequel I will mark some imprecise words like "carcinogen" by an asterisk,i.e.,carcinogen*,promoter*,extrapolation[*],dose[*], etc. This points out the importance of Pólya's recommendation III,the substitution of terms in Problem 1 by their (more precise) definitions. Indeed,we can distinguish at least five types of extrapolation[*] in carcinogenic risk assessment,namely (i)from one species to another, (ii)from one route of exposure to another, (iii)from one temporal pattern of exposure to another, (iv)from high doses to low doses, (v)from one cell type to another - but also from an increase of mutation rate to the incidence of a disease (see also Crump and Howe, 1985). It is difficult to extrapolate[*] from mouse to man without our outlook being obscured by the issues (ii),(iii) or (v). For the exact mathematical definition of extrapolation,the reader is referred to the Encyclopedia of Statistical Sciences(Vol. 2,p.599). The signification of dose[*] will be given in the next section.

2.The evolutionary-comparative conjecture. Let us replace conjecture C1 by another biological one : the evolutionary-comparative paradigm(Boxenbaum,1984). It essentially states that in pharmacology "drug disposition characterizations depend on species phenotypes which have evolved and are maintained or modified by the action of natural selection on genetically modifiable systems designed to regulate and protect the organism".

This conjecture induces a new perspective in comparative carcinogenesis : it would be plausible to assume that some differences across species may be a consequence of a specific evolutionary strategy "adopted by organisms for dealing with environmental xenobiotic loads"(Boxenbaum,1983,p.1060).

As a matter of fact,species differences in chemical carcinogenesis have been evidenced from the very beginning : indeed, as late as 1918,H.Tsutsui showed that rat and guinea pig are "resistant" to the painting of polycyclic hydrocarbon-containing oils and tars. The list of such observations about species-specific "anticarcinogenesis" is long enough (see,e.g.,Clayson, 1985,for some other examples). However,the case of 2-acetylaminofluorene(2-AAF) must be mentioned. The resistance of some species (guinea pig,Steppe lemming) to this aromatic amine can be explained by the absence in its metabolic pathway of the most mutagenic metabolite:N-hydroxy-AAF. The N-hydroxylation of AAF is catalyzed in the liver by P-450d, a cytochrome-P-450-associated mixed function oxidase,and further by a sulfotransferase; the level of hepatic sulfotransferase activity and the susceptibility to hepatocarcinogenesis following the exposure by 2-AAF was found to be directly proportional. The amount of N-hydroxy--AAF in the sensitive species varies 8-fold (e.g.,man<rabbit< <hamster),but even in humans its formation diversifies the amount by a factor of 10 (see Gillette et al.,1985). 2-AAF and N-hydroxy-AAF react generally with the C-8 position of guanine; the major adducts disappear from liver DNA with a half-life of about 7 days,but the minor adduct remains in DNA for a period of up to 8 weeks.

The evolutionary-comparative conjecture promotes objective knowledge : it obliges us to consider the other factors which are,in carcinogenesis,an indelible part of the original situations and to avoid "the monorail mistake"(de Bono,1971),that is the unilateral(non-scientific)thinking.

The empirical assertion illustrating the alternative lateral thinking is "Haynes' law" :

"Haynes' law"(Haynes,1986,p.248). In any well-balanced diet,for every mutagen there is an equal and opposite antimutagen.

(The Ames' statement(Ames,1986)is clearly unilateral : "There are a large number of carcinogens in every meal,all perfectly natural and traditional,and no human diet can be entirely free of carcinogens and mutagens.Nature is not benign.")

R.H.Haynes(1986) commented his "law" as follows : "Upon reflection,there may be more truth than humor in "Haynes' law"... The many pressures toward mutation are in fact balanced,to a remarkable degree,by antimutagenic devices and agents. However, being themselves composed of ordinary molecules,such systems cannot,for thermodynamic and other reasons,operate with 100 percent efficiency."

In both groups of events occurring during the interaction between a xenobiotic agent and an organism (e.g.,dispositional and reception events),evolutionary-adaptive modifications in the nature,sequence and realization become manifest,both groups depending on genetic structures involved in the regulation of essential processes and in the protection of the organism. One of the most common examples is the evolution of the cytochrome P-450 system(P-450) which plays a major role in the activation as well as the deactivation of chemical carcinogens. Its genetic polymorphism is evidenced with precision as well as the dependence of its isozymic composition on age,sex,and induction regimen(Vesell,1987). In 1979,E.Hodgson considered the key question whether P-450 is

-an ancient enzyme system of <u>monophyletic</u> origin (which has been modified for many different functions),or

-a class of heme pigments of <u>polyphyletic</u> origin (which vary considerably in other respects).

The actual interpretation is that initially there was only an ancestral P-450 gene family,more than 1.5 billion years ago, which had expanded via divergent evolution; the detoxification function is an additional one,appearing later in the evolution (Nebert and Gonzales,1987).

H.Boxenbaum(1983) applied a kind of thermodynamic order - disorder explanation to speculate about the complex properties and polymorphism of P-450. More generally,H.Boxenbaum suggested the existence of a highly coordinated program for the genetical control of pharmacokinetic processes,or a <u>plan</u>,namely "the pharmacokinetic ground plan" (1984). As part of this ground plan, smaller mammals have relatively larger drug-eliminating organs (viz.,liver,kidney) than larger mammals. The hypothesis is that mammalian species tend to dispose of drug molecules in accordance with their own needs,and these requirements may be regulated by, or correlated with,body size and longevity(Boxenbaum and Ronfeld, 1983). As we will note in the next paragraphs,this hypothesis allows the statement of a "theory" of pharmacokinetic similarity.

3.Understanding the problem(I). It clearly appears that the problem of quantitative extrapolation[*] can be solved only if we acquire knowledge in at least three complex fields:

(F1).Species differences of various kinds (e.g.,disposition and reception of xenobiotica,defence and tolerance,DNA repair with avoidance or fixation of error,etc.).

(F2).Basic mechanisms of human malignant neoplasias(with comparative carcinogenesis).

(F3).Theoretical biology of development and aging(relative to neoplasia interpreted as a biological process).

Beyond any reasonable doubt,the empirical problem P1 raised an inextricable scientific question ("animal extrapolation is a science" : Calabrese,1984),or,better,it is on the point of being substituted by a scientific one.However,as P.Diaconis (1981)noticed,in the analysis of scientific data "magical thinking" may subsist : "it provides approximate formulas (the simple descriptions) with little or no attempt to explain the

the formulas from more basic principles...People can imagine
patterns in data when there is nothing there."

This odd interaction between a scientist and his subject has
been named "the clever Hans phenomenon", in remembrance of Mr.
von Osten's horse(in Berlin,1904) who "solved" mathematical problems and "answered" verbal questions. It was rapidly discovered
(Pfungst,1907) that the clever Hans did not actually <u>understand</u>
the problems or questions that were posed nor did he calculate
the answers by <u>conceptual thought</u>. If no one knew the answers
in the horse's presence,the horse was unable to answer the questions and went on tapping and tapping indefinitely (Polanyi,
1958,p.169).

<u>4.Understanding the problem(II)</u>. Besides the accurate assertion
of facts in the fields F1-F3 above,two other questions must be
elucidated; the first one is of a pragmatic nature,but the
second one leads to a basic answer to the quantitative extrapolation.

(Q1).Can we extend("extrapolate") the data obtained from
(lucid) experiments on laboratory animal strains to heterogeneous human populations ? (Vide again Calabrese,1984 : no one
animal model can predict the response of such a diverse grouping
as humans.) For J.R.Gillette(1985),some investigators have -in
order to improve "predictive human pharmacokinetics"- sought
animal species that metabolize drugs similar to man : "but I
wonder what they mean".

His suspicion is based on the observation that the response
to a xenobiotic compound of any genetically homogeneous strain
of a rodent species cannot be extrapolated[*] to the entire human
population but only to a segment or stratum of this population.
This heterogeneity suggests the division of a defined human
population into four groups (called "oncodemes" by Knudson,1987),
according to the predominances in the pair nature-nurture.

———— NURTURE ————▶

NATURE ▼	1.Background oncodeme incidence determined by random mutations	2.Genetic oncodeme incidence determined by an inherited cancer proneness genotype
	3.Environmental oncodeme incidence determined by exposure to an environ- mental carcinogen[*]	4.Environmental-genetic oncodeme incidence determined by genetic susceptibility to an environmental carcinogen[*]

The consequences are clear : conventional tests and experiments might predict (if at all) only events in oncodeme 3.

(Q2).Is the 1-1 correspondence between a prototype and its model valid in biology ? That means,can small mammals be regarded as models ("small-scale replica") for large ones - or,in other words,is man a prototype with the laboratory mouse (even the megamouse) as an adequate model ?

The evident confusion between a physical model and a theoretical one must not hide the proper idea that the correspondence between a model and its prototype moots for examination the problem of measurement. Generally speaking,measurement is thought of as the process of locating (specifying the coordinates of) a point in some "frame of reference" and quantifying the coordinate system according to some convention of units. Of course,the everyday practice of measuring may need no explanation,but behind the practical activity the theoretical foundations are continuously tested for (see Yates and Kugler(1986) on two theories of measurement). In one of the principal steps of modelling (call it "the naming of variables"),we need clear statements about how the measurement of these variables is made and in what units the results will be expressed. As R.Carnap(1966) pointed out,"quantitative concepts are not given by nature ; they arise from our practice of applying numbers to natural phenomena".

Since J.B.Fourier(1822),J.Bertrand(1848)and J.C.Maxwell(1871), it is known that the measurable quantities which appear in the mathematical representation of physical laws,are in general not pure numbers,but rather have associated with them specific units called "dimensions". Let denote by (u) a standard unit; then the dimension of a quantity q can be denoted by $[q \cdot (u)]$, $q \in R$. The adoption of a different standard unit (u') or the different numerical assignment to the entities in (u),do not change the dimension. In addition,the dimension of any magnitude on the same scale is unchanged.

Yet,in the case of derived magnitudes,in the indirect and systematic measurement,we are changing the rule determining the scale as well as (perhaps) the unit and the basic assignment of numerical values (Kyburg,1984,p.163). For instance,if mass M, length L,and time T are considered the fundamental quantities (MLT class of systems of units,with M,L,and T as abstract positive numbers) in terms of which all else is referred to,then the dimensions of the derived variables can be found from those of the independent entities. Thus,the dimension formula for velocity is $[LT^{-1}]$, for acceleration $[LT^{-2}]$,and for force $[MLT^{-2}]$.

Such considerations led to the elaboration of similarity principles (geometrical,physical,biologica) and of dimensional analysis. The concept of similarity was applied in relation to physical phenomena : they are called _similar_ if they differ only with respect to the numerical values of those parameters which are "dimensional",while the numerical values of the corresponding "dimensionless" parameters must be _invariant_. The term "dimensionless" (or "pure") numbers is a rather misleading one and, consequently,R.E.Johnstone and M.W.Thring suggested in 1957 its replacement by the term "criterion of similarity". Their models dealt with models and scale-up methods in chemical engineering, because complex chemical systems cannot be scaled unless many variables are kept constant. In practice,any given physical model may be governed by numerous different similarity criteria simultaneously. Their invariance indicates that a model is physically similar to a prototype.

The initial question Q2 asks about biological similarity and its end is the understanding _whether_ and _how_ we might admit that mice should be analogous models for humans as far as chemical carcinogenesis is concerned. The facts briefly presented above as well as our ignorance revealed in the fields F1-F3, prevent us to cherish illusions about a prompt answer to Q2, and about an easy solution to Problem 1. Yet,theoretically,if all corresponding similarity criteria would be defined and measurable,and all general conditions of similarity satisfied,it would be possible to achieve an extended ("extrapolated") similarity analysis,under the alternative conditions (Stahl,1963):

(a)the similarity criteria have identical numerical values in the model and in the prototype,or

(b)the criteria are related to each other by defined functional equations which assign a numerical value to any given variable criterion as a function of fixed criteria for a given type of problem (e.g.,the dynamical similarity of a chemical carcinogen).

This project would require a vast mathematical investigation which obviously must start with the construction of an adequate theory of chemical carcinogenesis. Usually,it is not feasible to impose complete similarity (which must include geometric similarity) and,moreover,biological dimensional constants are not nearly so general in their significance as the basic physical constants. In almost all models there occur so-called scale effects,that is some disturbing influences on a parameter which is important for the model but it is negligible for the proto-type. A special skill is required rather for finding the theo-retical corrections to compensate the escapes from complete sim-ilarity than for justifying the departure from completeness.

5.Understanding dimensional analysis. The theory of dimensional analysis is the mathematical theory of dimensionally homogeneous functions (a generalization of Euler homogeneous functions). Following H.L.Langhaar(1951,p.14),the application of dimensional analysis to a practical problem is based on the hypothesis that the solution of the problem is expressible by means of a dimen-sionally homogeneous equation in terms of specified variables. This hypothesis is justified by the fact that the fundamental equations of classical physics are dimensionally homogeneous. Two definitions are indispensable.

Definition 1. An equation of the form

$$y = \Phi(x_1,x_2,\ldots,x_n) \quad , \quad n \in N \qquad (1)$$

is dimensionally homogeneous(dh) if,and only if,the relationship

$$K\Phi(x_1,x_2,\ldots,x_n) = \Phi(K_1 x_1, K_2 x_2,\ldots,K_n x_n) \qquad (2)$$

is an identity in the variables $x_1,x_2,\ldots,x_n,A,B,C$ (see Theorem 1 in Langhaar,1951),in which

$$K = A^u B^v C^z \quad , \quad A,B,C:\text{positive numbers}$$
$$K_i = A^{u_i} B^{v_i} C^{z_i} \quad , \quad 1 \le i \le n, \qquad (3)$$

and the dimensional matrix which designates the dimensions (for MLT class) is

	y	x_1	x_2	$\cdots$	x_n
M	u	u_1	u_2	$\cdots$	u_n
L	v	v_1	v_2	$\cdots$	v_n
T	z	z_1	z_2	$\cdots$	z_n

The symbol Φ in (1) may be viewed as an operator that is applied to the independent variables $x_1,x_2,\ldots,x_n$ to yield the proper value of the dependent variable y. Equation (1) is in-variant under the group transformations which are generated by all possible changes of the units in the MLT class, as defined in (3). For y differentiable and dh, see Eq.35 in H.L.Langhaar (1951,p.154); see also W.R.Stahl(1963,p.368)for the example of Navier-Stokes equation expressed by five dimensionless numbers.

Let variables $K_1, \ldots, K_n$ be defined by (3). Then the relations

$$x_i = K_i x_i^* , \quad 1 \le i \le n \qquad (4)$$

define a point transformation (the K-transformation) in the coordinate space S, namely a transformation that carries the point x_i^* to the point x_i.

Definition 2(Langhaar,1951,p.68). Let consider two functions

$$f = (x_1, x_2, \ldots, x_n)$$
$$f^* = (x_1^*, x_2^*, \ldots, x_n^*).$$

The function f^* is similar to the function f, provided that the ratio $K = f^*/f$ is a constant (and K is called the scale factor for the function f). The x_i's are obtained by applying (4).

Following a lemma given by H.L.Langhaar(Lemma 3,p.57), a dh dimensionless function

$$\pi = \Phi(x_1, x_2, \ldots, x_n) \qquad (5)$$

is constant in any K-space, that is, the set of all points that can be derived from a given point x_i^* by K-transformations; hence any dimensionless product of the x_i's is constant throughout each K-space.

These elementary definitions may, however, give us some suggestions how re-formulate Problem 1. The first ingredients are the following (see Barenblatt,1987):

1.Specify a system of independent variables $x_1, \ldots, x_n$ ("governing parameters") such that a relation of the form (1) can be assumed to hold.

2.Choose an appropriate class of systems unit and determine the dimensions of the dependent variable y ("governed parameter") and the independent variables $x_1, \ldots, x_n$ in this class. Mark those x's having independent dimensions and those x's whose dimensions are expressed in terms of products of powers of the dimensions of the former governing parameters. Then, rewrite (1) as

$$y = \Phi(x_1, \ldots, x_k, x_{k+1}, \ldots, x_n) \qquad (1')$$

in order to distinguish the two groups of x's (see Eq.2.1 in

Barenblatt,1987,p.31).

3.Express the dimensions of y and of x_m's(m=k+1,...,n)as products of powers of the dimensions of the x_i's(i=1,...,k).

4.Determine the similarity parameters and put the function (1') into a dimensionless form

$$\pi = \Phi(\pi_1,\pi_2,\ldots\pi_{n-k}). \qquad (6)$$

Thus,we can generally formulate the dimensional-analytical version of the empirical Problem 1 as follows:

Instance : There exists a dh relation (1') between the action (end-point) of a presumed carcinogen and the parameters which govern it.

Problem 2 : Determine a dh function,say,$\pi = \Phi(\pi^+)$, - where π^+ is a composite parameter (also including "dose") - for which the curve in dimensionless coordinates remains unchanged.

Cautions.(a)The determination of specific biological end-points of a carcinogen[*] is,strange to say,quite difficult(see Dunkel,1983). In principle,hyperplasia might be such a point (see Schulte-Hermann,1974) and two distinct types,the additive and the regenerative hyperplasias,have recently been described as the effect of non-genotoxic carcinogens(Loury et al.,1987). If one is going to consider biochemical end-points,kinetic modelling with multiresponse data (Ziegel and Gorman,1980) might be the appropriate mathematical investigation.

(b)The dimensional analysis of a growth equation is interest-ing in itself : W.R.Stahl(1963,p.455) gave a rough draft for the Bertalanffy equation,but with the exception of the sugges-tion of a self-similar solution and a hint on the possibility to associate local geometric factors,nothing more -to my knowl-edge- has been achieved.

(c)Dimensional analysis must be improved mathematically(see Rosen,1978,1983;Yates and Kugler,1986) because it cannot be applied to complex nonlinear and multiphasic processes.

6.Guessworking and sonking in carcinogenesis. Taking into ac-count all these difficulties,B.N.Ames(1986) states that the quantitative extrapolation[*] of risk from rodents to humans is a guesswork (see also Ames et al.,1987). "This is a controver-sial extrapolation -perceives Ames- based more on a desire for prudence than on scientific knowledge". I rely on Edith Efron (1984,Ch.13) as to the persuasive collection of critical com-ments by "foes" and "friends" to mouse-man extrapolation[*].

Ames' remark is a good example of the crucial distinction between cognitive problems (expressed by WHW-questions:"why,how, whether") and problems of action("what to do ?"). The cognitive (scientific) activity is truth-seeking and,hence,different from problem-solving. Yet,the quantitative extrapolation[*] remains an unsolvable problem(Gillette,1985) or only superficially "soluble",as long as a truthlike explanatory theory of animal and human carcinogenesis has not been established. If such a theory is not sufficently truthlike,"it may with good luck give a correct prediction in some particular cases,but not uniformly for an indefinitely large class of empirical problems"(Niiniluoto, 1985).

This uncertainty may lead to a "sonking" activity in carcinogenesis. The verb "to sonk" was coined by A.S.C.Ehrenberg as an acronym standing for the "scientification of non-knowledge", with the intention to criticize "a too facile writing down in pseudo-exact form,of relations which merely express our ignorance"(Kendall,1968). Indeed,there is a sonking activity in carcinogenesis and in cancer chemotherapy ; it can be avoided only if carcinogenesis is treated as a cognitive biological problem for which corresponding explanatory mathematical models are built up.

III.DO WE KNOW AN ALLIED PROBLEM
    AND WAS THERE A SOLUTION TO IT ?

1.Comparative pharmacokinetics. According to Pólya's recommendation II,one important step in solving a problem is the search for a similar or related one which has already been solved. The problem related to P1 that usually comes in sight,is the extrapolation in pharmacology. Efforts have been made in this field, particularly in the last decade,to achieve the simultaneous characterization of drug pharmacokinetics (PK,"what the body does to the drug") and pharmacodynamics (PD,"what the drug does to the body"),but the problem of quantitative prediction of drug toxicity is still tied up. One has so far been on the look out for similarity criteria for animal-man drug disposition (Ruelius,1987;Rahmani et al.,1988) and "comparative pharmacokinetics" as well as the prediction of species differences in the qualitative pattern of drug metabolism are "far from being an exact science"(Smith,1988).

However,the correspondence drug-carcinogen and toxicity-carcinogenicity had some positive consequences. Evidently, a carcinogen[*] is not a drug ; it is a xenobiotic compound, mostly a natural one rather than a man-made chemical substance (Gillette, 1979,Ames,1983,1986). It would then be appropriate to speak about xenokinetics(XK) and xenodynamics(XD).

The initiation of a carcinogenic process roughly and frequently entails that (1)the xenobiotic compound requires biotransformation (the so-called Phase I and Phase II reactions) in order to be chemically reactive; (2)the adducts between DNA and these reactive intermediates escape the usual DNA repair processes and induce nucleotide changes and DNA rearrangements; (3)the result of these complex processes leads to cellular-genetic reactions that may represent the initial conditions for carcinogenesis. As a sequel to the experimental results condensed on the points above,we notice that

(i)there are a few true enviromental carcinogens[*],most of the suspected ones being in reality procarcinogens which require the appropriate biotransformation. (The reader can contrast the progressive estimates of 65,80 and 90 percent of cancers due to environmental carcinogens ,in the 70's with the present opinion (Garner,1985) that "at the present time,the major causative agents,other than cigarette smoke,are unknown".)

(ii)the procarcinogens are converted into some chemically reactive forms (i.e.,short- and long-lived metabolites : Gillette,1982),one of them possibly being the ultimate carcinogen (often genotoxic).

(iii)the metabolites of procarcinogens may have different effects. The objectives of studies of drug disposition and pharmacokinetics(PK),as they are clarified by J.Gillette et al. (1985),can easily be transferred to xenobiotics (including procarcinogens),particularly if we also include cytotoxic effects. 2.The case Arley&Iversen. From its very beginning,the PK approach comprised mathematical modelling as an active and indispensable part so that it stands to reason that the principal objective of PK research concerns "the development of mathematical model descriptions of the dynamics of drug transference and drug effects in pharmacologically responding systems" (Smolen et al.,1972). Understandably,these models are mainly data-generated and must provide new data of practical interest.

The first stochastic model for carcinogenesis (Iversen and Arley,1950) may be viewed as a first and audacious attempt in this sense. Not having any available data about the disposition of genotoxic carcinogens,N.Arley and S.Iversen(1952) took advantage of the theoretical PK approach and introduced in their model the constants of elimination,adaptation and toxicity. The reader can look at Equations 14 and 15 in the mentioned paper to see the rather simple relationships they used (see also Eqs.9 and 10 in Arley,1961). According to the authors,the carcinogenic potency of a chemical compound is a function of

(1)pharmacologic variables,e.g.,the concentration of a carcinogen,

(2)environmental physical variables like temperature,and

(3)biological-cellular variables,namely

(a)the state of the tissue at the moment of exposure,and

(b)the number of cells susceptible to proliferate as malignant cells.

The use of "concentration" instead of dose[*] is worth noting; in the recent literature,S.Garattini accentuated this paramount distinction : "the dose can no longer be considered a reliable parameter for comparing toxic effects across animal species - the blood or tissue concentration may be a better index"(1982) because "comparing doses means comparing the amounts of a chemical outside the body"(1983).

In spite of its weakness (on which all pragmatic comments insisted),the Arley-Iversen model may be viewed as the trial model of a XK/XD approach in carcinogenesis. A glance at the recent pharmacologic literature (Sheiner et al.,1979;Dow et al. 1982;Meredith et al.,1983;Paalzow,1984) dealing with PK/PD models,suggests not only the inaccessible complexity of this problem but also the limits of the popular parallel approach pharmacology-chemical carcinogenesis.

3.The urethane story. In 1967,J.Neyman and E.Scott published a drastic analysis of their stochastic model constructed with the aim to answer "authoritatively" the question whether carcinogenesis is determined by one or two irreversible somatic mutations. The numerical results of their revised version of a two--stage mutation model (see also Schoenfelder and Hoel,1979) were compared with many laboratory data on lung carcinogenesis induced by urethane (e.g.,Shimkin et al.,1967;White et al.,1967). J.Neyman and E.Scott conjectured that the effects of urethane experimentally observed are possible if the first cancer cells are "second order" urethane mutants. (Nobody noticed that in the mentioned paper by M.B.Shimkin et al.(1967),the last comment is as follows : "It would seem,to a biologist,that this is a

complex continuum involving many steps. These steps do not cease
at the conversion of the alveolar liningcells to an organoid
mass of adenomatous cells."[Emphasis added]) A few years later,
Margaret White(1972) tried to answer experimentally the questions regarding (a)the dependence of urethane catabolism upon
the dose D, and (b)the carcinogenicity of urethane and its metabolites. The experimental results (see also Guillier,1972)
showed that

(i)the speed of elimination of urethane depends upon the dose
size;

(ii)the number of first order mutants(the "initial events")
is proportional to a quantity $E(D)$ [called "internal exposure
by C.L.Guillier(1972)],rather than to D for not too large doses
of urethane;

(iii)the ethyl moiety of urethane is more intimately involved
in "the process responsible for tumorigenic action" than is the
carbonyl moiety.

J.Neyman commented these results in two papers(1974,1982),
asking himself "who is the villain ?" ,but did not improve the
stochastic model correspondingly. However,he realized the complexity of XK/XD analysis in carcinogenesis when he ascribed
to the probability that the number of first order mutants increases by unity in a very small time interval t+h,a probability
depending on the number of molecules of the procarcinogen and its
its active metabolites at time t.

The second notable error in the Neyman-Scott model pertains
to the variable 3b considered by N.Arley and S.Iversen,in the
sense that the action of a ultimate carcinogen is not exerted
in a homogeneous,inert cell population but in a structured
(differentiated) and dynamical one. W.Klonecki(1979) refined
his 1976 branching model for urethane carcinogenesis according
to the observation that urethane has specific target cells
(i.e.,the type-II cells assumed to be the stem cells of the
alveolar epithelium) which are sensitive in cell cycle phase
G_1 (Kauffman,1974,1976).

4.The Lilliputian allometry. It is already known that one of
the common quantitative approaches in comparative biology(also
comparative physiology,comparative pharmacokinetics,etc.)is
scaling. Practically,this means the construction of a measure
for a variable which many phenomena may have in common.

When Cpt.Lemuel Gulliver was stranded in Lilliput,the Emper-
or of this country issued a decree precisely specifying the

quantity of food for the "Man-Mountain" : he shall have "a daily allowance of meat and drink sufficient for the support of 1728 of our subjects". This quantity was calculated by the Lilliputian mathematicians (the Lilliputians being "most excellent mathematicians,and arrived at a great perfection in mechanics") using the following rule : "having taken the height of my body by the help of a quadrant,and finding it to exceed theirs in the proportion twelve to one,they concluded from the similarity of their bodies that mine must contain at least 1728 of theirs, and consequently would require as much food as was necessary to support that number of Lilliputians".

Absolutely astonishing – the Lilliputians calculated the food requirement as proportional to a power of the body weight, W (that is,they "scaled" Gulliver nourishment in approximate proportion to $W^{3/4}$),thus anticipating by more than two centuries the scaling of M.Kleiber(1932) and S.Brody(1932) of the metabolic rates of eutherian mammals. Yet,if the Lilliputians had used Sarrus-Rameaux'(1837),Reubner's(1883)or Richet's(1889) "surface law", Gulliver would have received only 675 portions and would have starved miserably (Schmidt-Nielsen,1970) or entered hibernation(?).

5.Allometric scaling and pharmacokinetic similarity.It is well known that the basal metabolic rate of some mammals as related to their body mass forms,on a log-log scale,a straight line with a slope of 0.75. The mathematical expression of the famous "mouse-to-elephant curve" (determined in 1934 by S.Brody and,independently,byF.G.Benedict) became one of the few demonstrations of a "universal law" in biology,called the "allometric law". This is the power function

$$Y = aW^b \; , \; a>0 \; , \; b \in R_1 \qquad (7)$$

with domain W>0 and range Y>0. In physiology,Y represents a physiological variable (e.g.,cardiac output,renal plasma flow, etc.),W is the body weight,and a and b are two constants : a is the Y-intercept and b is the slope of the log-log plot. Normally, in solving for parameters a and b, a logarithmic transformation is used,yielding

$$\log Y = \log a + b \log W. \qquad (8)$$

Let us introduce the new variables U=log Y, X=log W, and A= =log a ; the relationship (8) becomes

$$U = bX + A,$$

which is a linear one.

The allometric "law" shared the fate of all empirical relationships : while some scientists,fascinated by the "ubiquitous" 0.75 power,suggested different explanations about its nature (e.g.,the "elastic similarity"),others collected data,showing the existence of many exceptions (see Economos,1982). In fact, most allometric data are confined to less than 10 percent of mammalian species (Prothero,1986). Clearly,the allometric approach is a black box ; as R.J.Smith(1980) pointed out,there is rarely a good theoretical basis for hypothesizing a power function,and simple untransformed linear equations often work just as well (see D'Arcy Thompson in his 1943 revised edition of the book "On Growth and Form").

The reader must realize that the critiques are addressed to the excessive and unreasonable use of the log-log representation where the distribution of points looks linear and the correlation coefficient is high. A log-log transformation is an efficient means of altering the distribution of data to meet the statistical assumptions of normality and homoscedasticity. However,mathematically deduced power functions are present in some pharmacological models (Wise et al.,1968;Wise,1974;Marcus, 1975,etc.). As M.A.Savageau(1979) pointed out,power-law relations are predicted for variables of a system in quasi-steady state. Simple allometry follows "naturally" from the "power--law formalism" (which is identified explicitly in the "biochemical systems theory" : Savageau et al.,1987) and the assumption of a single,temporally dominant process.

Generally speaking,when inter-species relationships are expressed (with good or bad reason) in an allometric form,the system is said to be "scaled". For example,creatinine clearance (C_1) "scales" the body weight as

$$C_1 = 8.2 \ W^{0.69},$$

and,similarly,methotrexate clearance (C_2) "scales" to W as

$$C_2 = 10.9 \ W^{0.69}.$$

Their ratio $C_1/C_2 = 1.33$ is considered invariant.

The theory of pharmacokinetic similarity (Boxenbaum and Ronfeld,1983) states that the disposition of drug molecules could be correlated between species if one uses an intrinsic biological property (e.g.,creatinine clearance,blood circulation

velocity,mean residence time in a compartment,etc.) as an equivalent time-scaling factor. In other words,two species obeying
the same dynamics of drug elimination are in a similar state at
equal moments of "biologic"(="pharmacokinetic")time,even though
the elimination has unequal rates when measured within a chronological time scale.

Since pharmacokinetic and physiologic events appear to be
correlated with W, it is possible to use W as a part of a coordinate system on which one bases a time function. For example,
the ratio t/W^{1-b} defines a new unit of pharmacokinetic time,the
kallynochron : it signifies the time required to clear drug
from plasma. The theoretical argument is that any process that
includes chronological time is size-dependent. By removing this
dependence,one scales the chronologic time to a pharmacokinetic
one : the latter should be interpreted as a species-dependent
unit of the chronologic time required to complete a species-
-independent pharmacokinetic event.

Another pharmacokinetic unit is the apolysichron,a species-
-independent measure of half-life,turnover time,and mean residence time. It is defined as $t/W^{b_2-b_1}$,where b_2 and b_1 are the
allometric exponents relating the volume of distribution and
the clearance,respectively,to W.

The power equation (7) has frequently been applied to the
prediction of drug pharmacokinetics,by defining Y as being the
renal clearance (see Dedrick et al.(1970) for methotrexate,
Dedrick et al.(1973) for arabinofuranosylcytosine,Boxenbaum
(1980,1982) for benzodiazepines,Sawada et al.(1984) for β-lactam,etc.). The latter authors compared two approaches,i.e.
(i)the Adolph-Dedrick approach which can be used to predict PK
parameters in man from the relationship between W and Y:PK
parameters in other animal species (e.g.,mouse,rat,rabbit,dog,
monkey),and (ii)the Boxenbaum approach based on the correlation
between PK parameters in a single species and those in man.

J.Mordenti(1986) used (7) with Y being the dosage variable
of ceftzoxime and found that (a)concerning the dose,as animals
decrease in size,the dose of ceftizoxime that is needed to
achieve the same peak concentration increases,and (b)concerning
the dose schedule,as animals decrease in size,the time between
doses decreases ; the need for more frequent injections in the
smaller animals is the result of the more rapid elimination of

the drug. Three other points are interesting in her paper,namely

(1) The use of W=body surface area is not recommended.

(2) The complexity of inter-species pharmacokinetics : "Nature has raised an enormous barrier to drug development by assigning the drug-metabolizing enzymes to various species in astonishingly diverse amounts. So great are these differences that it is often a matter of pure luck that animal experiments lead to clinically useful drugs."

(3) Extrapolation[*] of animal data in an attempt to predict the carcinogenic potential of chemical xenobiotica is "somewhat different" and depends upon other factors and processes (damage--repair,dose dependency of metabolic pathways,the change of carcinogenic activity during the disposition of the xenobiotic agent,etc.).

The last point shows the great distance between the regulatory,empirical Problem 1 and the serious scientific problem in studying procarcinogens and their disposition.

The allometric approach may be applied to PK models,provided that

(i) the PK process is of first order in each species;

(ii) the percentage of protein binding is similar and linear over the concentration range;

(iii) the elimination processes are "physical"(i.e. renal, biliary);

(iv) sufficient data exist for satisfactory linear regression.

Without some information about the biotransformation of xenobiotica in each species it is extremely difficult to extrapolate[*] toxicity data for chemical compounds that undergo metabolism.

Besides the allometric approach,a physiologic one has been suggested (Dedrick,1973) : a physiologic PK model must include mass balances,thermodynamics,transport and flow. The working hypothesis is that thermodynamic factors such as tissue-to--blood distribution ratios are more likely to be similar among mammalian species than intrinsic rates of metabolism (Dedrick, 1985). Consequently,the physiologic approach can be applied when

(i) the details of drug disposition are important;

(ii) the central compartment is not the site of action;

(iii) the chemical substance is highly lipid-soluble and extensively metabolized;

(iv) the protein binding is strong and nonlinear.

The corresponding mathematical model is obtained by writing mass balance equations (see Upton et al.,1988) for the sum of processes occurring in each compartment.

It has been believed that the allometric law can be derived by using dimensional analysis and various similarity rules based on physical considerations. This is not correct : the allometric relationship remains empirical,and it is now clear why I discussed the similarity principle and the allometric approach separately. J.P.Butler et al.(1987) demonstrated that the metabolic rate Y depends on several dimensionless variables (see Eq.3) but this does not imply that Y is proportional to 0.75 power or any other power of body mass W. "It does not imply that a power law relationship between Y and W exists at all". If one can distinguish between "intrinsic" and "empirical" scaling exponents,dimensional analysis can tell us certain things about intrinsic exponents "but without other information,it cannot tell us how a particular variable will scale observationally" (Butler et al.,1987).

IV.INSTEAD OF CONCLUSIONS

The somatic mutation theory of carcinogenesis remains "the main tenet for explaining the carcinogenic activity of chemicals"(Barrett et al.,1987). Maybe it is time to correct this theory. The existence of non-genotoxic xenobiotica and the mutation theory of atherosclerosis are the first perplexing questions. If carcinogens must be mutagens,then at least some of them might be atherosclerotic agents,too (compare with Wilson and Crouch,1987:"and we would not be surprised if... carcinogens were to produce chronic effects other than cancer"). Again,the correct definition of a carcinogen fails - as well as the precise indication of the type of mutation (other than conventional). Population geneticists (Crow,1986) suppose that in higher organisms with limited reproductive capacity,the species can better keep up with a changing environment by reshuffling existing alleles than by creating new ones by mutation.

The current dogma in oncology is the existence of a direct causal relation "environmental carcinogen → malignant tumour". Many arguments and evidences in the present paper suggest that

we positively deal with a random network of biotransformations
and cellular reactions of various order,where many casual pathways might induce carcinogenesis (see also Tautu,1975). This
conjecture insinuates gradually and is obliquely suggested by
looking at the superb linear dose-effect relations in chemical
carcinogenesis : the linearity may be valid only if the mutational process is accelerated and the induction of repair processes were not significant (Woodhead et al.,1985,cit.by Ames et
al.,1987). It seems that "carcinogenic" is a set of random paths
in the network above rather than an environmental procarcinogen
alone.

REFERENCES

Ames,B.N.(1983).Dietary carcinogens and anticarcinogens.
    Science,$\underline{221}$:1256-1264

Ames,B.N.(1986).Carcinogens and anticarcinogens. In:Antimu-
    tagenesis and Anticarcinogenesis Mechanisms(D.M.Shankel
    et al.eds.),p.7-35.Plenum Press,New York

Ames,B.N.,Magaw,R.,and Gold,L.S.(1987).Ranking possible carcino-
    genic hazards.Science,$\underline{236}$:271-280

Arley,N.(1961).Theoretical analysis of carcinogenesis. Proc.4th
    Berkeley Symp.Math.Statist.Probab.,Vol.IV,p.1-18.Univ.Cal-
    ifornia Press,Berkeley

Arley,N.,and Iversen,S.(1952).On the mechanism of experimental
    carcinogenesis.III.Further development of the hit theory of
    carcinogenesis. Acta Pathol.Microbiol.Scand.,$\underline{30}$:21-53

Ashby,J.(1983).The unique role of rodents in the detection of
    possible human carcinogens and mutagens. Mutation Res.,$\underline{115}$:
    177-213

Ashby,J.(1985).Fundamental structural alerts to potential
    carcinogenicity or noncarcinogenicity. Environ.Mutagen.,$\underline{7}$:
    919-921

Ashby,J.(1986).The prospects for a simplified and international-
    ly harmonized approach to the detection of possible human
    carcinogens and mutagens. Mutagenesis,$\underline{1}$:3-16

Ashby,J.(1988).Computer assisted short-term test battery design:
    Some questions. Environ.Molec.Mutagen.,$\underline{11}$:443-448

Ashby,J.,and Purchase,I.F.H.(1985).Significance of the genotox-
    ic activities observed in vitro for 35 of 70 NTP noncarcino-
    gens. Environ.Mutagen.,$\underline{7}$:747-758

Ashby,J.,and Tennant,R.W.(1988).Chemical structure,Salmonella
    mutagenicity and extent of carcinogenicity as indicators of
    genotoxic carcinogenesis among 222 chemical tests in rodents
    by the U.S.NCI/NTP. Mutation Res.,$\underline{204}$:17-115

Baláž,Š.,Šturdík,E.,Rosenberg,M.,Augustín,J.,and Škaára,B.(1988).
    Kinetic of drug activities as influenced by their physico-
    chemical properties:Antibacterial effects of alkylating

2-furyl ethylenes. J.Theor.Biol.,131:115-134

Barenblatt,G.I.(1987).Dimensional Analysis. Gordon and Breach, New York

Barrett,J.C.,Oshimura,M.,Tanaka,N.,and Tsutsui,T.(1987).Genetic and epigenetic mechanisms of presumed nongenotoxic carcinogens. In:Nongenotoxic Mechanisms in Carcinogenesis (B.E. Butterworth,T.J.Slaga eds.),p.311-324. Cold Spring Harbor Lab.

Benigni,R.,and Giuliani,A (1987).Carcinogenicity,mutagenicity, toxicity and chemical structure in a homogeneous data base. In:Drug Design and Toxicology(D.Hadzi,B.Jerman-Blažič eds.), p.346-348. Elsevier,Amsterdam

Boxenbaum,H.(1980).Interspecies variation in liver weight, hepatic blood flow,and antipyrine intrinsic clearance extrapolation of data to bezodiazepines and phenytoin. J.Pharmacokin.Biopharm.,8:165-176

Boxenbaum,H.(1982).Comparative pharmacokinetics of benzodiazepines in dog and man. J.Pharmacokin.Biopharm.,10:411-426

Boxenbaum,H.(1983).Evolutionary biology,animal behavior,fourth-dimensional space,and the raison d'être of drug metabolism and pharmacokinetics. Drug.Metab.Rev.,14:1057-1097

Boxenbaum,H.(1984).Interspecies pharmacokinetic scaling and the evolutionary-comparative paradigm. Drug.Metab.Rev.,15:1071-1121

Boxenbaum,H.,and Ronfeld,R.(1983).Interspecies pharmacokinetic scaling and the Dedrick plots. Amer.J.Physiol.,245:R768-R774

Brockman,H.E.,and DeMarini,D.M.(1988).Utility of short-term tests for genetic toxicity in the aftermath of the NTP's analysis of 73 chemicals. Environ.Molec.Mutagen.,11:421-435

Brusick,D.(1983).Evaluation of chronic rodent bioassays and Ames assay tests as accurate models for predicting human carcinogens. In:Application of Biological Markers to Carcinogen Testing(H.A.Milman,S.Sell eds.),p.153-163.Plenum Press,New York

Brusick,D.(1988).Evolution of testing strategies for genetic toxicity. Mutation Res.,205:69-78

Butler,J.P.,Feldman,H.A.,and Fredberg,J.J.(1987).Dimensional analysis does not determine a mass exponent for metabolic scaling. Amer.J.Physiol.,253:R195-R199

Calabrese,E.J.(1984).Suitability of animal models for predictive toxicology:Theoretical and practical considerations. Drug Metab.Rev.,15:505-523

Carnap,R.(1966).An Introduction to the Philosophy of Science. (Ed.by M.Gardner).Basic Books,New York

Claxton,L.D.,Stead,A.G.,and Walsh,D.(1988).An analysis by chemical class of Salmonella mutagenicity tests as predictors of animal carcinogenicity. Mutation Res.,205:197-225

Clayson,D.B.(1985).Problems in interspecies extrapolation. In: Toxicological Risk Assessment(D.B.Clayton,D.Krewski,I.Munro eds.),Vol.I,p.105-122. CRC Press,Boca Raton

Clayson,D.B.(1987).The need for biological risk assessment in reaching decisions about carcinogens. Mutation Res.,185:243-269

Crow,J.F.(1986).Population consequences of mutagenesis and anti-
     mutagenesis. In:Antimutagenesis and Anticarcinogenesis Mech-
     anisms(D.M.Shankel et al.eds.),p.519-530.Plenum Press,New York

Crump,K.S.,and Howe,R.B(1985).A review of methods for calculat-
     ing statistical confidence limits in low dose extrapolation.
     In:Toxicological Risk Assessment(D.B.Clayson,D.Krewski,I.
     Munro eds.),Vol.I,p.187-203. CRC Press,Boca Raton

Dawe,C.J.(1983).Comparative neoplasia. In:Cancer Medicine(J.F.
     Holland,E.Frei III eds.),p.209-256.2nd ed. Lea&Febiger,Phil-
     adelphia

De Bono,E.(1971).Practical Thinking. J.Cape,New York

Dedrick,R.L.(1973).Animal scale-up. J.Pharmacokin.Biopharm.,$\underline{1}$:
     435-461

Dedrick,R.L.,Bischoff,K.B.,and Zaharko,D.S.(1970).Interspecies
     correlation of plasma concentration history of methotrexate.
     Cancer Chemother.Rep.,Part 1,$\underline{54}$:95-101

Dedrick,R.L.,Forester,D.D.,Cannon,J.N.,ElDareen,S.M.,and Mellett,
     L.B.(1973).Pharmacokinetics of 1-β-D-arabinofuranosylcytosine
     (Ara-C)deamination in several species. Biochem.Pharmacol.,
     $\underline{22}$:2405-2417

Diaconis,P.(1981).Magical thinking in the analysis of scientific
     data. Ann.N.Y.Acad.Sci.,$\underline{364}$:236-244

Dow,J.,Laquais,B.,Tisne-Versailles,J.,Pourrias,B.,and Strolin
     Benedetti,M.(1982).Pharmacokinetics and pharmacodynamics of
     the antiarrhytmic compound MD 750819 in dogs with experimen-
     tally induced arrhytmias. J.Pharmacokin.Biopharm.,$\underline{10}$:283-296

Dunkel,V.G.(1983).Biological significance of end points. Ann.
     N.Y.Acad.Sci.,$\underline{407}$:34-41

Economos,A.C.(1982).On the origin of biological similarity.
     J.Theor.Biol.,$\underline{94}$:25-60

Efron,E.(1984).The Apocalyptics.Cancer and the Big Lie. Simon
     and Schuster,New York

Ehrenberg,A.S.C.(1968).The elements of lawlike relationships.
     J.Roy.Statist.Soc.Ser.A,$\underline{131}$:280-302

Ehrenberg,L.,Moustacchi,E.,Osterman-Golkar,S.,and Ekman,G.
     (1983).Dosimetry of genotoxic agents and dose-response rela-
     tionships of their effects. Mutation Res.,$\underline{123}$:121-182

Frierson,M.R.,Klopman,G.,and Rosenkranz,H.S.(1986).Structure-
     -activity relationships(SARs)among mutagens and carcinogens:
     A review. Environ.Mutagen.,$\underline{8}$:283-327

Garattini,S.(1982).Concluding remarks:Extrapolation of toxico-
     logical data from animals to man. In:Animals in Toxicolog-
     ical Research(I.Bartošek,A.Guaitani,E.Pacei eds.),p.201-208.
     Raven Press,New York

Garattini,S.(1983).Notes on xenobiotic metabolism. Ann.N.Y.
     Acad.Sci.,$\underline{407}$:1-25

Garner,R.C.(1985).Assessment of carcinogen exposure in man.
     Carcinogenesis,$\underline{6}$:1071-1078

Gillette,J.R.(1982).The problem of chemically reactive metabo-
     lites. Drug.Metab.Rev.,$\underline{13}$:941-960

Gillette,J.R.(1985).Biological variation:The unsolvable prob-
     lem in quantitative extrapolations from laboratory animals

and other surrogate systems to human populations. In:Risk Quantitation and Regulatory Policy(D.G.Hoel,R.A.Merrill,F.P. Perera eds.),p.199-209. Cold Spring Harbor Lab.

Gillette,J.,Weisburger,E.K.,Kraybill,H.,and Kelsey,M.(1985). Strategies for determining the mechanisms of toxicity. J.Toxicol.-Clin.Toxicol.,23:1-78

Grasso,P.,and Crampton,P.F.(1972).The value of the mouse in the carcinogenicity testing. Food Cosmet.Toxicol.,10:418-422

Guillier,C.L.(1972).Evaluation of the internal exposure due to various administered dosages of urethane to mice. Proc.6th Berkeley Symp.Math.Statist.Probab.,Vol.IV,p.309-315. Univ. California Press,Berkeley

Hart,R.W.,and Fishbein,L.(1985).Interspecies extrapolation of drug and genetic toxicity data. In:Toxicological Risk Assessment(D.B.Clayson,D.Krewski,I.Munro eds.),Vol.I,p.3-40. CRC Press,Boca Raton

Haseman,K.K.(1983).Patterns of tumor incidence in two-year cancer bioassay feeding studies in Fisher 344 rats. Fund.Appl.Toxicol. 3:1-9

Haynes,R.H.(1986).Introduction:Molecular basis of genomic stability and change. In:Antimutagenesis and Anticarcinogenesis Mechanisms(D.M.Shankel et al.eds.),p.245-249. Plenum Press, New York

Heddle,J.A.(1988).Prediction of chemical carcinogenicity from in vitro genetic toxicity. Mutagenesis 3:287-291

Hodgson,E.(1979).Comparative aspects of the distribution of cytochrome P-450 dependent mono-oxygenase systems:An overview. Drug.Metab.Rev.,10:15-33

Iversen,S.,and Arley,N.(1950).On the mechanism of experimental carcinogenesis. Acta Pathol.Microbiol.Scand.,27:773-803

Jeffery,A.M.(1987).DNA modification by chemical carcinogens. In:Mechanisms of Cellular Transformation by Carcinogenic Agents(D.Grunberger,S.P.Goff eds.),p.33-71. Pergamon Press, Oxford

Kauffman,S.L.(1974).Kinetics of alveolar epithelial hyperplasia in lungs of mice exposed to urethane. Lab.Invest.,30:170-175

Kauffman,S.L.(1976).Autoradiographic study of type II-cell hyperplasia in lungs of mice chronically exposed to urethane. Cell Tissue Kinet.,9:489-497

Kendall,M.G.(1968).On the future of statistics - a second look. J.Roy.Statist.Soc.Ser.A,131:182-192

Klonecki,W.(1979).A one-branching model of urethane carcinogenesis and its qualitative consistency with empirical findings. Math.Biosci.,43:23-39

Knudson,A.G.(1987).Genetic oncodemes and antioncogenes. In:Biochemical and Molecular Epidemiology of Cancer(C.C.Harris ed.), p.127-134. A.R.Liss,New York

Kuhn,T.S.(1961).The function of measurement in modern physical science. Isis,52:161-190 (Reproduced in "The Essential Tension",Univ.of Chicago Press,Chicago,1977)

Kyburg,H.E.(1984).Theory and Measurement. Cambridge Univ.Press, Cambridge

Langhaar,H.L.(1951).Dimensional Analysis and Theory of Models.
Wiley,New York

Loury,D.J.,Goldsworthy,T.L.,and Butterworth,B.E.(1987).The value
of measuring cell replication as a predictive index of tissue-
-specific tumorigenic potential. In:Nongenotoxic Mechanisms
in Carcinogenesis(B.E.Butterworth,T.J.Slaga eds.),p.119-136.
Cold Spring Harbor Lab.

Marcus,A.H.(1975).Power laws in compartmental analysis.I,II.
Math.Biosci.,$\underline{23}$:337-350;$\underline{35}$:27-45

Meredith,P.A.,Kelman,A.W.,Elliott,H.L.,and Reid,J.L.(1983).
Pharmacokinetic and pharmacodynamic modelling of trimazosin
and its major metabolite. J.Pharmacol.Biopharm.,$\underline{11}$:323-335

Mordenti,J.(1986).Dosage regimen design for pharmaceutical
studies conducted in animals. J.Pharm.Sci.,$\underline{75}$:852-857

Natarajan,A.T.,and Obe,G.(1986).How do in vivo mammalian assays
compare to in vitro assays in their ability to detect mutagens ? Mutation Res.,$\underline{167}$:189-201

Nebert,D.W.,and Gonzalez,F.J.(1987).P450 genes:structure,evo-
lution,and regulation. Ann.Rev.Biochem.,$\underline{56}$:945-993

Neyman,J.(1974).A view of biometry:An interdisciplinary domain
concerned with chance mechanisms operating in living organisms;illustration:urethan carcinogenesis. In:Reliability and
Biometry(F.Proschan,R.J.Serfling eds.),p.183-201. SIAM,Phil-
adelphia

Neyman,J.(1982).Avenue to understanding the mechanism of radiation effects:Extended serial sacrifice experimental methodology. In:Probability Models and Cancer(L.LeCam,J.Neyman eds.),
p.45-60. North-Holland,Amsterdam

Neyman,J.,and Scott,E.L.(1967).Statistical aspect of the problem
of carcinogenesis. Proc.5th Berkeley Symp.Math.Statist.Probab.
Vol.IV,p.745-776. Univ.of California Press,Berkeley

Niiniluoto,I.(1985).Paradigms and problem-solving in operations
research. In:Logic of Discovery and Logic of Discourse(J.
Hintikka,F.Vandamme eds.),p.145-159. Plenum Press,New York

Oser,B.L.(1981).The rat as a model for human toxicological evaluation. J.Toxicol.Environ.Health,8:521-534

Paalzow,L.K.(1984).Integrated pharmacokinetic-dynamic modeling
of drugs acting on the CNS. Drug Metab.Rev.,$\underline{15}$:383-400

Parodi,S.,Taningher,M.,and Santi,L.(1988).Utilization of the
quantitative component of positive and negative results of
short-term tests. Mutation Res.,$\underline{205}$:283-294

Polany,M.(1958).Personal Knowledge. Routledge&Kegan,London

Pólya,G.(1945).How to Solve It.A New Aspect of Mathematical
Method. Princeton Univ.Press,Princeton

Prothero,J.(1986).Methodological aspects of scaling in biology.
J.Theor.Biol.,$\underline{118}$:259-286

Rahmani,R.,Richard,B.,Fabre,G.,and Cano,J.-P.(1988).Extrapola-
tion of preclinical pharmacokinetic data to therapeutic drug
use. Xenobiotica,$\underline{18}$(Suppl.1):71-88

Rall,D.P.(1979).The role of laboratory animal studies in estimating carcinogenic risks for man. In:Carcinogenic Risks.
Strategies for Intervention(W.Davis,C.Rosenfeld eds.),p.179-
-189. Intern.Agency Res.Cancer,Lyon

Rodricks,J.V.,and Tardiff,R.G.(1983).Biological bases for risk assessment. In:Safety Evaluation and Regulation of Chemicals (F.Homburger ed.),p.77-84. Karger,Basel

Rosen,R.(1978).Dynamical similarity and the theory of biological transformations. Bull.Math.Biol.,$\underline{40}$:549-570

Rosen,R.(1983).Role of similarity principles in data extrapolation. Amer.J.Physiol.,$\underline{244}$:R591-R599

Rosenkranz,H.S.,and Ennever,F.K.(1988).Quantifying genotoxicity and non-genotoxicity. Mutation Res.,$\underline{205}$:59-67

Ruelius,H.W.(1987).Extrapolation from animals to man:predictions, pitfalls and perspectives. Xenobiotica,$\underline{17}$:255-265

Savageau,M.A.(1979).Allometric morphogenesis of complex systems: Derivation of the basic equations from first principles. Proc.Natl.Acad.Sci.USA,$\underline{76}$:6023-6025

Savageau,M.A.,Voit,E.O.,and Irvine,D.H.(1987).Biochemical systems theory and metabolic control theory.1,2. Math.Biosci.,$\underline{86}$:127--145;147-169

Sawada,Y.,Hanano,M.,Sugiyama,Y.,and Iga,T.(1984).Prediction of the disposition of β-lactam antibiotics in humans from pharmacokinetic parameters in animals. J.Pharmacokin.Biopharm., $\underline{12}$:241-261

Schmidt-Nielsen,K.(1970).Energy metabolism,body size,and problems of scaling. Fed.Proc.,$\underline{29}$:1524-1532

Schneiderman,M.A.,Mantel,N.,and Brown,C.C.(1975).From mouse to man-or how to get from the laboratory to Park Avenue and 59th Street. Ann.N.Y.Acad.Sci.,$\underline{246}$:237-248

Schoenfelder,C.A.,and Hoel,D.G.(1979).Properties of the Neyman--Scott carcinogenesis model at low dose rates. Math.Biosci., $\underline{45}$:227-246

Schulte-Hermann,R.(1974).Induction of liver growth by xenobiotic compounds and other stimuli. Crit.Rev.Toxicol.,$\underline{3}$:97-158

Sheiner,L.B.,Stanski,D.R.,Vozeh,S.,Miller,R.D.,and Ham,J.(1979). Simultaneous model of pharmacokinetics and pharmacodynamics: application to d-tubocurarine. Clin.Pharmacol.Ther.,$\underline{25}$:358--371

Shelby,M.D.,Zeiger,E.,and Tennant,R.W.(1988).Commentary on the status of short-term tests for chemical carcinogens. Environ. Molec.Mutagen.,$\underline{11}$:437-441

Shimkin,M.B.,Wieder,R.,Marzi,D.,Gubareff,N.,and Suntzeff,V.(1967) Lung tumors in mice receiving different schedules of urethane. Proc.5th Berkeley Symp.Math.Statist.Probab.,Vol.IV,p.707-719. Univ.of California Press,Berkeley

Smith,R.J.(1980).Rethinking allometry. J.Theor.Biol.,$\underline{87}$:97-111

Smith,R.L.(1988).The role of metabolism and disposition studies in the safety assessment of pharmaceuticals. Xenobiotica,$\underline{18}$ (Suppl.1):89-96

Smolen,V.F.,Turrie,B.D.,and Weigand,W.A.(1972).Drug input optimization:Bioavailability-effected time-optimal control of multiple simultaneous,pharmacological effects and their interrelationships. J.Pharm.Sci.,$\underline{61}$:1941-1952

Stahl,W.R.(1963).The analysis of biological similarity. Adv. Biol.Med.Phys.,$\underline{9}$:355-464

Tautu,P.(1975).Some examples of probability models in cancer
    epidemiology. Bull.Intern.Statist.Inst.,46(Book 2):144-158

Teichmann,B.,and Schramm,T.(1979).'Human' and 'animal' carcino-
    gens. In:Carcinogenic Risk.Strategies for Intervention(W.
    Davis,C.Rosenfeld eds.),p.203-206. IARC,Lyon

Tennant,R.W.et al.(1987).Prediction of chemical carcinogenicity
    in rodents from in vitro genetic toxicity assays. Science,
    236:933-941

Tennant,R.W.,Stasiewicz,S.,and Spalding,J.W.(1986).Comparison
    of multiple parameters of rodent carcinogenicity and in vitro
    genetic toxicity. Environ.Mutagen.,8:205-227

Upton,R.N.,Mather,L.E.,Runciman,W.B.,Nancarrow,C.,and Carapetis,
    R.J.(1988).The use of mass balance principles to describe
    regional drug distribution and elimination. J.Pharmacokin.
    Biopharm.,16:13-29

Vesell,E.S.(1987).Pharmacogenetic differences between humans
    and laboratory animals:implications for modelling. In:Human
    Risk Assessment-The Role of Animal Selection and Extrapolat-
    ion(M.V.Roloff et al.,eds.),p.229-237. Taylor&Francis,London

Weinstein,H.,Osman,R.,Topiol,S.,and Green,J.P.(1981).Quantum
    chemical studies on molecular determinants for drug action.
    Ann.N.Y.Acad.Sci.,367:434-451

White,M.R.(1972).Studies of the mechanism of induction of pul-
    monary adenomas in mice. Proc.6th Berkeley Symp.Math.Statist.
    Probab.,Vol.IV,p.287-307. Univ.California Press,Berkeley

White,M.,Grendon,A.,and Jones,H.B.(1967).Effects of urethane
    dose and time patterns on tumor formation. Proc.5th Berkeley
    Symp.Math.Statist.Probab.,Vol.IV,p.721-743. Univ.California
    Press,Berkeley

Williams,G.M.(1987).DNA reactive and epigenetic carcinogens.
    In:Mechanisms of Environmental Carcinogenesis(J.C.Barrett
    ed.),Vol.I,p.113-127. CRC Press,Boca Raton

Wilson,R.,and Crouch,E.A.C.(1987).Risk assessment and compari-
    sons:An introduction. Science,236:267-270

Wise,M.E.(1974).Interpreting both short- and long-term power
    laws in physiological clearance curves. Math.Biosci.,20:327-
    -337

Wise,M.E.,Osborn,S.B.,Anderson,J.,and Tomlinson,R.W.S.(1968)
    A stochastic model for turnover of radiocalcium based on the
    observed power laws. Math.Biosci.,2:199-224

Yates,F.E.(1979).Comparative physiology:compared to what ?
    Amer.J.Physiol.,237:R1-R2

Yates,F.E.,and Kugler,P.N.(1986).Similarity principles and
    intrinsic geometries:Contrasting approaches to interspecies
    scaling. J.Pharm.Sci.,75:1019-1027

Ziegel,E.R.,and Gorman,J.W.(1980).Kinetic modelling with multi-
    response data. Technometrics,22:139-151

BIOLOGICAL BASIS FOR INTERSPECIES EXTRAPOLATIONS OF

HALOGENATED SOLVENTS AND OF 1,3-BUTADIENE

Hermann M. Bolt and Reinhold J. Laib

Institut für Arbeitsphysiologie an der
Universität Dortmund, Ardeystrasse 67
D-4600 Dortmund 1, F.R.G.

INTRODUCTION

It is well established that species differences in toxicity and carcinogenicity of xenobiotics are often based on species-specific metabolism. Hence, the use of pharmacokinetic models considering relevant metabolic routes may considerably improve risk assessment procedures (Bolt, 1987; Travis, 1987). The biological basis for an appropriate interspecies extrapolation is knowledge of the biochemical mode of action and of the toxicologically relevant metabolic pathways. This will be exemplified by a discussion of major halogenated industrial solvents and of 1,3-butadiene. Long-term animal bioassays with these compounds have demonstrated considerable differences between the two most widely used animal species, mice and rats. This review will not consider 1,1,1-trichloroethane. This solvent is metabolized in man and in experimental animals to a very low extent only (up to 5-10% of the inhaled dose), and no positive carcinogenicity data have hitherto been obtained. However, the closely related compounds 1,1,2-trichloroethane and 1,1,2,2-tetrachloroethane which are extensively metabolized have produced liver tumors in mice (Haseman et al., 1984).

1,1,2-TRICHLOROETHANE AND 1,1,2,2-TETRACHLOROETHANE

1,1,2-Trichloroethane and especially 1,1,2,2-tetrachloroethane are notoriously hepatotoxic.

1,1,2-Trichloroethane is efficiently metabolized in the mouse to chloroacetic acid which, in part, is further transformed to sulfur-containing metabolites (Yllner, 1971a). Similarly, 1,1,2,2-tetrachloroethane is converted in the same species to dichloroacetic acid which is the major urinary metabolite (Yllner, 1971b). Studies on the hepatic microsomal metabolism of both compounds in vitro (using rat liver microsomes) have demonstrated the implication of cytochrome P-450 (Ivanetich and van den Honert, 1981). Comparative kinetic investigations on both compounds in rats and mice have not been published.

DICHLOROMETHANE (METHYLENE CHLORIDE)

Biochemical investigations into the metabolism of dichloromethane have revealed two distinct pathways (Ahmed and Anders, 1976; Anders et al., 1977; Kubic and Anders, 1978; Stevens et al., 1980). On one hand, cytoplasmic enzymes using glutathione as co-factor biotransform dichloromethane to formaldehyde, formic acid, and CO_2. On the other hand, microsomal monooxygenases catalyze transformation to CO (and CO_2). Both pathways imply formation of theoretical reactive intermediates. Covalent binding of such intermediates to protein has been observed.

Pharmacokinetic investigations in rats after oral dosage (McKenna and Zempel, 1981) or inhalation exposure (Rodkey and Collison, 1977; McKenna et al., 1982) have demonstrated that metabolism of dichloromethane, in principle, is dose-dependent and saturable. Saturation of the oxidative microsomal pathway (the one leading to CO) has been confirmed by exposures of rats to 500 - 1000 ppm dichloromethane (Kurppa and Vainio, 1981): the uniform CO-Hb concentrations (8 - 9%) found after these different exposures indicated that this pathway was saturated at a 500 ppm exposure level.

Current experiments show that species-dependent differences exist in extent of metabolism and distribution of metabolites between the two pathways of dichloromethane (Green et al., 1986). An involvement of the glutathione-S-transferase pathway in species-specific carcinogenicity has been suggested. Studies on the pharmacokinetics of dichloromethane (Gargas et al., 1986) have been incorporated into risk assessment models (Andersen et al., 1987). The subsequent paper by Trevor Green will cover these aspects. At present, methylene chloride is the best example of an efficient use of biochemistry and pharmacokinetics in the assessment of carcinogenic risk to man based on experimental animal data.

TRICHLOROETHYLENE

The metabolism of trichloroethylene has been extensively studied. The compound is initially biotransformed to its epoxide which (under biological conditions) rearranges to chloral (Henschler, 1977). Alternatively, a model which implies chlorine migration at an oxygenated trichloroethylene-cytochrome P-450 transition state has been proposed, based on studies in vitro (Miller and Guengerich, 1982). These models have been used for a comparative assessment of the carcinogenicity of haloethylenes (Bolt et al., 1982).

In addition to the "classical" metabolites trichloroethanol and trichloroacetic acid (which are formed via chloral) also dichloroacetic acid is formed to some extent (Hathway, 1980). Furthermore, trichloroethylene oxide, in aqueous solution, gives rise to some other degradation products (Henschler and Hoos, 1982). This finding led to a re-investigation of metabolic trichloroethylene pathways (Dekant et al., 1984). According to these studies (including those reported by Dekant et al., 1986), the solvent may be metabolized via different routes under formation of trichloroethanol, trichloracetic acid and dichloroacetic acid, of N-(hydroxyacetyl)aminoethanol, and of oxalic acid. Moreover, differences in metabolism between mice and rats were noted in that mice biotransformed trichloroethylene at a higher rate , with no apparent saturation kinetics up to (oral) doses of 2.4 g/kg. After prolonged administration of high trichloroethylene doses signs of hepatotoxicity were observed in this species (Dekant et al., 1984), consistent with earlier observations of others (Stoff et al., 1982; Parchman and Magee, 1982). Specific adducts of trichloroethylene metabolites to DNA (Stoff et al., 1982;

Parchman and Magee, 1982; Bergman, 1983) or RNA (Laib et al., 1979) have not been detected although covalent protein binding occurs (Bolt et al., 1977). In conjunction with weak or negative responses of trichloroethylene in mutagenicity assays, this was interpreted as lack of a systemic genotoxic potential (Stoff et al., 1982).

Very recently, the differential pharmacokinetics of trichloroethylene in rats and mice have been re-evaluated (Prout et al., 1985; Green and Prout, 1985). There were indications that the major trichloroethylene metabolite, trichloroacetic acid, stimulates peroxisomal activities in hepatocytes (Mitchell et al., 1984). It was found that the relative proportions of the major metabolites were similar in both species (Green and Prout, 1985). However, because of different saturability of metabolism in rats and mice high doses (1000 mg/kg and above, given orally) of trichloroethylene caused much higher levels of metabolites, especially of trichloracetic acid, in the mouse (Prout et al., 1985): the concentrations of trichloroethanol and trichloroacetic acid in the blood, under such conditions, were 4-fold (or 7-fold, respectively) higher in mice than in rats. It was inferred that such quantities of trichloroethylene-derived trichloroacetic acid could induce hepatic peroxisome proliferation in mice, but not in rats. This effect of trichloroethylene has been demonstrated (Elcombe et al., 1985).

On this basis, it was suggested that the species difference in hepatocarcinogenicity of trichloroethylene were due to a species difference in hepatic peroxisome proliferation and cell proliferation (Elcombe et al., 1985) which were ultimately based on pharmacokinetic differences. Later, it was confirmed that dichloroacetic acid and trichloroacetic acid could produce liver tumors in the B6C3F1 mouse (Herren-Freund et al., 1987). Very recently, the formation of cysteine conjugates of halogenated ethylenes (Hassall et al., 1984) has reached much interest. In view of the nephrocarcinogenicity of trichloroethylene in male rats, the beta-lyase mediated cleavage of such conjugates to reactive intermediates has been proven (Dekant et al., 1986; Vamvakas et al., 1987). S-1,2-Dichloro-vinyl-N-acetyl-cysteine has been identified as a metabolite of trichloroethylene from rat urine (Dekant et al., 1986a). Species differences in this important pathway are a matter of current investigations.

PERCHLOROETHYLENE (TETRACHLOROETHYLENE)

Perchloroethylene is metabolized much slower than trichloroethylene. The excretion product, trichloroacetic acid, is presumed to originate via an intermediary epoxide (tetrachlorooxirane) and its rearrangement product trichloroacetyl chloride (for review, see Reichert, 1983). Furthermore, after application of ^{14}C-labelled perchloroethylene to rats exhalation of significant amounts of $^{14}CO_2$ and urinary excretion of oxalic acid have been observed (Pegg et al., 1979). The same study also reported about covalent binding of perchloroethylene metabolites to proteins, but not to hepatic DNA. It has also been recognized that the pharmacokinetics of perchloroethylene in rats are dose-dependent, showing a saturable metabolism (Pegg et al., 1979; Filser and Bolt, 1979). Moreover, this has been confirmed for (B6C3F1) mice (Schumann et al., 1980; Bolt and Link, 1980), which is in contrast to what has been found in these animals with trichloroethylene (v.s.).

Quantitative differences in metabolism of tetrachloroethylene have been reported between rats and mice.

Ikeda and Ohtsuji (1972) reported about excretion rates of trichloroacetic acid in rats and mice exposed to (or injected with) perchloroethylene. Their finding of a higher metabolite excretion in mice was confirmed by Schumann et al. (1980) and by Bolt and Link (1980). Mice metabolize perchloroethylene (based on kg body weight) between 2.7 and 8.5 times faster than rats, dependent on particular experimental conditions.

These differences lead also to differences in covalent binding of reactive metabolites. Perchloroethylene is transformed to such metabolites by hepatic microsomal cytochrome P-450 (Costa and Ivanetich, 1980). In an experiment with oral and inhalation exposure of rats and mice to ^{14}C-perchloroethylene, the hepatic macromolecular (protein) binding was between 1.5 and 9.2-fold higher in mice than in rats, depending on experimental conditions (Schumann et al., 1980).

Under normal conditions (no pretreatment) even very high doses of perchloroethylene, up to 1 g/kg daily, cause only minimal effects on the liver (Schumann et al., 1980). However, phenobarbital pretreatment of rats which significantly elevates metabolism of the compound (Bolt and Link, 1980) leads to signs of hepatotoxicity when such animals receive trichloroethylene afterwards (see Cooper, 1978).

Mice which metabolize the compound much faster and to a higher extent than rats develop histopathological hepatic changes after an 11-day-treatment at doses as low as 100 mg/kg perchloroethylene (p.o.) daily (Schumann et al., 1980).

The covalent binding of chloroacetylchloride on membrane constituents has been made responsible in part for the parenchyme damaging effect of vinylidene chloride (Reichert et al., 1979). The general implication of intermediary haloacetylating metabolites in the metabolism of halogenated hydrocarbons (e.g. chloroform, carbon tetrachloride, 1,1,2-trichloroethane, vinylidene chloride and perchloroethylene), where species differences in toxicity exist between rats and mice, has been discussed (Laib, 1982). Dichloroacetylchloride is also a proposed intermediate in the metabolism of 1,1,2,2-tetrachloroethane (see above).

If all this knowledge is taken together, it seems likely that the higher metabolic rates in mice may lead to a species-selective toxicity of perchloroethylene towards the liver in mice. Because of the very limited capacity of humans to metabolize this compound (Ohtsuki et al., 1983) this would probably not be relevant for men.

Like trichloroethylene, perchloroethylene induces renal tubular damage in male rats. An NTP bioassay (exposure to 100 and 200 ppm in a 2 year study) has revealed some renal tubular cell adenomas and adenocarcinomas in these animals (NTP, 1986). Genotoxic intermediates may arise locally via glutathione conjugation and the beta-lyase pathway (Dekant, 1986). After application of ^{14}C-labelled perchloroethylene, the mercapturic acid S-1,2,2-trichlorovinyl-N-acetyl-cysteine comprised 1.6% of the urinary radioactivity in rats, but only 0.5% in mice (Dekant et al., 1986b). This points to quantitative differences in biotransformation of perchloroethylene, as far as the toxicologically relevant pathways are concerned.

1,3-BUTADIENE

1,3-Butadiene is a systemic carcinogen in rats and mice, but quantitatively it displays a much more potent carcinogenic activity in mice than in rats (Hazleton Laboratories Europe, 1981; Huff et al., 1985). Very recently new experimental findings on the toxicology, carcinogenicity and potential human health effects of this compound were discussed on an international basis (NIEHS, 1988).

The metabolism of 1,3-butadiene proceeds via a primary epoxidation to its mono-epoxide, 1,2-epoxybutene-3 (Malvoisin and Roberfroid, 1982). Pharmacokinetic and mechanistic investigations on 1,3-butadiene and its epoxide have been performed in rats and mice. These studies which have been summarized elsewhere in more detail (Laib et al., 1988) are given below.

Starting from different initial exposure concentrations between 100 and 5000 ppm, the time dependent decline of butadiene in closed all-glass chambers, occupied by rats or mice, was investigated (Kreiling et al., 1986; Bolt et al., 1984). The decline curves observed in these experiments for rats or mice indicate a saturable metabolism of butadiene in these both species. Below concentrations of about 1000 ppm, the metabolic elimination of butadiene by rats or mice can be described by first order kinetics. At higher atmospheric concentrations saturation kinetics become apparent. Saturation of butadiene metabolism is observed in rats and mice at atmospheric concentrations of about 2000 ppm and above. The pharmacokinetic parameters for distribution and metabolism of butadiene (Kreiling et al., 1986; Bolt et al., 1984) show that butadiene is metabolized by mice at about twice the rate of rats. In a lower concentration range, where first order metabolism applies, metabolic clearance per kg body weight was 7300 ml x h^{-1} for mice and 4500 ml x h^{-1} for rats. The actual rates of butadiene metabolism in both species can be calculated for the exposure concentrations utilized in the two long-term bioassays with rats (Hazleton Laboratories Europe, 1981) and mice (Huff et al., 1985) under the assumption that butadiene metabolism in mice and rats remains constant during chronic exposure. The data show that under these particular bioassay conditions mice metabolized about 35% more butadiene than rats.

Whereas major differences in the transformation rates from 1,3-butadiene into 1,2-epoxybutene-3 are not apparent between mice and rats, such differences do occur in the inactivation of its primary epoxide intermediate.

Inhalation Pharmacokinetics of 1,2-Epoxybutene-3

Comparative investigations of inhalation pharmacokinetics of 1,2-epoxybutene-3 in rats and mice revealed major differences in metabolism of this compound between both species (Kreiling et al., 1987; Filser and Bolt, 1984). When mice were exposed in the closed desiccator jar chamber to different initial concentrations of epoxybutene between 100 and 2000 ppm, the decline curves obtained show a clear saturation behaviour of epoxybutene metabolism (Kreiling et al., 1987). At lower concentrations the elimination of epoxybutene is directly proportional to its concentration in the gas phase of the system. At higher epoxybutene concentrations, the slopes of the concentration-time curves decrease, and saturation of epoxybutene metabolism becomes apparent. In contrast to these data, only monoexponential decline curves were observed when rats were exposed to different initial epoxybutene concentrations between 10 and 5000 ppm (Filser and Bolt, 1984).

Whereas in rats no indication of saturation kinetics of epoxybutene metabolism could be observed up to exposure concentrations of 5000 ppm, in mice saturation of epoxybutene metabolism becomes apparent at atmospheric concentrations of about 500 ppm. The pharmacokinetic parameters for distribution and metabolism of epoxybutene were determined (Kreiling et al., 1987; Filser and Bolt, 1984). In the lower concentration range, where first order metabolism applies (up to 500 ppm) epoxybutene is metabolized by mice at higher rates compared to rats (metabolic clearance per kg body weight, mice: 24900 ml x h^{-1}, rats: 13400 ml x h^{-1}). Under these conditions the actual steady-state concentration of epoxybutene in the mouse was estimated to be about 10 times that in the rat. The calculated maximal metabolic rate for epoxybutene was 350 μmol x h^{-1} x kg^{-1} in mice and 2600 μmol x h^{-1} x kg^{-1} in rats. A comparison of the metabolic elimination rates of epoxybutene in both species reveals that, at lower exposure concentrations, mice show a higher metabolic rate for epoxybutene than rats. Whereas metabolic elimination of inhaled epoxybutene in rats is linearly dependent on the atmospheric concentration at least up to exposure concentrations of about 5000 ppm, in mice saturation of epoxybutene metabolism becomes apparent at about 500 ppm. Therefore, with increasing exposure concentration the metabolic capacity for inactivation of epoxybutene becomes rate limiting in mice, but not in rats.

Exhalation of 1,2-Epoxybutene-3

Exhalation of epoxybutene into the atmosphere of the closed exposure system is observed when mice or rats are exposed to butadiene (Kreiling et al., 1987; Filser and Bolt, 1984). In both experiments butadiene concentrations were maintained above 2000 ppm which ensured that metabolism of butadiene proceeded under saturation conditions. Remarkable differences occur between both species. Whereas epoxybutene exhaled by rats under these conditions reaches a plateau concentration of about 4 ppm, epoxybutene exhalation by mice leads to an increase in epoxybutene concentration in the system up to about 10 ppm, where acute toxicity is observed in the animals. No toxicity was observed with rats using the same protocol.

The differences in epoxybutene exhalation and in toxicity of butadiene between mice and rats can be easily explained on the basis of the differences in pharmacokinetics. As metabolic elimination of epoxybutene in mice is a saturable process, the concentration of epoxybutene metabolically generated from butadiene gradually increases in the animal organism. Because exhalation of a volatile compound is proportional to its concentration in the animal this results in an increase in epoxybutene exhalation.

Depletion of Hepatic Non-Protein Sulfhydryl Compounds (NPSH)

After inhalation exposure of mice (B6C3F1) and rats (Sprague-Dawley, Wistar) remarkable species differences in extent and time course of depletion of liver NPSH contents are observed. Exposure of mice to concentrations of 2000 ppm butadiene resulted in a progressive depression of hepatic NPSH to a value of about 20% after 7 h and a practically total depletion of hepatic NPSH after 15 h. In rats hepatic NPSH content was depleted to values between 65% (Wistar) and 80% (Sprague-Dawley) after 7 h but showed no major changes when exposure to butadiene was continued for further 8 hours.

At the end of a 15 h exposure to the same concentration of butadiene mice show signs of acute toxicity. No such toxicity was observed after 15 h exposure to butadiene of either Wistar or Sprague-Dawley rats.

In addition to the higher production rate of epoxybutene from butadiene in mice, metabolism of epoxybutene is saturable in mice (B6C3F1) but not in rats (Sprague-Dawley). This leads, at high exposure concentrations of butadiene, to a continuous accumulation in mice of epoxybutene, as traced in the exhaled air of the animals. A comparison of the time course of hepatic NPSH depletion with the time course of epoxybutene concentrations in the closed system shows that both parameters are related to each other. For rats, where after an initial moderate decline, hepatic NPSH levels show no major changes, epoxybutene exhalation remained constant until exposure to butadiene was ended. For mice an increase in epoxybutene exhalation can be observed, until after about 10 hours of exposure to butadiene hepatic NPSH levels are depleted to about 10% of their initial values.

Epoxybutene is conjugated with glutathione (Malvoisin and Roberfroid, 1982) and can be metabolized by glutathione-S-transferase. Hepatic NPSH depletion by butadiene may be regarded as the combined result of spontaneous and enzyme-mediated conjugation of reactive butadiene intermediates with glutathione (Ketterer, 1986).

With regard to the chemical stability of reactive butadiene intermediates (Gervasi et al., 1985) and their accumulation in the mouse organism (Bond et al., 1986; Kreiling et al., 1987) it seems reasonable to assume that reductions of hepatic NPSH in mice may reflect the situation in target organs of this species.

Alkylation of Nuclear Proteins and DNA

After exposure of mice (B6C3F1) or rats (Wistar) to (^{14}C)-butadiene, radioactivity was covalently bound to liver nucleoprotein fractions and to total liver DNA of both species. Covalent binding of radioactivity to liver nucleoproteins of mice was about twice as high as in rats. This shows that in parallel to the higher metabolic rate of butadiene in the mouse, the formation rate of reactive protein-binding metabolites is proportionally increased in this species. Comparable amounts of (^{14}C)-butadiene derived radioactivity were associated with the liver DNA of both species. To which extend the total radioactivity bound to liver DNA of the animals represents DNA alkylation at specific DNA targets or metabolic incorporation into the physiological nucleosides is not yet clear. The formation in DNA of 7-(2-hydroxy-3-buten-1-yl) guanine and of 7-(1-hydroxy-3-buten-2-yl) guanine has been demonstrated after chemical reaction of epoxybutene with DNA in vitro (Citti et al., 1984). This supports the assumption that epoxybutene is the major reactive intermediate covalently bound to DNA.

We conclude that, in addition to the higher production rate of epoxybutene from butadiene in mice versus rats, limited detoxification and thus accumulation of this primary reactive intermediate may be a major determinant for the higher susceptibility of mice to butadiene induced carcinogenesis. The observations that, under exposure to high concentrations of butadiene, exhalation of epoxybutene by mice is 2-3 times that of rats, that hepatic NPSH content is practically completely depleted by inhalation exposure of mice to butadiene and that considerably higher blood levels of epoxybutene (2-5 times) and diepoxybutane (up to 3 times) in mice occur versus rats (Bond et al., 1986) are supportive of this view.

FINAL REMARKS

The reviewed investigations reveal that differences in species susceptibility to inhaled xenobiotics may frequently be related to differences in metabolism of this compound. Such species differences may be qualitative or quantitative in nature. An incorporation of such knowledge into processes of risk assessment is necessary to avoid misinterpretations of the risk to man.

ACKNOWLEDGEMENT

The financial support of the studies on butadiene by the Deutsche Forschungsgemeinschaft, Grant No. La 515/1-2 is gratefully acknowledged.

REFERENCES

Ahmed, A.E., and Anders, M., 1976, Metabolism of dihalomethane to formaldehyde and inorganic halides. I. In vitro studies, Drug. Metab. Disposition, 4:357-361.

Anders, M.W., Kubic, V.L., and Ahmed, A.E., 1977, Metabolism of halogenated methanes and macromolecular binding, J. Env. Pathol. Toxicol., 1:117-124.

Andersen, M.E., Clewell, J.E., Gargas, M.L., Smith, F.A., and Reitz, R.H., 1987, Physiologically based pharmacokinetics and the risk assessment process for methylene chloride, Toxicol. Appl. Pharmacol., 87:185.

Bergman, K., 1983, Interactions of trichlormethylene with DNA in vitro and with RNA and DNA in various mouse tissues in vivo, Arch. Toxicol., 54:181-193.

Bolt, H.M., 1987, Pharmacokinetic factors and their implication in the induction of mouse liver tumours by halogenated hydrocarbons, Arch. Toxicol., Suppl., 10:190.

Bolt, H.M., Laib, R.J., and Filser, J.G., 1982, Reactive metabolites and carcinogenicity of halogenated ethylenes, Biochem. Pharmacol., 31:1-4.

Bolt, H.M., and Link, B., 1980, Zur Toxikologie von Perchloräthylen, Verh. Dtsch. Ges. Arbeitsmed. (Gentner, Stuttgart), 2:463-470.

Bolt, H.M., Buchter, A., Wolowski, L., Gil, D.L., and Bolt, W., 1977, Incubation of ^{14}C-trichlorethylene vapor with rat liver microsomes: uptake of radioactivity and covalent protein binding of metabolites, Int. Arch. Env. Occup. Hlth., 39:102-111.

Bolt, H.M., Filser, J.G., and Störmer, F., 1984, Inhalation pharmacokinetics based on gas uptake studies. V. Comparative pharmacokinetics of ethylene and 1,3-butadiene in rats, Arch. Toxicol., 55:213-218.

Bond, J.A., Dahl, A.R., Henderson, R.F., Dutcher, J.S., Mauderly, J.L., and Birnbaum, L.S., 1986, Species differences in the disposition of inhaled butadiene, Toxicol. Appl. Pharmacol., 84:617-627.

Citti, L., Gervasi, P.G., Turchi, G., Belluci, G., and Bianchini, R., 1984, The reaction of 3,4-epoxy-1-butene with deoxyguanosine and DNA in vitro: synthesis and characterization of the main adducts, Carcinogenesis, 5:47-52.

Cooper, P., 1978, Trichloroethylene: hepatic effects, metabolism and elimination, Fd. Cosmet. Toxicol., 16:491-492.

Costa, A.K., and Ivanetich, K.M., 1980, Tetrachloroethylene metabolism by the hepatic microsomal cytochrome P-450 system, Biochem. Pharmacol., 29:2863-2869.

Dekant, W., 1986, Metabolic conversion of tri- and tetrachloroethylene: formation and deactivation of genotoxic intermediates. In: New Concepts and Developments in Toxicology, P.L. Chambers, P. Gehring, and F. Sakai, eds., pp. 211-221, Elsevier Science Publishers, Amsterdam, New York, Oxford.

Dekant, W., Schulz, A., Metzler, M., and Henschler, D., 1986, Absorption, elimination and metabolism of trichloroethylene: a quantitative comparison between rats and mice, Xenobiotica, 16:143-152.

Dekant, W., Vamvakas, S., Berthold, K., Schmidt, S., Wild, D., and Henschler, D., 1986, Bacterial beta-lyase cleavage and mutagenicity of cysteine conjugates derived from the nephrocarcinogenic alkenes trichloroethylene, tetrachloroethylene and hexachlorobutadiene, Chem. biol. Interact., 60:31-45.

Dekant, W., Metzler, M., and Henschler, D., 1986a, Identification of S-1,2-divinyl-N-acetyl-cysteine as a urinary metabolite of trichloroethylene: a possible explanation for its nephrocarcinogenicity in male rats, Biochem. Pharmacol., 35:2455-2458.

Dekant, W., Metzler, M., and Henschler, D., 1986b, Identification of S-1,2,2-trichlorovinyl-N-acetyl-cysteine as a urinary metabolite of tetrachloroethylene: bioactivation through glutathione conjugation as a possible explanation of its nephrocarcinogenicity, J. Biochem. Toxicol., 1(2):57-72.

Dekant, W., Metzler, M., and Henschler, D., 1984, Novel metabolites of trichloroethylene through dechlorination reactions in rats, mice and humans, Biochem. Pharmacol., 33:2021-2027.

Elcombe, C.R., Rose, M.S., and Pratt, I.S., 1985, Biochemical, histological, and ultrastructural changes in rat and mouse liver following the administration of trichloroethylene: possible relevance to species differences in hepatocarcinogenicity, Toxicol. Appl. Pharmacol., 79:365-376.

Filser, J.G., and Bolt, H.M., 1979, Pharmacokinetics of halogenated ethylenes in rats, Arch. Toxicol., 42:123-126.

Filser, J.G., and Bolt, H.M., 1984, Inhalation pharmacokinetics based on gas uptake studies. VI. Comparative evaluation of ethylene oxide and butadiene monoxide as exhaled reactive metabolites of ethylene and 1,3-butadiene in rats, Arch. Toxicol., 55:219-223.

Gargas, M.L., Clewell, H.J., and Andersen, M.E., 1986, Metabolism of inhaled dihalomethanes in vivo: differentiation of kinetic constants for two independent pathways, Toxicol. Appl. Pharmacol., 82:211.

Gervasi, P.G., Citti, L., Del Monte, M., Longo, V., and Benetti, D., 1985, Mutagenicity and chemical reactivity of epoxidic intermediates of the isoprene metabolism and other structurally related compounds, Mutation Res., 156:77-82.

Green, T., and Prout, M.S., 1985, Species differences in response to trichloroethylene. II. Biotransformation in rats and mice, Toxicol. Appl. Pharmacol., 79:404-411.

Green, T., Nash, J.A., and Proven, W.M., 1986, Comparative pharmacokine-tics of inhaled dichloromethane in rats and mice, Abstract, Annual Meeting of the Society of Toxicology (SOT).

Haseman, J.K., Crawford, D.D., Huff, J.E., Boorman, G.A., and McConnell, E.E., 1984, Results from 86 two-year carcinogenicity studies conducted by the National Toxicology Program, J. Toxicol. Env. Hlth., 14:621-639.

Hassall, C.D., Gandolfi, A.J., Duhamel, R.C., and Brendel, K., 1984, The formation and biotransformation of cysteine conjugates of halogenated ethylenes by rabbit renal tubules, Chem. Biol. Interact., 49:283-297.

Hathway, D.E., 1980, Consideration of the evidence for mechanisms of 1,1,2-trichloroethylene metabolism, including new identification of its dichloroacetic acid and trichloroacetic acid metabolites in mice, Cancer Lett., 8:263-269.

Hazleton Laboratories Europe, 1981, 1,3-Butadiene. Inhalation study in the rat. Report No. 2788-522/3, Hazleton Labs., Harrowgate, England.

Henschler, D., 1977, Metabolism of chlorinated alkenes and alkane as related to toxicity, J. Environ. Pathol. Toxicol., 1:125-133.

Henschler, D., and Hoos, R., 1982, Metabolic activation and deactivation mechanisms of di-, tri-, and tetrachloroethylenes, in: Snyder, R. et al. (eds.) Biological Reactive Intermediates - II, part A, Plenum Publishing Corporation, pp. 659-666.

Herren-Freund, S.L., Pereira, M.A., Khoury, M.D., and Olson, G., 1987, The carcinogenicity of trichloroethylene and its metabolites, trichloroacetic acid and dichloroacetic acid, in mouse liver, Toxicol. Appl. Pharmacol., 90:183-189.

Huff, J.E., Melnick, R.L., Solleveld, H.A., Hasemann, J.K., Power, M., and Miller, R.A., 1985, Multiple organ carcinogenicity of 1,3-butadiene in B6C3F1 mice after 60 weeks of inhalation exposure, Science, 277:548-549.

Ikeda, M., and Ohtsuji, H., 1972, A comparative study of the excretion of Fujiwara reaction-positive substances in urine of humans and rodents given trichloro- or tetrachloro-derivatives of ethane and ethylene, Brit. J. Ind. Med., 29:99-104.

Ivanetich, K.M., and van den Honert, L.H., 1981, Chloroethanes: their metabolism by hepatic cytochrome P-450 in vitro, Carcinogenesis, 2:697-702.

Ketterer, B., 1986, Detoxication reactions of glutathione and glutathione transferases, Xenobiotica, 16:957-973.

Kreiling, R., Laib, R.J., Filser, J.G., and Bolt, H.M., 1986, Species differences in butadiene metabolism between mice and rats evaluated by inhalation pharmacokinetics, Arch. Toxicol., 58:235-238 (1986).

120

Kreiling, R., Laib, R.J., Filser, J.G., and Bolt, H.M., 1987, Inhalation pharmacokinetics of 1,2-epoxybutene-3 reveal species differences between rats and mice sensitive to butadiene induced carcinogenesis, Arch. Toxicol., 61:7-11.

Kubic, V.L., and Anders, M.W., 1978, Metabolism of dihalomethanes to carbon monoxide. III. Studies on the mechanism of the reaction, Biochem. Pharmacol., 27:2349-2355.

Kurppa, K., and Vainio, H., 1981, Effects of intermittent dichloromethane inhalation on blood carboxyhemoglobin concentration and drug metabolizing enzymes in rat, Res. Commun. Chem. Pathol. Pharmacol., 32:535-544.

Laib, R.J., Stöckle, G., Bolt, H.M., and Kunz, W., 1979, Vinyl chloride and trichloroethylene: comparison of alkylating effects of metabolites and induction of preneoplastic enzyme deficiencies in rat liver, J. Cancer Res. Clin. Oncol., 94:134-147.

Laib, R.J., 1982, Specific covalent binding and toxicity of aliphatic halogenated xenobiotics, in: " Reviews on Drug Metabolism and Drug Interactions", Vol. 5, No. 1, Beckett, A.H. and Gorrod, J.W., eds., pp. 1-48, Freund Publishing House Ltd., London.

Laib, R.J., Filser, J.G., Kreiling, R., Vangala, R.R., and Bolt, H.M., 1988, Inhalation pharmacokinetics of 1,3-butadiene and 1,2-epoxybutene-3 in rats and mice, Environ. Hlth. Perspect., in press.

Malvoisin, E., and Roberfroid, M., 1982, Hepatic microsomal metabolism of 1,3-butadiene, Xenobiotica, 12:137-144.

McKenna, M.J., and Zempel, J.A., 1981, The dose-dependent metabolism of ^{14}C-methylene chloride following oral administration to rats, Fd. Cosmet. Toxicol., 19:73-78.

McKenna, M.J., Zempel, J.A., and Braun, W.A., 1982, The pharmacokinetics of inhaled methylene chloride in rats, Toxicol. Appl. Pharmacol., 65:1-10.

Miller, R.E., and Guengerich, F.P., 1982, Oxidation of trichloroethylene by liver microsomal cytochrome P-450: evidence for chlorine migration in a transition state not involving trichloroethylene oxide, Biochemistry, 21:1090-1097.

Mitchell, A.M., Bridges, J.W., and Elcombe, C.R., 1984, Factors influencing peroxisome proliferation in cultured rat hepatocytes, Arch. Toxicol., 55:239-246.

NIEHS, 1988, International Symposium on the Toxicology, Carcinogenesis, and Human Health Aspects of 1,3-Butadiene, National Institute of Environmental Health Sciences, Research Triangle Park, North Carolina, USA, April 12-13.

NTP, 1986, Toxicology and carcinogenesis of tetrachloroethylene (perchloroethylene) in F 344/N rats and B6C3F1 mice (inhalation studies), NTP-TR311, US Dept. of Health & Human Services, Washington, DC.

Ohtsuki, T., Sato, K., Koizumi, A., Kumai, M., and Ikeda, M., 1983, Limited capacity of humans to metabolize tetrachloroethylene, _Int. Arch. Occup. Environ. Hlth._, 51:381-390.

Parchman, I.G., and Magee, P.N., 1982, Metabolism of ^{14}C-trichloroethylene to [14]CO_2 and interaction of a metabolite with DNA of rats and mice, _J. Toxicol. Environ. Hlth._, 9:797-813.

Pegg, D.G., Zempel, J.A., Braun, W.H., and Watanabe, P.G., 1979, Disposition of tetrachloro(^{14}C)ethylene following oral and inhalation exposure in rats, _Toxicol. Appl. Pharmacol._, 51:455-474.

Prout, M.S., Provan, W.M., and Green, T., 1985, Species differences in response to trichloroethylene. I. Pharmacokinetics in rats and mice, _Toxicol. Appl. Pharmacol._, 79:389-300.

Reichert, D., 1983, Biological actions and interactions of tetrachloroethylene, _Mutation Res._, 123:411-429.

Reichert, D., Werner, H.W., Metzler, M., and Henschler, D., 1979, Molecular mechanism of 1,1-dichloroethylene toxicity: excreted metabolites reveal different pathways of reactive metabolites, _Arch. Toxicol._, 42:159-169.

Rodkey, F.L., and Collison, H.A., 1977, Biological oxidation of ^{14}C-methylene chloride to carbon monoxide and carbon dioxide by the rat, _Toxicol. Appl. Pharmacol._, 40:33-38.

Schumann, A.M., Quast, J.F., and Watanabe, P.G., 1980, The pharmacokinetics and macromolecular interactions of perchloroethylene in mice and rats as related to oncogenicity, _Toxicol. Appl. Pharmacol._, 55:207-219.

Stevens, J.L., Ratnayake, J.H., and Anders, M.W., 1980, Metabolism of dihalomethanes to carbon monoxide. IV. Studies in isolated rat hepatocytes, _Toxicol. Appl. Pharmacol._, 55:484-489.

Stoff, W.T., Quast, J.F., and Watanabe, P.G., 1982, The pharmacokinetics and macromolecular interactions of trichloroethylene in mice and rats, _Toxicol. Appl. Pharmacol._, 62:137-151.

Travis, C.C., 1987, Interspecies extrapolations in risk analysis, _Toxicology_, 47:3.

Vamvakas, S., Dekant, W., Berthold, K., Schmidt, S., Wild, D., and Henschler, D., 1987, Enzymatic transformation of mercapturic acids derived from halogenated alkenes to reactive and mutagenic intermediates, _Biochem. Pharmacol._, 36:2741-2748.

Yllner, S., 1971a, Metabolism of 1,1,2-trichloroethane-1,2-^{14}C in the mouse, _Acta pharmacol. toxicol._, 30:248-256.

Yllner, S., 1971b, Metabolism of 1,1,2,2-tetrachloroethane-1,2-^{14}C in the mouse, _Acta pharmacol. toxicol._, 29:499-512.

SPECIES-SPECIFIC INHALATION PHARMACOKINETICS OF 2-NITROPROPANE, METHYL ETHYL KETONE, AND n-HEXANE

Winfried Kessler, Barbara Denk, and Johannes G. Filser*

GSF, Institut für Toxikologie

Ingolstädter Landstr. 1, D-8042 Neuherberg, FRG

INTRODUCTION

2-Nitropropane (2-NP), methyl ethyl ketone (MEK), and n-hexane (HEX) are used in large quantities for industrial processes. They are components of solvent mixtures and are present as thinners in commercial products like glues, paints, and laquers. Because of their high volatility persons are mainly exposed via inhalation of the vapors.

2-NP was a strong liver carcinogen in inhalation studies with Sprague-Dawley rats (SD rats) at 207 ppm (Lewis et al., 1979) and at 200 ppm (Griffin et al., 1980), resp.; all exposed rats developed liver carcinomas. In contrast, no evidence of toxicity was found at concentrations of 27 ppm (Lewis et al., 1979) and of 25 ppm (Griffin et al., 1980). Considerable sex differences were observed: in an acute toxicity test at 580 ppm no females died whereas all males died (Lewis et al., 1979). In a subchronic toxicity study (200 ppm, 6 months) glutamic-pyruvic transaminase was elevated in serum of males but not in females (Griffin et al., 1980). In a long-term study hepatocellular carcinomas developed at 100 ppm after 12 months in males and after 18 months in females (Griffin et al., 1980). The induction of DNA repair synthesis in isolated rat hepatocytes following treatment in vivo was considerably more effective in those from males than in those from females (Andrae et al., 1988). The mechanisms leading to the observed differences have not been clarified; sex specific pharmacokinetics have not been investigated.

For MEK, no data on carcinogenicity are available. Chronic animal studies with guinea pigs, rats, and cats did not lead to any pathological or toxicological changes (reviewed in: Deutsche Forschungsgemeinschaft, 1976). However, MEK increased the neurotoxicity of HEX, 2-hexanone, and 2,5-hexanedione (Duckett et al., 1974, Saida et al., 1976, Altenkirch et al., 1978, Ralston et al., 1985). This has also been observed in humans (Altenkirch, 1977, Couri and Milks, 1982). Furthermore, MEK enhanced the hepatotoxicity of carbon tetrachloride (Traiger and Bruckner, 1976). In guinea pigs and rats, MEK was metabolized reductively to 2-butanol presumably by alcohol dehydrogenase and oxidatively to 3-hydroxy-2-butanone presumably by cytochrome P-450-dependent monooxygenases. The latter compound was further reduced to 2,3-butanediol (DiVicenzo et al., 1976, Dietz et

---

*To whom correspondence should be sent

al., 1981). Metabolites of MEK in urine of man were 3-hydroxy-2-butanone (Miyasaka et al., 1982, Perbellini et al., 1984) and 2,3-butanediol (Liira et al., 1988). Up to now, two studies on inhalation kinetics of MEK in man have been published (Perbellini et al., 1984, Liira et al., 1988). However, no such data are available for the rat.

HEX was not carcinogenic in animal bioassays (Sice, 1966, Ranadive et al., 1972, for review see Deutsche Forschungsgemeinschaft, 1982). However, it is neurotoxic in humans and in experimental animals: sensory polyneuropathy and polyneuropathy characterized by symmetrical, predominantly dis-

tal motor deficits are observed (reviewed by Couri and Milks, 1982). The same symptoms have been found in workers exposed to 2-hexanone (Mendell et al., 1974). HEX is metabolized in man and animals to 2,5-hexanedione (HDO) via 2-hexanol, 2,5-hexanediol, 2-hexanone, and 5-hydroxy-2-hexanone (Perbellini et al., 1980). In the experimental animal, these compounds produced peripheral neuropathies, HDO being most potent (Schaumburg and Spencer, 1976, Perbellini et al., 1978, Spencer et al. 1978, Krasavage et al., 1980). This diketone is the ultimate toxic agent as has been demonstrated by DeCaprio et al. (1983) and Anthony et al. (1983). HDO reacts covalently with primary amino groups of neurofilamental proteins resulting in pyrrolic adducts. This reaction is regarded to be the first step leading to neurotoxicity. (DeCaprio et al., 1985, 1988). Pyrrolidation of proteins has also been found in other tissues by measuring the absorption of a characteristic dye after reaction with 4-dimethylaminobenzaldehyde (DeCaprio et al., 1983). Excretion of substances behaving like pyrroles has been demonstrated in urine of rats after inhalation of HEX (Filser et al., 1987a).

An assessment of toxic or carcinogenic risks of these substances is mainly hampered by the difficulty of extrapolating results obtained from animal experiments to man. A necessary prerequisite is the knowledge of the pharmacokinetics of each substance in the experimental animals and in man. We studied the pharmacokinetics of inhaled vapors of 2-NP, MEK, and HEX in the rat. In case of 2-NP no pharmacokinetic data in man are available. Since the pharmacokinetics of HEX (Römmelt and Dirnagl, 1977, Perbellini et al., 1986, Filser et al., 1987b) and of MEK (Perbellini et al., 1984, Liira et al., 1988) in man are known, we compared the pharmacokinetic parameters in man with those obtained in rats. Finally we discuss the usefulness of pharmacokinetics of inhaled vapors in the extrapolation from one species to another.

MATERIALS AND METHODS

Animals

Exposures to HEX and MEK were performed with male Wistar rats, 180-220 g, and exposures to 2-NP with male and female Sprague-Dawley rats (SD rats), 160-190 g (inbred strains, GSF, Neuherberg, FRG). Before experiments, animals were housed in a temperature-controlled room and provided with standard rat chow (Altromin 1324, Altromin GmbH & Co.KG, Lage, FRG) and tap water ad libitum.

Chemicals

Chemicals and gases were obtained from following sources: HEX (p.a.), MEK (p.a.), and sodium diethyldithiocarbamate (p.a.) (dithiocarb) from Merck, Darmstadt, FRG; 2-NP 98% from Aldrich Chemie, Steinheim, FRG; Tenax 60-80 mesh from Serva, Heidelberg, FRG; Dräger-Sorb 800 from Dräger-Werk AG, Lübeck, FRG; nitrogen, hydrogen, and oxygen from Linde AG, München, FRG.

Methods

In order to determine inhalation pharmacokinetics rats were housed for the time period indicated in closed all-glass exposure chambers of 6.4 l containing 135 g soda lime and equipped with an automatic oxygen supply as described by Lieser (1983). Each experimental group was composed of six rats, two rats per chamber. The animals were exposed to varying initial atmospheric concentrations of the respective substances as outlined in the figures. Solvents were injected into the gas phase of the chambers as vapors in order to achieve low concentrations and as liquids in order to achieve high concentrations in the atmosphere. Evaporation period did not exceed 10 min. During exposure time the decline of concentrations in the gas phase of the closed exposure chambers was monitored continously. Since 2-NP reacts intensively with soda lime rats were placed in exposure chambers of 21 l not containing soda lime. Every 2 h rats were quickly transferred into an empty chamber and the former 2-NP concentration in the gas phase was adjusted. Some experiments with MEK were carried out after IP administration of 3.6 µl MEK in 1 ml olive oil/kg body weight. Subsequently, rats were placed in the exposure chambers (groups of three rats, one rat per chamber). Concentrations of the exhaled vapors in the atmosphere of the chamber were followed during the time course of the experiment.

To inhibit monooxygenases of the endoplasmic reticulum animals were pretreated 15 min before exposure by IP administration of dithiocarb 200 mg/kg dissolved in saline (Siegers et al. 1978).

Analyses of atmospheric concentrations of the solvents were done using a Shimadzu GC-8A gas chromatograph equipped with a 1 ml injection loop and a flame ionisation detector. The compounds were separated isothermally on a stainless steel column (2.5 m) packed with Tenax 60-80 mesh. For each substance separation conditions were developed.

Determination of the Ostwald's partition coefficients olive oil/air and water/air was done at 37°C according to Hallier et al. (1981). Using these data the thermodynamic partition coefficient (body/air) was estimated as described by Filser and Bolt (1984) assuming the body to be composed of 70% aqueous and 10% fatty compartments for rats (Altman and Dittmer, 1964), and of 60% aqueous and 16% fatty compartments for male humans (Documenta Geigy, 1973).

Mathematical analysis of the experimental concentration-time curves was done adapting the pharmacokinetic two-compartment model which had been developed for first-order kinetics (Filser and Bolt, 1981; 1983). To describe different metabolic processes we introduced k*el (fig. 1.). Three equations used for k*el are presented in fig. 2. Equations A and C describe one and two saturable processes, resp., according to Michaelis-Menten kinetics. Equation B describes two processes, a saturable one according to Michaelis-Menten kinetics and a non-saturable one according to first-order kinetics. Calculation of inhalation kinetics was performed using a computer software package specially developed. After insertion of eq. A, B, or C for k*el in the second differential equation (fig. 1.), both differential equations were integrated iteratively over the exposure time. The obtained curves were plotted and compared with the measured data. The best fit was used to calculate the thermodynamic partition coefficient (body/air), concentration ratio in steady state (body/air), Kmapp., and Vmax. Clearances of uptake from the atmosphere, of metabolism, and of exhalation were calculated in relation to the atmospheric concentration for an open exposure system (V1 being infinitely large). The actual rate of uptake, metabolism, or exhalation is given by the product of the respective clearance value with the actual atmospheric concentration.

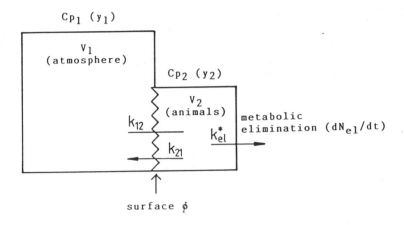

Differential equations related to the pharmacokinetic model:

Atmosphere: $V_1 \cdot \dfrac{dy_1}{dt} = -k_{12} \cdot V_1 \cdot y_1 + k_{21} \cdot V_2 \cdot y_2.$

Animal: $V_2 \cdot \dfrac{dy_2}{dt} = k_{12} \cdot V_1 \cdot y_1 - (k_{el}^* + k_{21}) \cdot V_2 \cdot y_2$

Fig. 1. Pharmacokinetic two-compartment model and differential
equations for the exposure system.
Cp1: compartment 1;   Cp2: compartment 2;
y1: concentration in the atmosphere;
y2: concentration in the organism;
V1: volume of the gas phase;   V2: volume of the animal;
k12: microconstant of the uptake process;
k21: microconstant of the exhalation process;
k*el: microconstant of the metabolic elimination
         (concentration dependent)

eq.A : $k_{el}^* = \dfrac{V_{max}}{V_2 \cdot (Km_{app.} + y_2)}$

eq.B : $k_{el}^* = \dfrac{V_{max}}{V_2 \cdot (Km_{app.} + y_2)} + k_{el}$

eq.C : $k_{el}^* = \dfrac{V_{max_1}}{V_2 \cdot (Km_{app.1} + y_2)} + \dfrac{V_{max_2}}{V_2 \cdot (Km_{app.2} + y_2)}$

Fig. 2. Equations for k*el related to the pharmacokinetic model.
Vmax: maximal rate of metabolism;   Kmapp.: apparent
Michealis-Menten constant for a saturable pathway
(= concentration in Cp2 at Vmax/2);   kel: microconstant
for non-saturable pathway according to first-order kinetics

RESULTS AND DISCUSSION

2-Nitropropane

The Ostwald's partition coefficients of 2-NP were 128 for water/air and 710 for olive oil/air at 37°C. From these data the thermodynamic partition coefficient for rats was estimated to be 161. A similar value of 180 for this coefficient was obtained from the inhalation kinetics of 2-NP in SD rats (table 1.) as evaluated from experimental data (fig. 3.a, b). These data forced us to express for both sexes k*el as a function composed of two different metabolic processes (eq.B, fig. 2.): a saturable one of low capacity and high affinity according to Michaelis-Menten kinetics and a non-saturable one following first-order kinetics. This procedure resulted in calculated curves fitting the measured data (fig. 3.a, b). The calculated kinetic parameters (table 1.) demonstrated that uptake processes were equal in both sexes. The clearance of uptake was remarkably high and even coincided with the ventilation rate in this species (Guyton, 1947). The sums of the rates of both metabolic processes were similar in both sexes below 100 ppm. At concentrations below 10 ppm clearances of metabolism reached maximal values approximating the clearance of uptake. Obviously, at low concentrations the ventilation rate limited the clearance of metabolism. These findings explain the low value of the concentration ratio in steady state compared to the thermodynamic partition coefficient (table 1.). Only small amounts of unchanged 2-NP were exhaled as calculated from the ratio of the clearance of exhalation to the clearance of uptake (18% females, 13% males). Moreover, first-order metabolism was similar in both sexes, although striking sex differences existed in the kinetics of the saturable metabolic pathway. In females Kmapp. which is

Table 1. Sex-Specific Pharmacokinetic Parameters of 2-NP in SD Rats (250 g)

Parameter	Value (female rat)	Value (male rat)	Dimension
Thermodynamic partition coefficient (body/air)	180	180	nl gas/ml tissue ppm in atmosphere
Concentration ratio in steady state (body/air)[1]	30	23	nl gas/ml tissue ppm in atmosphere
Clearance of uptake (related to atmosph.conc.)	180	180	ml/min
Clearance of exhalation[1] (related to atmosph.conc.)	32	24	ml/min
Clearance of metabolism[1] (related to atmosph.conc.)	150	160	ml/min
Clearance of non-saturable metabolic pathway[1](related to atmosph.conc.)	25	32	ml/min
Vmax	0.48	0.21	μmol/min
Kmapp.	2900	900	nl gas/ml tissue

1: valid for atmospheric concentrations less than 10 ppm

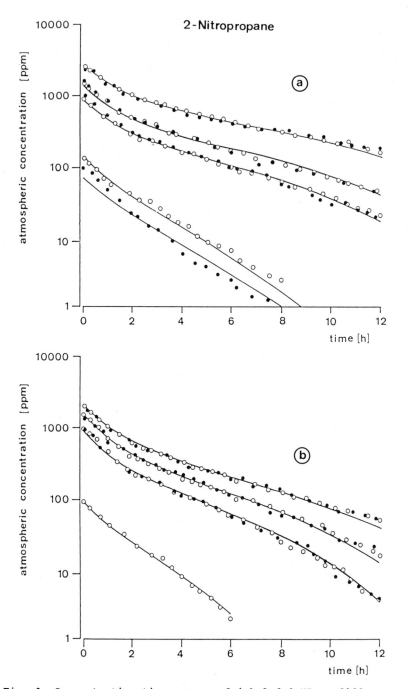

Fig. 3. Concentration-time curves of inhaled 2-NP at different
initial concentrations in the gas phase of a closed
exposure chamber occupied by two SD rats.
(a) females, (b) males
Dots: measured values; lines: calculated curves using
the kinetic data shown in table 1.

related to the concentration in the body was 3.2 times and Vmax 2.3 times higher than in males. At steady state, the atmospheric concentration of 2-NP at Vmax/2 was 71 ppm in females and 28 ppm in males. The rates of the different metabolic processes in males and females are given in fig. 4. Since 2-NP is metabolized partly by a saturable pathway, the lines calculated for the non-saturable pathways are curved. In females more 2-NP is metabolized by the non-saturable pathway at concentrations above 180 ppm, in males at concentrations above 60 ppm. Because of the non-saturable pathway, the accumulation of inhaled 2-NP cannot reach the thermodynamic

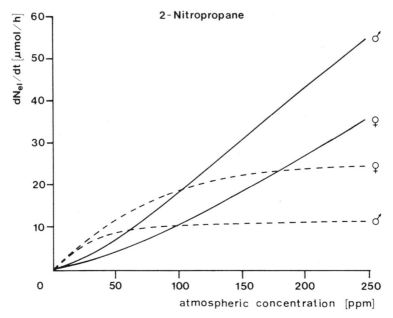

Fig. 4. Rate of metabolism (dNel/dt) at steady state of 2-NP in a SD rat of 250 g dependent on the atmospheric concentration, calculated for an open exposure system. Dashed lines: saturable metabolic pathway; solid lines: non-saturable metabolic pathway

partition coefficient. With increasing atmospheric concentrations of 2-NP, the concentration ratio in steady state amounted from 30 (females) and 23 (males) at concentrations below 10 ppm to 80 (females) and 65 (males) at concentrations above 400 ppm (females) and 200 ppm (males) (data not shown). With respect to the higher sensitivity of male rats to hepatotoxicity (Lewis et al., 1979), carcinogenicity (Griffin et al., 1980), and genotoxicity (Andrae et al., 1988), we conclude that these effects are not the result of 2-NP itself which accumulates in females to a higher degree than in males. They are probably due to the first order metabolic process. In contrast, the saturable metabolic process also observed in male SD rats by Nolan et al. (1982) is more likely to be leading to less toxic or carcinogenic metabolites, since at the same concentration of 2-NP this pathway is slower in males than in females.

Methyl ethyl ketone

The Ostwald's partition coefficients at 37°C of MEK for water/air and olive oil/air were 134 and 131, respectively. Using a different method Sato and Nakajima (1979) determined them to be 254 and 263, Perbellini et al. (1984) 193 and 191, respectively. Since the distributions in oil and water are equal it can be concluded that in the organism MEK is equally distributed within aqueous and fatty compartments. This is corroborated by thermodynamic partition coefficients found in different human tissues (Perbellini et al., 1984). We estimated a thermodynamic partition coefficient for rats of 107. From the gas uptake studies using Wistar rats (fig. 5.) it was calculated to be 103 (table 2.). For man, the value of this partition coefficient can be estimated by the ratio of the MEK-concentration in peripheral blood to the concentration in the alveolar air which was determined to be between 104 and 116 by Perbellini et al. (1984). Kinetic parameters for rats (table 2.) were calculated from the experimental data using eq.A (fig. 2.) which describe one saturable metabolic pathway according to Michaelis-Menten. The calculated concentration-time curves are shown in fig. 5. Below 180 ppm, concentration ratio in steady state of MEK was only 14 compared to the thermodynamic partition coefficient of 103 being indicative that metabolism is limited by the transport to the enzymes. This conclusion was supported by the findings of exhalation experiments after IP administration of MEK to by-pass lung uptake. The exhaled amounts of MEK were only 20% of those expected from the outcome of the inhalation experiments. In further inhalation studies, dithiocarb (200 mg/kg), an inhibitor of cytochrome P-450-dependent monooxygenases, was administered IP before exposure. This treatment resulted in an inhibition of the MEK-metabolism of 21% if related to atmospheric concentrations below 180 ppm. Due to this inhibitory effect on the metabolizing enzymes the concentration ratio in steady state being 33 was 2.3 times higher than in untreated animals. Relating this inhibition not to concentrations in the atmosphere but to equal concentrations in the organism its value was calculated to be 66%. This relatively low value compared to other substances, metabolized by monooxygenases exclusively (Siegers et al., 1978, Bolt et al., 1984, Robertson et al., 1985), can be explained assuming that only the oxidative of the two metabolic pathways (see above) was inhibited by dithiocarb. The clearance of uptake from the gas phase was found to be 62 ml/min. The clearance of metabolism (below 180 ppm) was 53 ml/min i.e. 40% of the pulmonary ventilation of the rat: pulmonary retention was 40%. The clearance of exhalation was 8.4 ml/min i.e. 14% of the clearance of uptake: 14% of the absorbed dose are exhaled as the unchanged substance. Since with respect to the distribution of MEK the whole body can be regarded as one homogenous compartment, the concentration ratio in steady state equals the enrichment in blood. By dividing the value of the clearance of uptake by the value of the concentration ratio in steady state the clearance of uptake can be related to the concentration in blood. This clearance value is calculated to be 4.4 ml/min i.e. 10% of the blood flow through the lung (45 ml/min, Sapirstein et al., 1960) and 26% of the blood flow through the liver (17 ml/min, Boxenbaum, 1980) of the adult rat. Since the clearance of metabolism is 86% of the clearance of uptake it has to be deduced that below 180 ppm the transport through the lung is the step limiting the rate of metabolism. This conclusion is supported further by the outcome of the IP experiments.

Our data obtained in rats can be compared with those published for man. Exposed workers revealed a pulmonary retention of 70% at concentrations of up to 100 ppm (Perbellini et al., 1984). Liira et al. (1988) obtained a pulmonary retention of 53% in male volunteers at a concentration of 200 ppm. In the rat it was determined to be 40% (see above). Assuming a pulmonary ventilation rate of 8 l/min in man, the clearance of metabolism related to the atmospheric concentration can be estimated to be 5.6 l/min

Table 2. Pharmacokinetic Parameters for MEK in Wistar Rats (250 g)

Parameter	Value	Dimension
Thermodynamic partition coefficient (body/air)	103	$\dfrac{\text{nl gas/ml tissue}}{\text{ppm in atmosphere}}$
Concentration ratio in steady state (body/air)[1]	14	$\dfrac{\text{nl gas/ml tissue}}{\text{ppm atmosphere}}$
Clearance of uptake (related to atmosph.conc.)	62	ml/min
Clearance of exhalation[1] (related to atmosph.conc.)	8.4	ml/min
Clearance of metabolism[1] (related to atmosph.conc.)	53	ml/min
Vmax	2.5	µmol/min
Kmapp.	17,000	nl gas/ml tissue

1: valid for atmospheric concentrations less than 180 ppm

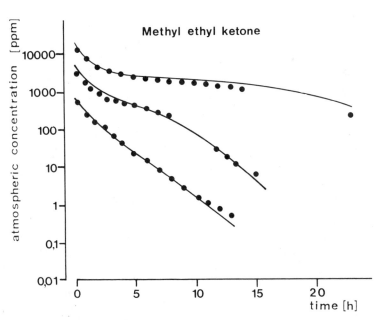

Fig. 5. Concentration-time curves of inhaled MEK at different initial concentrations in the gas phase of a closed exposure chamber occupied by two Wistar rats. Dots: measured values (means of 3 values obtained from concentration-time curves achieved with identical exposure conditions); lines: calculated curves using the kinetic data shown in table 2.

(Perbellini et al., 1984) and 4.2 l/min (Liira et al., 1988). Related to the blood concentration, Liira et al. (1988) gave a clearance of metabolism of 0.44 l/min at rest and of 0.33 l/min at temporary exercises. These are between 25% and 19% of the blood flow through the liver (1.8 l/min, Boxenbaum, 1980). The enrichment in blood (ratio of concentration in venous blood to concentration in alveolar air) was calculated using the data of Liira et al. (1988) to be 13 at rest which coincides with the value obtained by us for the rat. At temporary exercise it was 20 and in occupationally exposed workers 31-35 (Perbellini et al., 1984). In contrast to the increase of the enrichment in blood at working conditions the clearance of metabolism related to the concentration in blood decreased (Liira et al., 1988). The rate of metabolism is the clearance of metabolism related to the concentration in blood multiplied with the blood-concentration. This rate increased only by 11% at temporary exercise at 200 ppm compared to conditions at rest. Such a compensative effect was also found in rats after administration of dithiocarb to inhibit MEK-metabolizing enzymes (see above). The amount of MEK exhaled unchanged related to the amount absorbed was found to be 3% (Liira et al., 1988) and 30% (Munies and Wurster, 1965) in man, 30% in dog (Schwarz 1898), and 14% in rat (see above). From their results on inhalation kinetics of MEK in man Liira et al. (1988) inferred "that pulmonary ventilation is indeed the rate limiting step of uptake" which is in agreement with our findings in rat.

n-Hexane

HEX revealed Ostwald's partition coefficients of 1 for water/air and of 81 for olive oil/air at 37°C whereas Perbellini et al. (1985) obtained 146 for olive oil/air using a different method. With our values the thermodynamic partition coefficient was estimated to be 9 for rats and 13.6 for men which are similar to the values of 9.6 and 11 obtained for rats, and of 12 obtained for men from gas uptake studies (table 3.). In order to describe the concentration-time curves measured in Wistar rats (fig. 6.) we had to express k^*_{el} by two independent kinetics according to Michaelis-Menten (eq.C, fig. 2). This procedure resulted in the smooth curves plotted in fig. 6. One of the two pathways was of high capacity but low affinity, the other one of low capacity but high affinity (table 3.). The atmospheric concentrations at Vmax/2 correspondent to Kmapp. are 4000 ppm and 240 ppm, respectively. The first metabolic process (lower Vmax, lower Kmapp.) seemed to lead to the ultimate neurotoxic metabolite (HDO), because the excretion rate of this metabolite in urine reached half of its maximum when rats were exposed to 250 ppm HEX (Fedtke and Bolt, 1987, Filser et al. 1987a). It seems likely that the two separate saturation kinetics of inhaled HEX observed by us can be attributed to different species of cytochrome P-450-linked monooxygenases with different substrate specificities. This is in accordance with the conclusion of Frommer et al. (1974) who investigated the hydroxylation pattern of HEX in rat liver microsomes. Saturation of HEX-metabolism was observed by Baker and Rickert (1981) and Hilderbrand and Andersen (1981) in Fischer 344 rats and by Filser et al. (1987) in SD rats (table 3.). Hilderbrand and Andersen (1981) described the biotransformation of HEX by Michaelis-Menten kinetics dependent on the concentration in the atmosphere. They found values similar to those determined by us for one of the two metabolic pathways: Vmax was estimated 0.4 µmol/min for a rat of 250 g, Km corresponded to a HEX-concentration of 163 ppm. Under the experimental conditions used by these authors the second metabolic process was not observed. Clearance of uptake from the atmosphere (table 3.) was found to be 24 ml/min (SD rat) and 35 ml/min (Wistar rat). In male Fischer 344 rats, Andersen (1981) reported a "maximum first-order rate constant" of 0.24/(h·kg) obtained in a chamber of 31 l. The clearance of uptake can roughly be estimated from the product of the chamber volume with the given rate constant yielding 31 ml/min per

Table 3. Pharmacokinetic Parameters for HEX in Rat (250 g) and Man (79 kg)

Parameter	Man	Value SD rat	Wistar rat	Dimension
Thermodynamic partition coefficient (body/air)	12	9.6	11	$\frac{\text{nl gas/ml tissue}}{\text{ppm in atmosphere}}$
Concentration ratio in steady state (body/air)	2.3[1]	1.6[2]	1.2[3]	$\frac{\text{nl gas/ml tissue}}{\text{ppm in atmosphere}}$
Clearance of uptake (related to atmosph.conc.)	2800	24	35	ml/min
Clearance of exhalation (related to atmosph.conc.)	530[1]	4.2[2]	3.8[3]	ml/min
Clearance of metabolism (related to atmosph.conc.)	2200[1]	20[2]	31[3]	ml/min
Vmax1	–	–	0.3	µmol/min
Vmax2	–	–	2.4	µmol/min
Kmapp.1	–	–	290	nl gas/ml tissue
Kmapp.2	–	–	24,000	nl gas/ml tissue

Data for man and SD rat are from Filser et al. (1987b)
1: determined for atmospheric concentrations up to 2 ppm
2: valid for atmospheric concentrations up to 300 ppm
3: valid for atmospheric concentrations up to 150 ppm

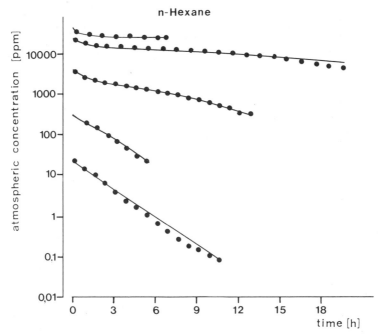

Fig. 6. Concentration-time curves of inhaled HEX at different
initial concentrations in the gas phase of a closed
exposure chamber occupied by two Wistar rats.
Dots: measured values (means of 3 values obtained
from concentration-time curves achieved with identical
exposure conditions);   lines: calculated curves using
the kinetic data shown in table 3.

one rat of 250 g. From the data given by Dahl et al. (1988), who used the
same rat strain but a different exposure system, a higher value of
38 ml/min can be calculated. At concentrations below 300 ppm (SD rats) and
150 ppm (Wistar rats) concentration ratios in steady state were 1.6 and
1.2, respectively (table 3.). These values are much lower than could be
expected from the thermodynamic partition coefficients: only a small accumulation of HEX was observed. Furthermore, the clearances of metabolism
were only slightly lower than those of uptake from the gas phase (83% in
SD rats and 89% in Wistar rats). This means that most of HEX entering the
body was metabolized and minor amounts were exhaled unchanged (17% in SD
rats and 11% in Wistar rats). Pulmonary retention (for calculation see
MEK) was obtained to be 15% (SD rats) and 23% (Wistar rats). In the rat
the partition coefficient blood/air was determined to be 0.88 (Böhlen et
al., 1973). By dividing the value of the clearance of uptake by 0.88 this
parameter can be related to the concentration in blood. It was calculated
to be 27 ml/min (SD rat) and 40 ml/min (Wistar rat). These values correspond to 60% and 89% of the the blood flow through the lung (see above).
Using the same procedure the clearance of metabolism related to the blood
flow through the liver was estimated to be 135% (SD rat) and 200% (Wistar
rat). Apparently the liver was not the only organ metabolizing HEX. At
lower concentrations the rate of metabolism seemed not to be limited by
the metabolic capacity but by transport to the metabolizing enzymes. This
conclusion is corroborated by the low concentration ratio in steady state
compared to the thermodynamic partition coefficient.

As for MEK a comparison of the data obtained in the rat with those published for man can be done. We determined clearance of metabolism to be 2.2 l/min in a man of 79 kg at concentrations below 2 ppm (table 3.). Pulmonary retention calculated from this value (see above) was 28%. Römmelt and Dirnagl (1977) and Brugnone et al. (1978) published retentions of 20% (at 100 ppm) and of 34% (at 1 ppm). In rats, retention values were between 15% and 23% (see above). Using the data of retention and a pulmonary ventilation of 8 l/min for man the clearance of metabolism related to the atmospheric concentration is calculated to be 1.6 l/min (Brugnone et al., 1978) and 2.7 l/min (Römmelt and Dirnagl, 1977). The partition coefficient blood/air in man was determined to be 0.8 (Perbellini et al., 1985). The clearance of uptake (table 3.) related to the concentration in blood (see above) gave a value 3.5 l/min i.e. 70% of the blood flow through the lung (rats: 60 - 89%). Relating the values obtained for the clearance of metabolism (1.6 l/min, 2,2 l/min, and 2.7 l/min) to the concentration in blood, values of 2.0 l/min, 2.8 l/min, and 3.4 l/min are yielded. These are between 110 - 190% of the blood flow of 1.8 l/min through the liver and are similar to results obtained in rats. For both species it can be concluded that metabolism was limited by transport processes, probably by the blood flow through the lung. This interpretation was supported by the findings of the low accumulation of HEX in steady state (2.3, table 3.) and of the small amount of HEX exhaled (19% of the amount taken up, calculated from table 3.) as observed in rats too. Using concentration-time courses of HEX in venous blood of humans obtained experimentally by Veulemans et al. (1982), Perbellini et al. (1986) presented a physiologicomathematical model to predict pharmacokinetics of HEX in man. The authors assumed that metabolism of HEX took place exclusively in the liver. However, the results presented here indicate that in rat and man the liver is not the only HEX-metabolizing organ.

General conclusions

In the low concentration range metabolism of the three inhaled compounds studied was not limited by metabolic capacity but by transport to the metabolizing enzymes. Transport limitation of the metabolism of some inhaled substances was first observed by Filser and Bolt (1979). Pulmonary uptake, pulmonary retention, accumulation in the body, exhalation and rate of metabolism of MEK and HEX, resp., were comparable in rat and man, if related to physiological processes as ventilation rate or blood flow. In the rat the ventilation rate limited metabolism of 2-NP at concentrations below 10 ppm. Since no data are available on the pharmacokinetics in man, we do not know if this observation holds true for man also.

Often toxicity or carcinogenicity is not simply caused by the very compound taken up but by its reactive metabolites. Their concentrations are determined by the rates of production and of decomposition both of which are frequently enzymatic processes. The capacity of toxication and detoxication enzymes might be the reason for the sex differences found with 2-NP and species differences as it was observed e.g. for butadiene in mice and rats (Kreiling et al., 1986). As far as the species-specific pharmacokinetics of the ultimate toxic or carcinogenic metabolite are not evaluated species extrapolation is not justified.

ACKNOWLEDGEMENT

The financial support of the studies on HEX and MEK by the Umweltbundesamt, FRG, Grant No. UBA-FB 106 06 043 are gratefully acknowledged.

REFERENCES

Abdel-Rahman, M. S., Hetland, L. B., and Couri, D., 1976, Toxicity and metabolism of methyl n-butyl ketone, Am. Ind. Hyg. Assoc. J., 3:95

Altenkirch, H., Mager, J., Stoltenburg, G., and Helmbrecht, J., 1977, Toxic polyneuropathies after sniffing a glue thinner, J. Neurol., 214:137

Altenkirch, H., Stoltenburg, G., and Wagner, H. M., 1978, Experimental studies on hydrocarbon neuropathies induced by methyl ethyl ketone (MEK), J. Neurol., 219:159

Altenkirch, H., Wagner, H.M., Stoltenburg, G., and Spencer, P.S., 1982, Nervous system responses of rats to subchronic inhalation of n-hexane and n-hexane + methyl ethyl ketone mixtures, J. Neurol. Science, 57:209

Altman, P. L. and Dittmer, D. S., 1964, "Biology Data Book, vol. 3", Federation of American Societies for Experimental Biology, Washington

Andersen, M., E., 1981, A physiologically based toxicokinetic description of the metabolism of inhaled gases and vapors: Analysis at steady state, Toxicol. Appl. Pharmacol., 60:509

Andrae, U., Homfeldt, H., Vogl, L., Lichtmannegger, J., and Summer, K. H., 1988, 2-Nitropropane induces DNA repair synthesis in rat hepatocytes in vitro and in vivo, Carcinogenesis, 9:811

Anthony, D. C., Boekelheide, K., Anderson, C.W., and Graham, D. G., 1983, The effect of 3,4-dimethyl substitution on the neurotoxicity of 2,5-hexanedione. II. Dimethyl substitution accelerates pyrrole formation and protein crosslinking, Toxicol. Appl. Pharmacol., 71:372

Baker, T. S. and Rickert, D. E., 1981, Dose-dependent uptake, distribution, and elimination of inhaled n-hexane in the Fischer-344 rat, Toxicol. Appl. Pharmacol., 61:414

Böhlen, P., Schlunegger, U. P., and Läuppi, E., 1973, Uptake and distribution of hexane in rat tissues, Toxicol. Appl. Pharmacol., 25:242

Bolt, H, M., Filser, J. G., and Störmer, F., 1984, Inhalation pharmacokinetics based on gas uptake studies V. Comparative pharmacokinetics of ethylene and 1,3-butadiene in rats, Arch. Toxicol., 55:213

Boxenbaum, H., 1980, Interspecies variations in liver weight, hepatic blood flow, and antipyrine intrinsic clearance: extrapolation of data to benzodiazopines and phenytoin, J. Pharmocokinet. Biopharmac., 8:165

Brugnone, F., Perbellini, L., Grigolini, L., and Apostoli, A., 1978, Solvent exposure in a shoe factory. I. n-Hexane and acetone concentration in alveolar and environmental air and in blood, Int. Arch. Occup. Environ. Health, 40:241

Couri, D., and Milks, M., 1982, Toxicity and metabolism of the neurotoxic hexacarbons n-hexane, 2-hexanone, and 2,5-hexanedione, Ann. Rev. Pharmacol., 22:145

Dahl, A. R., Damon, E. G., Mauderly, J. L., Rothenberg, S. J., Seiler, F. A., and McClellan, R. O., 1988, Uptake of 19 hydrocarbon vapors inhaled by F344 rats, Fundament. Appl. Toxicol., 10:269

DeCaprio, A. P., Strominger, N. L., and Weber, P., 1983, Neurotoxicity and protein binding of 2,5-hexanedione in the hen, Toxicol. Appl. Pharmacol., 68:297

DeCaprio, A. P., and O'Neill, E. A., 1985, Alterations in rat axonal cytoskeletal proteins induced by in vitro and in vivo 2,5-hexanedione exposure, Toxicol. Appl. Pharmacol., 78:235

DeCaprio, A. P., Briggs, R. G., Jackoswki, S. J., Kim, J. C. S., 1988, Comparative neurotoxicity and pyrrole-forming potential of 2,5-hexanedione in the rat, Toxicol. Appl. Pharmacol., 92:75

Deutsche Forschungsgemeinschaft, 1976, 2-Butanon, in: "Toxikologisch-arbeitsmedizinische Begründung von MAK-Werten," D. Henschler, ed., VCH, Weinheim

Deutsche Forschungsgemeinschaft, 1982, n-Hexan, in: "Toxikologisch-arbeitsmedizinische Begründung von MAK-Werten", D. Henschler, ed., VCH, Weinheim

Dietz, F. K., and Traiger, G. J., 1979, Potentiation of CCl4 hepato-toxicity in rats by a metabolite of 2-butanone: 2,3-butanediol, Toxicol., 14:209

Dietz, F. K., Rodriguez-Giaxola, M., Traiger, G. J., Stella, V. J., and Himmelstein, K. J., 1981, Pharmacokinetics of 2-butanol and its metabolites in the rat, J. Pharmacokin. Biopharm., 9:553

DiVicenzo, G. D., Kaplan, C. J., and Dedinas, J., 1976, Characterization of the metabolites of methyl n-butyl ketone, methyl isobutyl ketone, and methyl ethyl ketone in guinea pig serum and their clearance, Toxicol. Appl. Pharmacol., 36:511

Documenta Geigy, 1973, "Wissenschaftliche Tabellen", 7. ed., Ciba-Geigy, Basel

Duckett, S., Williams, N., and Francis, S., 1974, Peripheral neuropathy associated with inhalation of methyl n-butyl ketone, Experientia, 30:1283

Fedtke, N. and Bolt, H. M., 1987, The relevance of 4,5-dihydroxy-2-hexanone in the excretion kinetics of n-hexane metabolites in rat and man, Arch. Toxicol., 61:131

Filser, J. G. and Bolt, H. M., 1979, Pharmacokinetics of halogenated ethylenes in rats, Arch. Toxicol., 42,123

Filser, J. G. and Bolt, H. M., 1981, Inhalation kinetics based on gas uptake studies I. Improvement of kinetic models, Arch. Toxicol., 47:279

Filser, J. G. and Bolt, H. M., 1983, Inhalation pharmacokinetics based on gas uptake studies IV. The endogenous production of volatile compounds, Arch. Toxicol., 52:123

Filser, J. G., and Bolt, H. M., 1984, Inhalation pharmacokinetics based on gas uptake studies VI. Comparative evaluation of ethylene oxide and butadiene monoxide as exhaled reactive metabolites of ethylene and 1,3-butadiene in rats, Arch. Toxicol., 55:219

Filser, J. G., Heilmaier, H. E., Summer, K. H., and Greim, H., 1987a, Spektralphotometrischer Test zur Bestimmung der 2,5-Hexandion-belastung aus dem Urin von Ratten, in: "Bericht über die 27. Jahrestagung der Deutschen Gesellschaft für Arbeitsmedizin e.V., Band 1", K. Norpoth, ed., Gentner Verlag, Stuttgart

Filser, J. G., Peter, H., Bolt, H. M., and Fedtke, N., 1987b, Pharmacokinetics of the neurotoxin n-hexane in rat and man, Arch. Toxicol., 60:77

Frommer, U., Ullrich, V., and Orrenius, S., 1974, Influence of inducers and inhibitors on the hydroxylation pattern of n-hexane in rat liver microsomes, FEBS Letters, 41:14

Griffin, T. B., Coulston, F., and Stein, A. A., 1980, Chronic inhalation exposure of rats to vapors of 2-nitropropane at 25 ppm, Ecotoxicol. Environ. Safety, 4:267

Guyton, A. C., 1947, Respiratory volumes of laboratory animals, Am. J. Physiol., 150:70

Hallier, E., Filser, J. G., and Bolt, H. M., 1981, Inhalation pharmacokinetics based on gas uptake studies II. Pharmacokinetics of acetone in rats, Arch. Toxicol., 47:293

Hilderbrand, R. L., and Andersen, M. E., 1981, In vivo kinetic constants for the metabolism of inhaled hydrocarbon toxicants as determined by gas uptake methods, Toxicologist, 1:86

Krasavage, W. J., O'Donoghue, J. L., DiVincenzo, G. D., and
    Terhaar, C. J., 1980, The relative neurotoxicity of methyl
    n-butyl ketone, n-hexane and their metabolites, Toxicol. Appl.
    Pharmacol., 52:433
Kreiling, R., Laib, R. J., Filser, J. G., and Bolt, H. M., 1986, Species
    differencesin butadiene metabolism between mice and rats evaluated
    by inhalation pharmacokinetics, Arch. Toxicol., 58:235
Lewis, T. R., Ulrich, C. E., and Busey, W. M., 1979, Subchronic
    inhalation toxicity of nitromethane and 2-nitropropane,
    J. Environ. Pathol. Toxicol., 2:233
Liira, J., Riihimäki, V., and Pfäffli, P., 1988, Kinetics of methyl
    ethyl ketone in man: absorption, distribution and elimination in
    inhalation exposure, Int. Arch. Environ. Health, 60:195
Lieser, K., 1983, "Tierexperimentelle Pharmakokinetik von 1,3-Butadien",
    Inauguraldissertation im Fachbereich Medizin der Universität
    Mainz
Miyasaka, M., Kumai, M., Koizumi, A., Watanabe, T., Kurasako, K.,
    Sato, K., and Ikeda, M., 1982, Biological monitoring of
    occupational exposure to methyl ethyl ketone by means of
    urinalysis for methyl ethyl ketone itself, Int. Arch. Occup.
    Environ. Health, 50:131
Munies, R., and Wurster, D. E., 1965, Investigations of some factors
    influencing percutaneous absorption. III. Absorption of methyl
    ethyl ketone, J. Pharmacol. Sci., 54:1281
Nolan, R. J., Unger, S. M., and Muller, C. J., 1982, Pharmacokinetics
    of inhaled [14C]-2-nitropropane in male Sprague-Dawley rats,
    Ecotoxicol. Environ. Safety, 6:388
Perbellini, L., DeGrandis, D., Semenzato, F., Rizzuto, N., and
    Simonati, A., 1978, An experimental study on the neurotoxicity of
    n-hexane metabolites: hexanol-1 and hexanol-2, Toxicol. Appl.
    Pharmacol., 46:241
Perbellini, L., Brugnone, F., and Pavan, I., 1980, Identification of the
    metabolites of n-hexane, cyclohexane, and their isomers in men's
    urine, Toxicol. Appl. Pharmacol., 53:220
Perbellini, L., Brugnone, F., Mozzo, P., Cocheo, V., and Caretta, D.,
    1984, Methyl ethyl ketone exposure in industrial workers. Uptake
    and kinetics, Int. Arch. Occup. Environ. Health, 54:73
Perbellini, L., Brugnone, F., Caretta, C., and Maranelli, G., 1985,
    Partition coefficients of some industrial aliphatic hydrocarbons
    (C5-C7)in blood and human tissues, Br. J. Ind. Med., 42:162
Perbellini, L., Mozzo, P., Brugnone, F., and Zedde, A., 1986,
    Physiologico-mathematical model for studying human exposure to
    organic solvents: kinetics of blood/tissue n-hexane concentrations
    and of 2,5-hexanedione in urine, Br. J. Ind. Med., 43:760
Robertson, L. W., Regel, U., Filser, J. G., and Oesch, F., 1985,
    Absence of lipid peroxidation as determined by ethane exhalation
    in rats treated with 2,3,7,8-tetrachlorodibenzo-p-dioxin (TCDD),
    Arch. Toxicol., 57:13
Römmelt, H., and Dirnagl, K., 1977, Pulmonale Resorption von sechs
    Kohlenwasserstoffen in Abhängigkeit von der Konzentration in der
    Atemluft, Münch. med. Wschr., 119:367
Saida, K., Mendell, J. R., and Weiss, H. S., 1976, Peripheral nerve
    changes induced by methyl n-butyl ketone and potentiation by
    methyl ethyl ketone, J. Neuropath. Exp. Neurol., 35:207
Schaumburg, H. H., and Spencer, P. S., 1976, Degeneration in central
    and peripheral nervous systems produced by pure n-hexane: An
    experimental study, Brain, 99:183
Schwartz, L., 1898, Über die Oxydation des Acetons und homologer Ketone
    der Fettsäurereihe, Arch. Exp. Pathol. Pharmakol. 40:168

Siegers, P. C., Filser, J. G., and Bolt, H. M., 1978, Effect of ditiocarb on metabolism and covalent binding of carbon tetrachloride, Toxicol. Appl. Pharmacol., 46:709

Spencer, P. S., Bischoff, M. C., and Schaumburg, H. H., 1978, On the specific molecular configuration of neurotoxic aliphatic hexacarbon compounds causing central-peripheral distal axonopathy, Toxicol. Appl. Pharmacol., 44:17

Traiger, G. J., and Bruckner, J. V., 1976, The participation of 2-butanone in 2-butanol-induced potentiation of carbon tetrachloride hepatotoxicity, J. Pharmacol. Exp. Ther., 196:493

Veulemans, H., Van Vlem, E., Jansses, H., Masschelein, R., and Leplat, A., 1982, Experimental human exposure to n-hexane study of the respiratory uptake and of n-hexane: study of the respiratory uptake and elimination, and of n-hexane concentrations in peripheral venous blood, Ind. Arch. Occup. Environ. Health, 49:251

OVERVIEW OF PROMOTION AS A MECHANISM IN CARCINOGENESIS

Monique Castagna and Isabelle Martelly

Institut de Recherches Scientifiques sur le Cancer
7, rue Guy Mocquet
94802 Villejuif Cedex France

INTRODUCTION

Considerable evidence has accumulated that cancer is a multifactorial and multistep process. Cancer does not result from a simple exposure to a single exogenous factor but rather from a complex interaction between exogenous and/or endogenous factors. The model of chemical carcinogenesis in mouse skin designed by Berenblum (1) and Mottram (2) has led to the characterization of two stages in carcinogenesis, initiation and promotion, caused by two different classes of agents, the initiators and the promoters. More recently, models of cultured cells have provided evidence that cell transformation by chemical carcinogens, U.V. light or X-rays, requires at least two steps. As a result of probability-based studies J. Little and co-workers have emphasized that the initial step is a frequent event since 100 % of the progeny of methylcholanthrene-treated cells are potentially transformed or "initiated" cells. However, a very small minority of the progeny of initiated cells actually yields transformed colonies, suggesting that a second step occurs which is a very rare event. This second step behaves like a spontaneous mutation in that it has small but constant probability of occurring each time an initiated cell divides (3). The requirement for two genetic events in the process of cancer appears to be in agreement with the results of transfection experiments, which indicate that at least two cooperating oncogenes are needed to convert embryo fibroblasts in primary cultures into tumor cells (4). Likewise, the model of transgenic mice in which oncogenes were expressed from tissue-specific promoters, has allowed to state that the expression of oncogen appears to result in hyperplasia with tumors arising as a rare clonal outgrowth, suggesting also the occurrence of secondary events.

Initiators essentially include chemicals as well as a number of other agents which generate genetic damage (i.e. point mutations, deletions, insertions, translocations or amplifications), such as U.V. light, ionizing radiation, various retroviruses and DNA containing viruses. Promoters, which are mostly chemicals as well as agents causing chronic tissue injury, are not carcinogenic by themselves but increase the probability of an "initiated" cell to become malignant. Despite their lack of carcinogenicity, tumor promoters play an important role in the etiology of cancer. With the exception of occupational exposure, initiators are present at harmless doses in the environment and have to be associated with promoters, which dramatically lower their threshold of action, for causing morbidity (5).

In contrast with initiators which elicit irreversible alterations, promoters reversibly modify the cellular phenotype. In cultured cells these agents evoke a pleiotropic response depending largely on the target cell. In some cell lines, phorbol ester 12-0-tetradecanoyl phorbol 13-acetate (TPA), reversibly evokes several properties associated with the tumor phenotype, including changes in cell morphology, high saturation density, low calcium requirement and inhibition of terminal differentiation. For instance, when TPA is applied to quail myoblasts, either normal or RSV-tsNY68 mutant-transformed cells, at the non-permissive temperature, morphological changes occur and myogenic differentiation is prevented. Alternatively, reciprocal effects are observed in some other cell lines, generally malignant, in which TPA induces cells to differentiate and inhibits cell growth (as reviewed in 6).

At variance with initiators, promoters do not directly affect DNA. The molecular target responsible for epigenetic changes in carcinogenesis was unknown up to very recently. The finding that protein kinase C, an enzyme which plays a key role in signal transduction, was the major and possibly the exclusive target for phorbol ester tumor promoters, has provided a substantial advance in the understanding of the mechanism of action of these agents (7-10).

PHOSPHOINOSITIDE PATHWAY

In multicellular organisms, cells respond to the environment and communicate with each other by extracellular messengers. Information is transferred from one cell to others in such a way that the cell specific function is integrated at the level of the whole organism. Two major strategies, eventually implicating protein phosphorylation, are used for transducing extracellular signals into the cell, which are schematically drawn in fig. 1. Upon binding to specific receptors, a set of hormones and neurotransmitters generates cyclic AMP which serves as a second messenger and triggers protein phosphorylation through activation of a cyclic AMP-dependent protein kinase, while two GTP-binding proteins negatively or positively modulate the response. Alternatively, the transduction of a large number of ligands controlling growth and cellular functions, including neurotransmitters, regulatory peptides, hormones, releasing factors, platelet activators and growth factors requires the mediation of two second messengers : 1,2-diacylglycerol (DG) and inositol-1,4,5-trisphosphate (IP_3), which are formed as a result of phosphatidylinositol 4,5-bisphosphate breakdown The former triggers activation of protein kinase C, a phospholipid and Ca^{2+}-activated enzyme which phosphorylates a large variety of proteins located in all the subcellular components, including the nucleus. The latter evokes Ca^{2+} mobilization from internal stores, thereby the free Ca^{2+} concentration rises, affecting Ca^{2+}-dependent fluxes as well as cellular processes under the control of Ca^{2+} and/or calmodulin-dependent enzymes. The two second-messenger-mediated sets of events contribute to the mobilization of the whole target cell in order to fully achieve the physiological response. The synergistic action of the two branches has been experimentally shown in many cell types such as platelets, mast cells, neutrophils, hepatocytes, pituitary cells, pancreatic islets and acini. A GTP-binding protein, functionally similar to those which have been involved in the adenylate cyclase system, modulate signal transduction at this step.

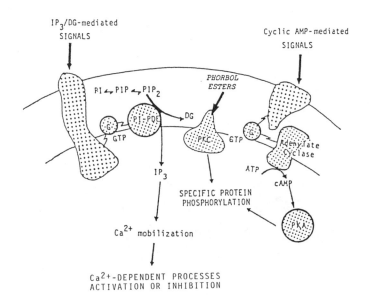

Fig.1 - <u>Proposed models of signal transduction involving IP$_3$/DG and cyclic AMP as second messengers.</u> Abbreviations : PKA, cyclic AMP-dependent protein kinase ; PKC, protein kinase C ; PI-PDE, phosphatidylinositol phosphodiesterase ; PI, phosphatidylinositol PIP, phosphatidylinositol 4-phosphate ; PIP$_2$, phosphatidylinositol 4,5-bisphosphate; IP$_3$, inositol-1,4,5-trisphosphate ; DG, diacylglycerol ; G, G-protein.

Of importance is the fact that protein kinase C can switch the phosphoinositide pathway on or off. Negative feedback control includes down-regulation of surface receptors, inhibition of receptor-mediated phosphoinositide hydrolysis, activation of inositol trisphosphate 5'-phosphomonoesterase, which hydrolyzes IP$_3$ and increased expression of growth inhibitors such as interferon β2, tumor growth factor β, tumor necrosis factor.

Generally, the adenylate cyclase pathway and the phosphoinositide pathway are not independent and control each other. Cyclic AMP-mediated signals negatively control the phosphoinositide pathway in platelets, neutrophils and lymphocytes. Conversely, IP$_3$/DG-mediated signals block the adenylate cyclase system in avian erythrocytes and Leydig cells, for instance. Also, both pathways potentiate each other in various cell types such as pinealocytes, pituitary and lacrymal gland cells.

These aspects of transmembrane signaling have been recently reviewed (6, 11).

PROTEIN KINASE C AS A TARGET FOR PHORBOL ESTERS

In 1982, we showed in a cooperative study with Nishizuka and co-workers, that phorbol esters directly activated protein kinase C in platelets as well as in the reconstituted system <u>in vitro</u> (7). Phorbol esters bind at nanomolar concentrations to the enzyme which turns out to be the previously characterized high-affinity binding site for these agents (12). Diacylglycerol competes with phorbol esters for the binding site. Thus, these tumor promoters usurp the place of second messenger diacylglycerol in the phosphoinositide pathway and, as a result, mimic the effects of physiological ligands.

It should be pointed out that phorbol-ester-mediated protein kinase C activation does not seem to require Ca^{2+}, as shown in <u>in vitro</u> (13) as well as <u>in vivo</u> experiments. The latter have been performed in platelets previously loaded with 100 uM quin 2, a potent Ca^{2+} chelator which lowers Ca^{2+} concentration to approximately 20 uM. Activation of protein kinase C in those cells by TPA was unaffected, as shown by the degree of phosphorylation of the 43 kDa protein, the major substrate of this enzyme in platelets (fig. 2).

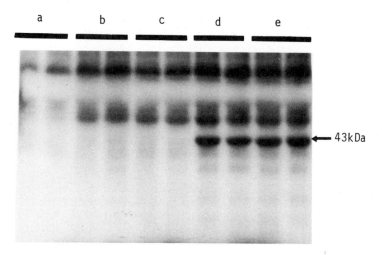

Fig.2 - <u>Autoradiogram of SDS-PAGE electrophoresis of platelet proteins.</u>
10^8 cells were washed and ^{32}P-labeled as described in ref.20, the incubated at 37°C for 20 min (left wells) or 40 min. (right wells) in a Ca^{2+}-free Tyrode solution containing 0.2 mM EGTA (lanes a), as well as 0.1 mM quin 2 (lanes b), 10 % DMSO (lanes c), 0.1 mM quin 2 + 0.1 µg ml^{-1} TPA (lanes d), or 10 % DMSO + 0.1 µg ml^{-1} TPA (lanes e). TPA was present in samples d and e during the last two min of the incubation.

The relationship between the potency of phorbol ester-related promoters to activate protein kinase C and their biological activity in animal models has been examined. A good correlation has been generally found between enzyme activation and tumor promotion with the exception of mezerein and phorbol retinoyl acetate (PRA), potent hyperplasiant and inflammatory agents, which are as potent as TPA in enzyme activation although having a weak tumor promoting action. These results emphasize that a tumor promoter appears to not be exclusively a cell proliferating agent. Similar discrepancy has already been reported between the effects of various protein kinase C activators. Indeed, the cell permeable dioctanoylglycerol and bryostatins, both potent activators of the enzyme, failed to mimic the long-term effects of phorbol ester TPA, such as induction of differentiation or tumor promotion (14, 15). Seemingly, protein kinase C activators and physiological ligands trigger quantitatively and qualitatively different protein kinase C-mediated responses which may be related to their specific properties, differing in several respects :
1 - the half-life of diacylglycerol is less than 1 min in platelet whereas phorbol esters such as TPA are slowly metabolized in the cells and are able to evoke a more sustained activation.

2 - protein kinase C activators acting at the enzyme step, bypass the upper part of the phosphoinositide pathway, subsequently these agents are unable to mobilize Ca^{2+} from internal stores the way physiological ligands can.

3 - it has been shown that phorbol esters can bypass some regulatory mechanisms which control the phosphoinositide pathway, as illustrated in platelets where cyclic nucleotides inhibit thrombin-mediated-but not phorbol-ester-mediated protein kinase C activation (16).

4 - phorbol esters are amphiphatic compounds which diffuse rapidly in all cellular compartments and as a consequence should evoke a different localization of protein kinase C compared to physiological ligands and other activators, thereby providing additional substrates to the enzyme. Moreover, the phorbol-ester-mediated alterations in membrane dynamic properties and increase in lipid microviscosity already reported (17), may also cause changes in the protein substrates surrounding the enzyme.

It is attractive to suggest that these distinctive features may account, at least partly, for the promoting action of phorbol esters.

IMPLICATION OF PROTEIN KINASE C IN TUMOR PROMOTION.

Although protein kinase C is presumably the exclusive target for tumor promoting phorbol esters, direct evidence for these agents exerting their promoting effects through activation of this enzyme is still missing.

Table I - <u>Promoting agents other than diterpene esters.</u>

Fatty acids
Fatty acid methyl esters
Surface-active agents
Cantharidin
Anthralin
Limonene and citrus oil
Undecane and other linear alkanes
Cigarette smoke condensate
Iodoacetic acid
1-Fluoro-2,4-dinitrobenzene
Flame retardants
Teleocidin and dihydroteleocidin B
Lyngbyatoxin A
Aplysiatoxin
Thapsigargin
Psoralen
Palytoxin
Phenobarbital
Benzoyl peroxide
Estrogens
Halogenated aromatics and aliphatics
Chloroform
Carbon tetrachloride
2,3,7,8-tetrachlorobenzo-p-dioxin
Bile acids
Saccharin and cyclamate
1,25 dihydroxyvitamin D3
dl-tryptophan and metabolites
Cyclophosphamide
Calculi
Wounding
Plastics
Asbestos

The potency of some promoters chemically unrelated to phorbol esters from the list included in Table I, to activate protein kinase C, has been examined by us and others. Promoters from the series of indol alkaloïds and polyacetates isolated by Sugimura and co-workers, such as teleocidin B, lyngbyatoxin A and aplysiatoxin, have been shown to be competitive inhibitors of phorbol ester binding and potently activate the enzyme. Several studies have also shown that unsaturated fatty acids directly activate the enzyme in vitro : the reaction not requiring phospholipid and Ca^{2+}. Similarly, we have shown that oleic acid is able to activate protein kinase C in intact platelets, the 43 kDa protein being used as an index of activity. For comparison purposes, the autoradiography of phosphoproteins from platelets treated with thrombin was displayed in fig. 3. Retinoic acid which suppresses the malignant phenotype of cultured cells, has also been associated with an increased risk of cancer in humans, as reviewed in ref. 18. It has been reported that retinoic acid activate protein kinase C, this reaction occurring in phospholipid-free conditions (19). Likewise, chloroform reveals as a potent activator of protein kinase C in in vitro and in vivo tests (20). Interesting by these drugs, do not compete for the phorbol ester binding site. At variance with fatty acids and retinoic acid, the reaction is greatly enhanced in the presence of phospholipids, although Ca^{2+} is not require for activation. Structurally related compounds, carbon tetrachloride and methylene chloride, similarly activate the enzyme. Benzene, which causes leukemia in humans and many cancers in laboratory animals, has been considered as having a promoting action. This drug evokes a protein kinase C activation which shares all the properties of that mediated by chloroform and derivatives (21).

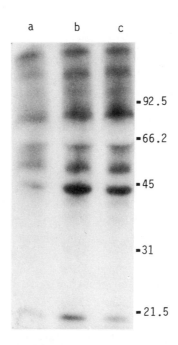

Fig.3 - Autoradiogram of SDS-PAGE electrophoresis of ^{32}P-labeled platelet proteins. Cells were stimulated for 1 min as described in ref. 20 by adding 0.5 % DMSO (a), one unit thrombin (b), or 200 µg ml^{-1} oleic acid.

In the same respect, we have recently investigated the effects of bile acids on protein kinase C activation. Epidemiological studies have shown a positive correlation between the risk of colon cancer and the levels of secondary bile acids in the feces. In addition, bile salts behave as tumor promoters in experimental colon carcinogenesis (22-24). Sodium deoxycholate at concentrations elicits protein kinase C activation in a phospholipid-free reaction. The dose-response curve of enzyme activation by sodium deoxycholate is given in fig. 4a. In addition, the effect of phosphatidylserine have been tested : at a concentration as low as 1.6 µg ml^{-1}, phosphatidylserine dramatically activates the

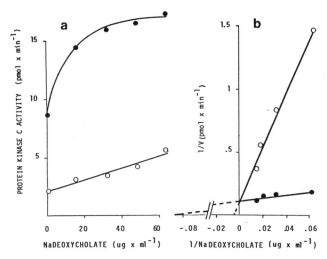

Fig.4 - <u>Protein kinase C activation by sodium deoxycholate</u> in the absence (○) or in the presence of 1.6 ug ml^{-1} phosphatidylserine (●). Rat brain protein kinase C was assayed as in (20) and expressed as pmol ml^{-1} (a). Reciprocal plot of protein kinase C activation as a function of sodium deoxycholate concentrations (b).

reaction (fig. 4a) and decreases the apparent Ka from 216 to 11 µg ml^{-1} (fig. 4b). In contrast, sodium deoxycholate at grading doses of phosphadidylserine does not affect the apparent Ka but markedly increases the Vmax. of the reaction (fig. 5). Sodium deoxycholate does not require Ca^{2+} for activity, since a similar response may be obtained in 0.5 mM EGTA (data not shown). A variety of bile salts have been tested for their effects on the enzyme. It appears that the order of potency is deoxycholate $\geqslant$ chenodeoxycholate $>$ taurodeoxycholate $>$ taurocholate $>$ cholate, as shown in Table II.

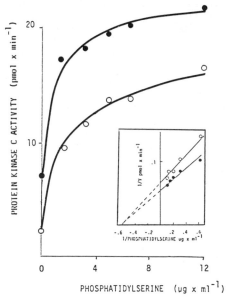

Fig.5 - <u>Protein kinase C activation by phosphatidylserine</u> in the absence (o) or in the presence of 78 ug ml⁻¹ sodium deoxycholate (●). Protein kinase C was assayed as in legend to fig. 4. Insert : Reciprocal plot of protein kinase C activation as a function of phosphatylserine concentrations.

Table II - Effects of various bile salts on Ca^{2+} or TPA-activated protein kinase C.

Bile salts[a]	$CaCl_2$ [b]		TPA[b]	
	pmol	% of controls	pmol	% of controls
Untreated	0.9	100	2.6	100
Cholate	1.2	133	4.2	162
Taurocholate	1.2	133	4.8	185
Chenodeoxycholate	2.3	256	4.9	188
Taurodeoxycholate	3.6	400	9.1	350
Deoxycholate	4.2	467	7.5	288

[a] Bile salts were added at the concentration of 100 μM.
[b] $CaCl_2$ was present at 0.5 mM and TPA at 100 ng ml⁻¹.

All together the presented results suggest that some structurally unrelated tumor promoters can activate protein kinase C with different requirements for phospholipid and Ca^{2+}, presumably through interaction at different sites of the molecule. It should be pointed out that protein kinase C is actually a family of isoforms which display different requirements for activation (25). It is attractive to suggest that the heterogenous distribution of these different forms may account for the tissue specificity of some tumor promoters. In contrast, we have shown that some well-characterized tumor promoters such as anthralin, tetrachlorodibenzodioxin, phenobarbital, estradiol, palytoxin, benzoyl peroxyde and 1,25-dihydroxyvitamin D3 do not activate the enzyme. However, the possibility that these promoters which are directly uneffective on protein kinase C activation may affect the phosphoinositide pathway upstream or downstream from the enzyme, is still to be explored.

COOPERATION BETWEEN INITIATORS AND PROMOTERS

The link between these two classes of agents responsible for two-stage carcinogenesis has gained some clarity. Over the past few years, this critical interrelation has become cooperation between oncogenes and promoters. Diethylnitrosamine and aflatoxin B_1, raise the expression of oncogenes in hepatocellular carcinoma (26). Likewise, activation of H-ras oncogenes in mammary carcinoma induced by N-methyl-N-nitrosurea (NMU) was due to a specific G-A transition, thereby providing evidence that NMU is directly responsible for mutations that activate ras gene in these cells. Balmain and co-workers have identified activated H-ras oncogene in pre-neoplastic skin papillomas initiated with dimethylbenzanthracene. Furthermore, these authors have transfected an activated ras gene into epidermal cells ; this introduction failed to complete the carcinogenic process unless TPA was applied. In addition, oncogene-induced transformation of various cell lines was enhanced by tumor promoters. Along the same line, it has been demonstrated that rat embryo fibroblasts containing ras oncogene became transformed by subsequent treatment with phorbol esters (as reviewed in 27).

It turns out that oncogene products and promoters share the same site of action since all the oncogene proteins, the function of which are known, belong to the signaling pathways. Sis gene specifies B chain of growth factor PDGF and gives rise to an autocrine cell stimulation. Erb B and fms are truncated forms of cell surface receptors for growth factors EGF and CSF-1, which elicit constitutive activity. Neu is a point-mutated cell surface receptor which encodes for an unknown ligand. It is predicted that crk oncogene encodes for phospholipase C (28). Moreover, as a result of transfection or microinjection experiments, it has been shown that the products of oncogenes ros, src, fos, fms, activate the basal rate of phosphoinositide breakdown. Ras product, presumably a G protein stimulating phospholipase C activity, displays an altered guanosine triphosphatase activity which normally stops ligand-mediated cell activation.

Protein kinase C and phorbol esters appear to controlled post-translationally some proto-oncogene products, such as c-fos and c-K-ras (29, 30). The enzyme and its potent activators rapidly alter gene expression. A program of gene expression similar to that induced by growth factor PDGF or transforming genes, was reported (31). Some inducible genes have been characterized including some nuclear proto-oncogenes c-fos, c-myc and presumably c-jun. A feedback loop limiting proliferation was suggested since IP_3/DG pathway activation leads to an elevated expression of growth inhibitors such as transforming growth factor ß and interferon ß-2 (33).

At present, the most important issue is to understand how extracellular messengers control the transcriptional machinery. Multiple trans acting regulatory proteins recognize cell type specific-enhancers elements. It is of interest that phorbol esters enhance the expression of transcription factor AP1 encoded by proto-oncogene c-jun which interacts with TPA-inducible enhancer elements (34). Furthermore, it is worth pointing out that erbA oncogene encodes for the thyroïd hormone receptor which presents large homologies with a family of transcription factors which are receptors for progesterone and glucocorticoïds as well as dihydroxyvitamin D3, estradiol, tetrachlorodibenzodioxin and retinoic acid (35).

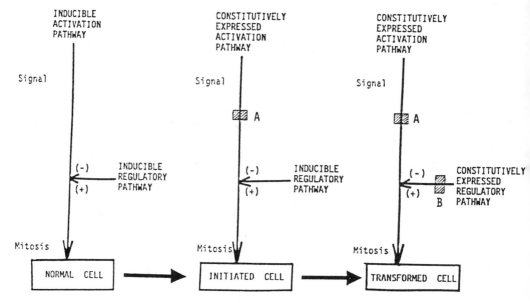

Fig.6 - <u>A proposed model for conversion of reversible to irreversible and uncontrolled cell activation.</u> A and B are constitutively expressed or repressed proto-oncogene proteins.

CONCLUSION

Two subversive mechanisms affecting signaling pathways appear to play a major role in transformation. First, the constitutive expression of a growth factor gene in a cell that synthesizes its receptor generates an autocrine stimulation. Second, genetic alterations in oncogenes generate truncated proteins which induce a persistent activation of the signaling pathway leading to cell proliferation.

Oncogene proteins contribute to the constitutive activation of the signaling pathways. A naive model for conversion of reversible (inducible) to irreversible (constitutive) cell activation is presented in fig. 6. At the initiated stage one protein is constitutively expressed (or repressed), but the pathway remains under positive or negative control. At variance at the transformed stage an additional protein of the regulatory pathways is constitutively expressed (or repressed), and then, the cell becomes irreversibly activated. It can be hypothesized that tumor promoters favor the second genetic event which "awakens" the initiated cell. It may be reasonably assumed that this second event depends greatly on the nature of the first genetic event, the cell phenotype and the applied tumor promoter.

It should be emphasized that phorbol esters alter the pattern of phosphorylated substrates of protein kinase C in a qualitatively and quantitatively different manner than the enzyme activators devoid of promoting effects. Taking into account the fact that the carcinogenic process takes months in laboratory animals and years in man to be completed, it may be further anticipated that protein kinase C activity, depending on the cell phenotype, may qualitatively differ in relation to the time of exposure to tumor promoters when the cell progresses to transformation.

It may be assumed that a better understanding of the physiology of the signaling pathways from the cell surface to the nucleus and their regulation in a specific target cell, will contribute to elucidate the functions of proto-oncogene proteins and the large variety of mysfunctions which lead to cell transformation.

Acknowledgments   This work has been supported by the Ligue Nationale Française contre le Cancer. The authors want to thank Mme Maillot for her excellent technical assistance.

REFERENCES

1 - Berenblum, I., 1941, The cocarcinogenic actions of croton resin.
       Cancer Res., 1 : 44.
2 - Mottram J.C., 1944, A developing factor in developing blastogenesis.
       J. Pathol. Bacteriol., 56 : 181.
3 - Kennedy A.R., Cairns, J. and Little, J.B., 1984, Timing of the steps
       in transformation of C3H-10T1/2 cells by X-irradiation.
       Nature, 307 : 85.
4 - Land, H., Parada, I.F. and Weinberg, R.A., 1983, Tumorigenic
       conversion of primary embryo fibroblasts requires at least two
       cooperating oncogenes.
       Nature, 304 : 596.
5 - Boutwell, R.K., 1974, The function and mechanism of promoters of
       carcinogenesis.
       C.R.C. Crit. Rev. Toxicol., 2 : 419.
6 - Castagna, M., 1987, Phorbol esters as signal transducers and tumor
       promoters.
       Biology of the Cell, 59 : 3.
7 - Castagna, M., Takai, Y., Kaibuchi, K., Sano, K., Kikkawa, U. and
       Nishizuka, Y., 1982, Direct activation of calcium-activated,
       phospholipid-dependent protein kinase by tumor promoting phorbol
       esters.
       J. Biol. Chem., 257 : 7847.
8 - Aschendel, C.I., Staller, J.M. and Boutwell, R.K., 1983, Identifi-
       cation of a calcium and phospholipid-dependent phorbol ester binding
       activity in the soluble fraction.
       Biochem. Biophys. Res. Commun., 111 : 340.
9 - Kraft, A.S. and Anderson, W.B., 1983, Phorbol esters increase the
       amount of Ca^{2+}, phospholipid-dependent protein kinase associated
       with plasma membrane.
       Nature, 305 : 621.
10 - Niedel, J.E., Kuhn, L.J. and Vandenbark, G.R., 1983, Phorbol diester
       receptor copurifies with protein kinase C.
       Proc. Natl. Acad. Sci. USA, 80 : 36.
11 - Nishizuka, Y., 1986, Studies and perspectives of protein kinase C.
       Science, 233 : 305.
12 - Driedger P. and Blumberg, P.M., 1980, Specific binding of phorbol
       ester tumor promoters.
       Proc. Natl. Acad. Sci. USA, 77 : 567.
13 - Couturier, A., Bazgar, S. and Castagna, M., 1984, Further
       characterization of tumor promoter-mediated activation of protein
       kinase C.
       Biochem. Biophys. Res. Commun., 121 : 448.
14 - Kreutter, D., Caldwell, A.,B. and Morin, M.J., 1985, Dissociation
       of protein kinase C activation from phorbol ester-induced
       maturation of HL60 leukemia cells.
       J. Biol. Chem., 260 : 5977.

15 - Kraft, A.S., Smith, J.B. and Berkov, R.I., 1986, Bryostatin an
     activator of the calcium phospholipid-dependent protein kinase,
     blocks phorbol ester-induced differenciation of human promyelocytic
     leukemia cells HL60.
          Proc. Natl. Acad. Sci., USA, 83 : 1334.
16 - Yamanishi, J., Takai, Y., Kaibuchi, K., Sano, K., Castagna, M. and
     Nishizuka, Y., 1983, Synergistic functions of phorbol ester and
     calcium in serotonin release.
          Biochem. Biophys. Res. Commun., 112 : 778.
17 - Castagna, M.,Rochette-Egly, C., Rosenfeld, C. and Mishal, Z., 1979,
     Altered lipid microviscosity in lymphoblastoid cells treated with
     12-O-tetradecanoyl phorbol 13-acetate, a tumor promoter.
          Febs lett., 100 : 62.
18 - Paganini-Hill, A., Chao, A., Ross, R.K. and Henderson, B.E., 1987,
     Vitamin A, ß-carotene, and the risk of cancer : A prospective
     study.
          J. Natl. Cancer Inst., 79 : 443.
19 - Ohkubo, S., Yamada, E., Endo, R., Itoh, H. and Hidaka, H., 1984,
     Vitamin A acid induced activation of Ca^{2+}-activated, phospholipid
     dependent protein kinase from rabbit retina.
          Biochem. Biophys. Res. Commun., 118 : 460.
20 - Roghani, M., Da Silva, C. and Castagna, M., 1987, Tumor promoter
     chloroform is a potent protein kinase C activator.
          Biochem. Biophys. Res. Commun., 142 : 738.
21 - Roghani, M., Da Silva, C., Guvelli, D. and Castagna, M., 1987,
     Benzene and toluene activate protein kinase C.
          Carcinogenesis, 8 : 1105.
22 - Reddy, B.S. and Wynder, E.L., 1973, Large lowel carcinogenesis :
     fecal constituants of populations with diverse incidence rates of
     colon cancer.
          J. Natl. Cancer Inst., 50 : 1437.
23 - Narisawa, RT., Magadia, N.E., Weisburger, J.H. and Wynder, E.L.,
     1974, Promoting effects of bile acids on colon carcinogenesis after
     intrarectal instillation of N-methyl-N-nitrosoguanidine in rats.
          J. Natl. Cancer Inst., 53 : 1093.
24 - Kaibara, N., Yurugi, E. and Koga, S., 1984, Promoting effect of bile
     acids on the chemical transformation of C3H 10T1/2 fibroblasts
     in vivo.
          Cancer Res., 44 : 5482.
25 - Ono, Y., Fujii, T., Ogita, K., Kikkawa, U., Igarashi, K. and
     Nishizuka, Y., 1988, The structure, expression and properties of
     additional members of the protein kinase C family.
          J. Biol. Chem., 263 : 6927.
26 - Tashiro, F., Morimura, S., Hayashi, K., Makino, R., Kawamura, H.,
     Horikoshi, N., Nemoto, K., Ohtsubo, K., Sugimura, R. and Ueno, Y.,
     1986, Expression of the c-Ha-ras and c-myc genes in aflatoxin B1-
     induced hepatocellular carcinomas.
          Biochem. Biophys. Res. Commun., 138 : 858.
27 - Barbacid, M., 1986, Oncogenes and human cancer; cause or conseqence?
          Carcinogenesis, 7 : 1037.
28 - Mayer, B.J., Hamaguchi, M. and Hanafusa, H., 1988, A novel viral
     oncogene with structural similarity to phospholipase C.
          Nature, 332 : 272.
29 - Ballester, R., Furth, M.E. and Rosen, O.M., 1987, Phorbol ester and
     protein kinase C-mediated phosphorylation of the cellular Kirsten
     ras gene product.
          J. Biol. Chem., 262 : 2688.
30 - Barber, J.R. and Verma, I.M., 1987, Modification of fos proteins :
     phosphorylation of c-fos, but not v-fos, is stimulated by 12-tetra-
     decanoylphorbol 13-acetate and serum.
          Mol. Cell. Biol., 7 : 2201.

31 - Rabin, M.S., Doherty, P.J. and Gottesman, M.M., 1986, The tumor
     promoter phorbol 12-myristate 13-acetate induces a program of
     altered gene expression similar to that induced by platelet-derived
     growth factor and transforming oncogenes.
         Proc. Natl. Acad. Sci., USA, 83 : 357.
32 - Varmus, H.E., 1987, Oncogenes and transcriptional control.
         Science, 238 : 1337.
33 - Sehgal, P.B., Walther, Z. and Tamm, I., 1987, Rapid enhancement of
     ß2-interferon/B-cell differentiation factor BSF-2 gene expression
     in human fibroblasts by diacylglycerols and the calcium ionophore
     A23187.
         Proc. Natl. Acad. Sci., USA, 84 : 3663.
34 - Lef, W., Mitchell, P. and Tjian, R., 1987, Purified transcription
     factor AP-1 interacts with TPA-inducible enhancer elements.
         Cell, 49 : 741.
35 - Petkovich, M., Brand, N.J., Krust, A. and Chambon, P., 1987, A human
     retinoic receptor which belongs to the family of nuclear receptors.
         Nature, 330 : 444.

HEPATOCARCINOGENESIS BY NON-GENOTOXIC COMPOUNDS

R. Schulte-Hermann, W. Parzefall, W. Bursch, and
I. Timmermann-Trosiener

Institute of Tumorbiology-Cancer Research
University of Vienna, Borschkegasse 8a
A - 1090 Vienna

Abstract

Many compounds have been found to produce liver tumors after long-term treatment of experimental animals, mostly rodents, without exhibiting detectable genotoxic activity or potential. These agents include phenobarbital, certain estrogens and progestins, hypolipidemic and other drugs as well as environmental pollutants such as DDT, hexachloro-cyclohexane, phthalate plasticizers etc. After short-term treatment the agents induce liver growth and increases of certain enzymes which probably represents enhanced expression of specific gene programs. Mechanisms involved include stimulation of cell proliferation and inhibition of cell death (apoptosis).

In addition to negative tests for genotoxicity these agents generally are also negative when assayed for tumor initiating activity in the liver; however, many but not all compounds show tumor promoting activity. Tumor promotion may be due to overexpression of gene programs in initiated/preneoplastic cells in the liver; inhibition of death of preneoplastic cells by promoters seems to cause rapid growth of preneo-plastic lesions. Possible implications for risk assessment are discussed.

INTRODUCTION

Non-genotoxic carcinogens produce tumors without exhibiting detectable genotoxic activity or potential as would be identified as mutation at the level of the gene, chromosome or genome, as chemical alteration of the DNA, as induction of DNA repair etc. In a variety of organs, mostly in animal experiments, tumors were found to form during treatment with non-genotoxic carcinogens; most frequently the liver appears to be involved (Schulte-Hermann, 1985). Several mechanisms can be considered through which non-genotoxic carcinogens could lead to tumor formation. Some are listed in Table 1. It is obvious that the mechanisms possibly involved may be quite heterogeneous. Their elucidation will be crucial for a reliable risk assessment. Below some aspects relevant to mechanisms and risk evaluation of non-genotoxic liver carcinogens will be presented.

Table 1. Some mechanisms through which non-genotoxic compounds may lead to tumor formation

1) Initiation through undetected genotoxic effects
2) Initiation through indirect genotoxic effects (e.g. errors during cell replication, oxygen radical formation)
3) Initiation through non-genotoxic ("epigenetic") mechanisms
4) Promotion of initiated or preneoplastic cells that occur "spontaneously"
5) Induction of progression of preneoplastic cells that occur "spontaneously"

Table 2. Some liver tumor promoters and their acute effects on the liver (see Schulte-Hermann 1985 for references)

Class	Growth	Induction of enzymes/proteins
1) Phenobarbital (PB) Hexachlorocyclohexane (HCH)	+	P_{450}-PB, "phase II" enzymes
2) TCDD	+	P_{450}-MC, "phase II" enzymes
3) Progesterone Cyproterone acetate	+	P_{450}-PCN, "phase II" enzymes
4) Estradiol esters Ethinylestradiol	+	– blood clotting factors, angiotensinogen
5) Clofibrate Diethylhexyl-phthalate	+	P_{450}-clof, peroxisomal enzymes
6) CCl$_4$	+	

RESULTS AND DISCUSSION

I. Effects of non-genotoxic carcinogens on normal liver

Short-term effects of non-genotoxic carcinogens in normal liver may provide a clue for the elucidation of the mechanisms of action of these agents. We have therefore studied these effects in some detail.

Examples of non-genotoxic liver carcinogens active on experimental animals are provided in Table 2. According to their acute effects on the liver they have been grouped into 6 different classes. Class 1 to 5 includes drugs, environmental pollutants and hormones which produce no signs of major cytotoxicity in the liver but induce a variety of presumably adaptive responses as indicated by the increases in specific functions and in growth. Group 6 exemplifies cytotoxic agents which cause regenerative hyperplasia in the

liver. Thus, all of the agents listed, although exhibiting divergent effects on hepatic functions, share the ability to induce liver growth and/or hepatocyte proliferation.
Studies by ourselves and other groups on liver growth induced by compounds of class 1 to 5 have yielded the following results:

1) Liver enlargement reflects a true growth response as indicated by proportional increases of the main cell constituents protein, RNA, lipid, glycogen, and water (Schulte-Hermann, 1974; Kunz et al., 1966; Argyris and Magnus, 1968).

2) Enhanced cell multiplication is indicated by increases in DNA synthesis and mitosis. The total DNA content of the organ usually is enhanced, the increase may be relatively less or more (as shown recently for estrogens) than that of total liver mass. In rat liver no change in cellular ploidy was found, while mouse liver may exhibit considerable increases in cellular ploidy. In both species binuclearity decreases, while nuclear ploidy increases (Schulte-Hermann, 1974; Kunz et al., 1966; Argyris and Magnus, 1968; Schulte-Hermann et al., 1980).

3) The growth response is dose-dependent and self limited. Active liver growth and cell multiplication are restricted to the early phase of treatment with an inducer. During prolonged action of a growth stimulus liver size and DNA are maintained at an enhanced level, and the rate of cell proliferation returns to normal. Obviously an effective feedback mechanism inhibits steady growth and counterbalances mitogenic activities of the compounds (Schulte-Hermann, 1974; Argyris and Magnus, 1968; Schulte-Hermann and Schmitz, 1980).

4) Liver enlargement is reversible following elimination of inducer. The hyperplasia may also be rapidly reversible if mitogens of sufficiently short biological halflife were used for induction of liver growth. Regression of hyperplasia appears to be effected by cell death through apoptosis (see below) (Schulte-Hermann, 1974; Bursch et al., 1986).

5) The role of cell death in the control of cell number in the liver has recently been studied in detail by our group. The type and mechanisms of cell death involved appears to differ from the well known necrosis as occuring after CCl_4 or severe hypoxia, but rather resembles forms of cell death in excessive tissues e.g. during ontogenesis in interdigit webs, during insect metamorphosis, or in endocrine dependent organs. Recently the term apoptosis has been proposed (Wyllie et al., 1980). Apoptosis exhibits a sequence of characteristic morphologic stages (Wyllie et al., 1980; Bursch et al., 1985). In the liver it can be inhibited by hepatomitogens and by feeding (Bursch et al., 1985; Schulte-Hermann et al., 1988). Apoptosis is a rapid process; its morphological signs disappear from liver tissue with a halflife of about 2 hours. The incidence of apoptosis is very low in normal liver (less than 1 per 1000 hepatocytes) but increases dramatically during severe starvation or during regression of mitogen induced hyper-

plasia (up to 6 per 100 hepatocytes) (Schulte-Hermann et al., 1988). The remainders of cells dying through apoptosis are phagocytosed by intact hepatocytes and Kupffer cells. The enzyme transglutaminase appears to be expressed in apoptotic hepatocytes; this can possibly be of use as a marker of apoptosis. The results of these studies have been published in detail elsewhere (Bursch et al., 1985; Schulte-Hermann et al., 1988).

In summary the non-genotoxic hepatocarcinogens are either hormones or have hormone-like effects on the liver in that they induce a balanced growth response associated with increases in specific hepatic functions. They trigger the expression of certain gene programmes in the liver.

II. Effects of non-genotoxic carcinogens on tumor development and on putative preneoplastic foci in the liver

As first shown by Peraino and later confirmed and extended by various other groups most of the compounds shown in table 2 accelerate the development of liver tumors in animals previously exposed to a brief or even a single treatment with an initiating carcinogen (Schulte-Hermann, 1985; Peraino et al., 1971; Moore and Kitagawa, 1986). It is therefore now generally accepted that the respective agents have tumor promoting activity in the liver - with the exception of class 5 compounds (peroxisome proliferators) with which experimental evidence of tumor-promoting activity is still equivocal (see below). For the other compounds the promotion concept was greatly supported by finding enhancement of the growth rate of putative preneoplastic liver foci. To investigate the mechanisms underlying this effect we have used two model compounds, namely phenobarbital (PB) and alpha-hexachlorocyclohexane (alpha-HCH), to study cell proliferation and cell death as well as phenotypes of these foci.

We induced formation of foci by single doses of diethyl-nitrosamine or N-nitrosomorpholine to young adult rats. Cell proliferation in foci and in surrounding liver was measured by ^{3}H-thymidine autoradiography and by mitotic counts. It was found that the foci exhibited enhanced rates of proliferation at all stages investigated and even when they first became detectable in the liver by a positive gamma-glutamyl-transferase reaction and/or by clearness of cytoplasm, namely 3 weeks after initiation, i.e. at a very early stage of development (Schulte-Hermann et al., 1981).

Single doses of non-genotoxic carcinogens further increased the already enhanced levels of proliferative activity in foci (Schulte-Hermann et al., 1981). However, somewhat unexpectedly this additional increment largely disappeared during prolonged treatment and during continuous administration of the promoters little or no enhancement of cell proliferation in foci over the basal level was observed (Schulte-Hermann et al., 1982). These findings suggested that not only cell proliferation determines the rate of foci growth. Consequently we studied cell death in foci and indeed found evidence of frequent apoptosis in liver foci of rats not treated with a promoter. Administration of PB decreased the incidence of apoptosis, withdrawal of PB led to a dramatic increase and retreatment decreased apoptosis again (Bursch et al., 1984). These results led to the following conclusions:

1) Under our experimental conditions foci cells appear to have a shorter life span than normal liver cells. This partially counterbalances the enhanced proliferative activity of early foci so that little net growth of foci occurs in the absence of promotion.

2) Tumor promoters, by inhibiting apoptosis in foci, can accelerate foci growth in the absence of an additional enhancement of cell proliferation.

3) Apoptosis may allow the liver to eliminate initiated or preneoplastic cells. This may constitute one of the organism's defense lines against cancer development. Tumor promoters may interfere with this protective mechanism.

Apoptosis has also been observed in liver tumors. Furthermore we observed apoptosis in an estrogen-dependent hamster kidney tumor demonstrating that the phenomenon is not restricted to carcinogenesis in the liver. Remarkably also in this hamster kidney tumor the incidence of apoptosis seemed to increase after withdrawal of the growth stimulus diethylstilbestrol (a synthetic estrogen), and to decrease dramatically after retreatment with this agent. Mitotic activity showed the opposite behaviour (Bursch et al., 1988).

These findings show that the effects of non-genotoxic carcinogens on cell proliferation and cell death must be taken into account in attempts to elucidate their mechanism of action. However, other actions may also be important.

Not all non-genotoxic liver carcinogens promote growth of putative preneoplastic foci in rat liver, at least not of the type mentioned so far. Peroxisome proliferators are one of the important exceptions. Even though all of these compounds are potent liver mitogens their promoting activity has not (yet) been convincingly demonstrated (Schulte-Hermann, 1985; Stäubli et al., 1984; Reddy and Lalwai, 1983). Thus, a hepatomitogenic activity seems to be a necessary but not sufficient property for tumor promotion in the liver. Analogous findings have previously been reported for skin.

Therefore something else in addition to mitogenesis appears to be required for tumor promotion in the liver, and it is suggested that induction of specific gene programs is required. In fact, it appears that the putative preneoplastic foci studied so far are committed for overexpression of that gene program (or a closely related one) inducible in normal liver by PB (Schulte-Hermann, 1985; Schulte-Hermann et al., 1986). The same program is not induced and even repressed partially by peroxisome proliferators, and this might provide a clue to understand the failure to promote foci growth. Furthermore, some findings suggest existence of another type of foci with a different commitment, and these might be promotable by peroxisome inducers (Schröter et al., 1985); this hypothesis still requires further experimental support.

In conclusion many tumor promoters are hormones or have hormone-like mechanisms of action in that they induce or reinforce expression of specific phenotypic differentiation programs.

How can promoters alone produce liver tumors? As mentioned in table 1, one possible mechanism is promotion of spontaneously appearing preneoplastic foci. In fact various groups of workers have reported the occurence of such foci in the liver of animals never exposed to experimental carcinogenic challenges. The incidence of "spontaneous" foci increases with age, being 100% in rats 2 years old in one study. These foci have been found to be promotable by PB and other promoters (Schulte-Hermann, 1985; Ward, 1983; Schulte-Hermann et al., 1983).

III. Some aspects relevant to risk assessment

The findings described above suggest that the carcinogenicity of promoting compounds may depend on the presence or absence of initiated or preneoplastic cells in the target tissue. Thus the question relevant for risk assessment of tumor promoters in humans may be: Do foci develop "spontaneously" in humans as they apparently do in the rat? When do they develop, and how many may be formed? Unfortunately, these questions have found little attention so far.

Furthermore the findings illustrate the limited reliability of the long term carcinogenicity bioassay of chemical compounds. These bioassays do not discriminate between initiating and promoting properties of a test agent. Tumor promoting activity would not be detected in the absence of initiating activity or of initiated cells in the target tissue. On the other hand a pure promoter would be classified as a complete (initiating) carcinogen when initiating cells develop spontaneously. Therefore tests for initiating and promoting activity may be required for correct interpretation of results of long-term carcinogenicity studies.

One such test uses formation or growth of liver foci in rats as an endpoint to detect either initiating or promoting activity in a discriminating way. In addition this test allows a quantitative estimation of the promoting activity of a test compound. The test has proven useful in recent years. In Germany it has recently been used to check the present limit values of hexachlorocyclohexane isomers in milk and other food (Schröter et al., 1987).

Another important result of the studies presented above is the high correlation between induction of liver growth and hepatocarcinogenic potential of non-genotoxic agents. Tests for induction of liver growth may therefore be used to predict carcinogenic activity or potential in this class of compounds. Pertinent information can be obtained during routine toxicological testing, i.e. during the first animal experiments with a new compound.

As an example we have recently studied induction of liver growth by a series of 16 different steroids. Generally a good correlation with tumor promoting or carcinogenic potential was found. Among the agents tested estradiol and ethinyl estradiol were the most effective inducers of liver growth with an extrapolated threshold in the range of 1 ug/kg body weight (Ochs et al., 1986; Schulte-Hermann et al., 1988). With these agents induction of liver growth therefore appears by far more sensitive than other tumor related parameters such as DNA or protein binding.

Induction of cell growth, of DNA synthesis and of mitosis are endpoints accessible in vitro. Recent studies suggest that isolated hepatocytes from animals or humans can soon be used to identify potential promoters by means of induction of DNA synthesis (Parzefall et al., 1985; Bieri et al., 1984; Parzefall et al., 1988).

Finally, risk assessment of carcinogenic compounds is still largely based on the assumption of non-existence of a threshold. Hypothetically, a single molecule of a genotoxic compound could damage a critical gene and thereby lead to initiation; furthermore, dose-time-response studies with genotoxic carcinogens (Druckrey, 1967) favor the no-threshold concept. No such evidence exists in the case of non-genotoxic carcinogens. In contrast, in a number of cases alternative concepts have been well supported by experimental evidence, and the apparent hormonal or hormone-like mechanism of action of tumor promoters suggests that a threshold dose for promotion may well exist.

REFERENCES

Argyris, T.S., Magnus, D.R., 1968, The stimulation of liver growth and demethylase activity following phenobarbital treatment. Dev. Biol. 17:187.
Bieri, F., Bentley, P., Waechter, F., Stäubli, W., 1984, Use of primary cultures of adult rat hepatocytes to investigate mechanisms of action of nafenopin, a hepatocarcinogenic peroxisome proliferator. Carcinogenesis 5:1033.
Bursch, W., Düsterberg, B., Schulte-Hermann, R., 1986, Growth, regression and cell death in rat liver as related to tissue levels of the hepatomitogen cyproterone acetate. Arch. Toxicol. 59:221.
Bursch, W., Lauer, B,. Timmermann-Trosiener, I., Barthel, G., Schuppler, J., Schulte-Hermann, R., 1984, Controlled death (Apoptosis) of normal and putative preneoplastic cells in rat liver following withdrawal of tumor promoters. Carcinogenesis 5:453.
Bursch, W., Liehr, J., Sirbasku, D., Schulte-Hermann, R., 1988, Role of cell death for growth and regression of hormone-dependent H-301 hamster kidney tumors. in: "Chemical Carcinogenesis: Models and Mechanisms", F. Feo, P. Pani, A. Columbano, R. Garcea (eds.), Plenum press, in press.
Bursch, W., Taper, H.S., Lauer, B., Schulte-Hermann, R., 1985, Quantitative histological and histochemical studies on the occurrence and stages of controlled cell death (apoptosis) during regression of rat liver hyperplasia. Virch. Arch. Cell Pathol. 50:153.

Druckrey, H., 1967, Quantitative aspects in chemical carcinogenesis. UICC Monogr. 7:60.

Kunz, W., Schaude, G., Schmid, W., Siess, M., 1966, Leber-vergrößerung durch Fremdstoffe. Naunyn-Schmiedeberg's Arch. Pharmak. exp. Path. 254:470.

Moore, M.A., Kitagawa, T., 1986, Hepatocarcinogenesis in the rat: the effect of promoters and carcinogens in vivo and in vitro. Int. Rev. Cytol. 101:125.

Ochs, H., Düsterberg, B., Günzel, P., Schulte-Hermann, R., 1986, Effect of tumor promoting contraceptive steroids on growth and drug metabolizing enzymes in rat liver. Cancer Res. 46:1224.

Parzefall, W., Galle, P.R., Schulte-Hermann, R., 1985, Effect of calf and rat serum on the induction of DNA synthesis and mitosis in primary cultures of adult rat hepatocytes by cyproterone acetate and epidermal growth factor. In Vitro Cell. & Developmental Biology 21:665.

Parzefall, W., Monschau, P., Schulte-Hermann, R., 1988, Induction by cyproterone acetate of DNA synthesis and mitosis in primary cultures of adult rat hepatocytes in serum free medium. Biochem. Biophys. Res. Comm., submitted. Peraino, C., Fry, R.J.M., Staffeldt, E., 1971, Reduction and enhancement by phenobarbital of hepatocarcinogenesis induced in the rat by 2-acetylaminofluorene. Cancer Res. 31:1506.

Reddy, J.K., Lalwai, N.D., 1983, Carcinogenesis by hepatic peroxisome proliferators: Evaluation of the risk of hypolilpidemic drugs and industrial plasticizers to humans. Crit. Rev. Toxicol. 12:1.

Schröter, H., Gerbracht, U., Schulte-Hermann, R., Effects of hypolipidemic agents on 2 different types of putative preneoplastic foci in rat liver. Naunyn Schmiedeberg's Arch. of Pharmacol. 329:26 (1985).

Schröter, C., Parzefall, W., Schröter, H., Schulte-Hermann, R., 1987, Dose-response studies on the effects of a-, β- and g-hexachlorocyclohexane on putative preneoplastic foci, monooxygenases, and growth in rat liver. Cancer Res. 47:80.

Schulte-Hermann, R., 1974, Induction of liver growth by xenobiotic compounds and other stimuli. Crit. Rev. Toxicol. 3:97.

Schulte-Hermann, R., 1985, Tumor promotion in the liver, Arch. Toxicol. 57:147.

Schulte-Hermann, R., Bursch, W., Fesus, L., Kraupp, B., 1988, Cell death by apoptosis in normal, preneoplastic and neoplastic tissue. in: "Chemical Carcinogenesis: Models and Mechanisms", F. Feo, P. Pani, A. Columbano, R. Garcea, eds., Plenum Press, in press.

Schulte-Hermann, R., Schmitz, E., 1980, Feedback inhibition of hepatic DNA synthesis. Cell Tissue Kinet. 13:371.

Schulte-Hermann, R., Timmermann-Trosiener, I., Schuppler, J., 1982, Response of liver foci in rats to hepatic tumor promoters. Toxicol. Pathol. 10:63.

Schulte-Hermann, R., Timmermann-Trosiener, I., Schuppler, J., 1983, Promotion of spontaneous preneoplastic cells in rat liver as a possible explanation of tumor production by non-mutagenic compounds. Cancer Res. 43:839.

Schulte-Hermann, R., Timmermann-Trosiener, I., Schuppler, J., 1986, Facilitated expression of adaptive responses to phenobarbital in putative pre-stages of liver cancer. Carcinogenesis 7:1651.

Schulte-Hermann, R., Ochs, H., Bursch, W., Parzefall, W., 1988, Quantitative structure-activity studies on effects of sixteen different steroids on growth and monooxygenases of rat liver. Cancer Res. 48:2462.

Schulte-Hermann, R., Ohde, G., Schuppler, J., Timmermann-Trosiener, I., 1981, Enhanced proliferation of putative preneoplastic cells in rat liver following treatment with the tumor promoters phenobarbital, hexachlorocyclohexane, steroid compounds and nafenopin. Cancer Res. 41:2556.

Schulte-Hermann, R., Hoffmann, V., Landgraf, H., 1980, Adaptive responses of rat liver to the gestagen and anti-androgen cyproterone acetate and other inducers. III. Cytological changes. Chem.-Biol. Interactions 31:301.

Stäubli, W., Bentley, P., Bieri, F., Fröhlich, E., Waechter, F., 1984, Inhibitory effect of nafenopin upon the development of diethylnitrosamine-induced enzyme-altered foci within the rat liver. Carcinogenesis 5:41.

Ward, J.M., 1983, Increased susceptibility of livers of aged F344/NCr rats to the effects of phenobarbital on the incidence, morphology, and histochemistry of hepatocellular foci and neoplasms. J. Natl. Cancer Inst. 71:815.

Wyllie, A.H., Kerr, J.F.R., Currie, A.R., 1980, Cell death: the significance of apoptosis. Int. Rev. Cytol. 68:251.

THE ROLE OF INHIBITED INTERCELLULAR COMMUNICATION IN CARCINOGENESIS:

IMPLICATIONS FOR RISK ASSESSMENT FROM EXPOSURE TO CHEMICALS*

J.E. Trosko and C.C. Chang

Michigan State University

East Lansing, Michigan 48824

Introduction: A Crisis in Paradigms

With the reality that humans cannot live without chemicals and that the number of new chemicals to which we are exposed is increasing, the justified concern over the potential harm of any one or mixture of these chemicals to human health is also growing every day (Steering Committee, 1984). In addition, the harsh reality is that these chemicals cannot all be tested, in an absolute fashion, for their potential toxicity as an acute toxicant, teratogen, carcinogen, neuro- or reproductive toxicant. Constraints, such as (a) our lack of basic understanding of the mechanisms by which chemicals might lead to various toxic endpoints; (b) the reliance on short-term assays and animal model surrogates for human exposure; (c) limited resources (human, financial, technical) to perform the toxicological tests; and (d) imprecise ability due to species, genetic, developmental stage, sex and nutritional/occupational/ environmental background, to extrapolate from short-term test or animal bioassay results to the unique individual human situation, put great uncertainties in any risk assessment process.

In recent years, concern over this major problem has led to an accelerated attention to, and development of, concepts, techniques and strategies to attack this problem. Among the massive research activity in the fields of toxicology stimulated by this concern, the introduction of the concepts of "carcinogenesis as mutagenesis" (Ames et al., 1973) and of "genotoxicity" (Ehrenberg et al., 1973) has to be viewed as the major spark that ignited the energies of many scientists for the last fifteen years.

The paradigm that mutagens can induce cancers has, in our opinion, paralyzed our ability to develop a understanding of the process of carcinogenesis and of the practical issue of risk assessment after exposure to chemical agents (Trosko and Chang, in press). From experimental studies, _in vitro_ and _in vivo_, and from genetic predispositions to human cancer, it is obvious that mutations (genes and chromosomal) can play a role in carcinogenesis (Trosko et al., 1985). However, equally obvious is the realization that (a) not all toxic chemicals are mutagenic and (b) carcinogenesis is _more_ than mutagenesis (Trosko, in press; Trosko, 1984). It is this fact that we believe has been glaringly neglected in the design of the NTP bioassay protocol to test chemicals for their carcinogenic potential, in the design and interpretation of short-term assays, and the interpretation of results testing the concordance of the short-term results to the bioassay results (Trosko, in press).

The basis for our opinion can be illustrated by the recent evaluation of the results of the National Toxicology Program to test the mutagenicity/carcinogenicity of 300 chemicals (Tennant et al., 1987). Three of the "most potent carcinogens produced no genetic toxicity in any of the four short-term tests studied" (Tennant et al., 1987). The question is "Why?"

Carcinogenesis: A Multistep Process Involving Both Mutagenic and Epigenetic Processes

Carcinogenesis has been viewed, in both experimental animal studies and during the clinical course of tumor development in human beings, to consist of multiple and distinct phases (Fialkow, 1974; Foulds, 1975; Cairns, 1975). Conceptually, these stages have been classified as initiation/promotion/progression (Boutwell, 1974; Pitot et al., 1981; Weinstein et al., 1984). Although these operational concepts, derived from whole animal studies, do not specify any particular mechanism, it appears that the underlying cellular and molecular mechanisms of initiation and promotion are very different (Trosko and Chang, 1983; Trosko et al., 1983; Trosko and Chang, 1985).

Because initiation, by operational definition, is an irreversible event, and because many known mutagens are good initiators, it has been postulated that mutagenesis is the cellular basis for initiation (Trosko and Chang, 1978). On the other hand, promotion appears to be an interruptible or reversible process in its early phase. Because agents or conditions which can stimulate a sustained stimulation of growth of an initiated cell (surgery, wounding, cell death, normal growth or exposure to mitogenic chemicals), mitogenesis appears to be a necessary, if not sufficient, factor in tumor promotion (Trosko et al., 1983) [Fig. 1].

Based on phenomenological observations, it has been hypothesized that initiation is the process by which a single normal stem cell is irreversibly altered, such that it cannot terminally differentiate (see later discussion). However, as long as it is surrounded by, and communicating with, normal cells, it can be suppressed from further growth and expression of its altered genotype. Until and unless, it is released from the suppressing effects of its normal neighbors by agents or conditions which can inhibit gap junctional communication, this initiated cell will remain in a quiescent or latent state (Yotti et al., 1979).

If intercellular communication is inhibited by endogenous (i.e., growth factors, hormones) or exogenous factors (i.e., cytotoxicants, non-cytotoxicant modulators of gap junctions), these initiated cells can proliferate (self-renew, but not differentiate). If these inhibitors are removed before a "critical mass" of the initiated cells is attained, the clonal expansion is stopped or even reversed (Reddy and Fialkow, 1987). If during the promotion process, a single initiated cell acquires a phenotype, via either another genetic (Trosko and Chang, 1980; Potter, 1981; Moolgavkar and Knudson, Jr., 1981; Hennings et al., 1983; Reddy and Fialkow, 1983; O'Connell et al., 1986; Taguchi et al., 1984; Jaffe et al., 1987; Chu et al., 1987) or epigenetic (Kerbel et al., 1984) alteration, which makes it independent of exogenous promoters, it can be said to have reached the progression stage.

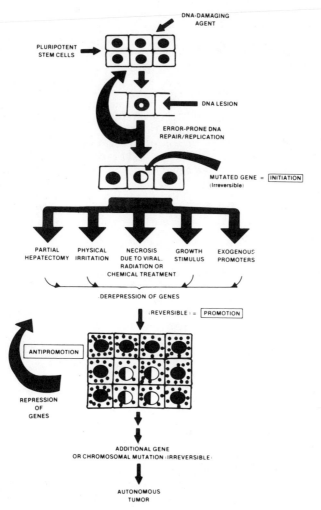

Fig. 1 Multiple modes by which initiated cells can be promoted. Promotion is conceptualized as a process allowing cells with a specific carcinogen-induced mutation to multiply, enabling them to reach either a "critical mass" in order to become resistant to the antiproliferative influences of normal cells or to increase the chance that one of these mutated cells would accumulate a second mutation. [From Trosko, J.E. and C.C. Chang (Trosko and Chang, 1980) with permission from Churchill Livingstone Medical J.].

Promotion, from this view, can then be seen as a rate-limiting step (Trosko and Chang, 1983). Without the _mitogenic_ stimulus of the promotion process, the probability of a single initiated cell to acquire the additional genetic/phenotypic changes for resisting the anti-mitogenic influences of the normal contact inhibiting cells would be very low. Expansion of the initiated clone increases the probability of acquiring those needed changes and decreases the anti-suppressing effects of contacting normal cells.

Carcinogenesis as a Disease of Differentiation in a Stem or Progenitor Cell

Several basic assumptions about the nature of carcinogenesis have to be made explicit. The first is the assumption that cancer is a "stem cell disease" or a "disease of differentiation" (Markert, 1968; Pierce, 1980; Potter, 1978). In contradistinction to this idea is that cancers might be derived from "retro- or de-differentiation of a differentiated cell. A second assumption is that cells of a tumor are of a clonal origin, in spite of the known genotypic and phenotypic heterogeneity in the late-stage tumor (Nicolson, 1987). Another subtle assumption is that only a few cells in an organism are susceptible to the transformation process (Nakano et al., 1985). Obviously, the opposite assumption is that all cells are subject to carcinogenic transformation.

From our vantage point, it seems that these three assumptions can be integrated by assuming that the number of stem cells in any tissue would be small, in comparison, to their daughter progenitor/ differentiated daughter cells, and any block in their ability to terminally differentiate but not self-renew, would give rise to a clonal-derived tumor.

T'so and his coworkers have shown that only a few, "contact-insensitive" cells of the Syrian hamster embryo seem to be susceptible to transformation (Nakano et al., 1985). Chang et al (Chang et al., 1987) have also identified, in human fetal kidney epithelial tissues, a small subpopulation of presumptive stem cells which are characterized as having no gap junctional communication. In addition, several workers have provided evidence that the carcinogenic initiation event inhibits some cells from terminally differentiating (Yuspa and Morgan, 1981; Kawamura et al., 1985; Scott and Maercklein, 1985; Miller et al., 1987). Taken together, one could speculate that carcinogenesis is that process in which a few target cells (stem or non-terminally differentiated progenitor cells) are the targets for the initiation event.

If a mutation is induced in one of these cells which prevents terminal differentiation, but not self-renewal, these cells could be the progenitors for the potential tumor [Fig. 2]. However, if the initiated stem/progenitor cell is surrounded by, and communicating with its normal neighbors, either by mechanisms of molecular signals received from the differentiated daughter cells (i.e., negative growth regulators) or from gap junctional communication with normal cells, then these initiated cells are held in check.

Upon exposure to agents or conditions which could block these negative suppressing factors (i.e., down-regulating receptors; decreasing gap junctions), then both the normal and initiated stem cell could escape "contact-inhibition" and proliferate. The normal stem cell could, after proliferation, terminally differentiate and eventually be removed from the tissue [especially open system tissues such as the lining of the intestine or the epidermis]. The initiated stem cell, however, would be unable to terminally differentiate. Therefore, there

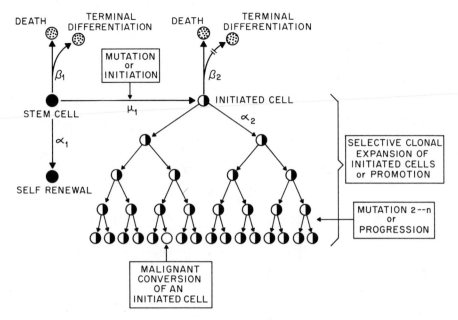

Fig. 2   The initiation/promotion/progression model of carcinogenesis.
β_1 = rate of terminal differentiation and death of stem cell; β_2
= rate of death, but not of terminal differentiation of the
initiated cell ($\dashv\mapsto$) α_1 = rate of cell division of stem cells;
α_2 = rate of cell division of initiated cells; μ_1 = rate of the
molecular event leading to initiation (i.e., possibly mutation);
μ_2 = rate at which second event occurs within an initiated cell.
[From Trosko et al (Trosko et al., in press), with permission
from Alan R. Liss, Inc., New York].

would be a "selective accumulation" or clonal expansion of these
dysfunctional, but not yet neoplastic cells. The papilloma of the skin,
enzyme altered foci of the liver and the polyps of the colon might all
represent this pre-malignant phase of carcinogenesis.

If during the clonal expansion of these undifferentiable initiated
cells, additional genetic or epigenetic alterations occur, the
acquisition of the phenotype needed [namely, the stable inhibition of
suppressing factors from normal cells received by intercellular
communication mechanisms], would now allow a single cell within this
clone of initiated cells to be tumor promoter independent. In closed
tissue systems, such as the liver or kidney, tight control of stem cells
must exist.   One might speculate that the terminally differentiated
cells of the stem-cell lineage could produce a negative growth regulator
which prevents the stem cell from dividing [Fig. 3].

One can explain the controlled regeneration which happens after
partial hepatectomy in the rat by this model. After removal of the
differentiated hepatocytes which might produce a negative growth
regulator, the source of this negative regulator is now gone. This
would allow the stem cells to start to proliferate, allowing some of
their daughter cells to differentiate into hepatocytes. When the number
of hepatocytes increases to a critical size, the amount of negative
growth regulators produced by the hepatocytes can now suppress the stem
cells. This would result in the regenerated liver being essentially the
same size of the original liver.   If any of the stem cells were
initiated, they would self-renew but not differentiate. These would give
rise to the enzyme-altered foci seen after initiation/partial hepatectomy and promotion (Goldsworthy et al., 1984).

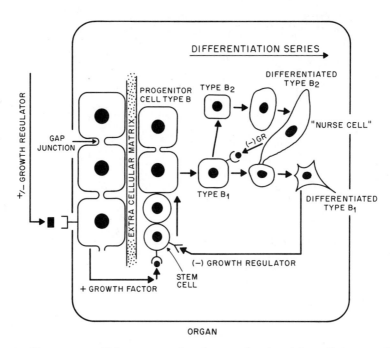

Fig. 3 A diagram to illustrate the interrelationship of intercellular
communication by positive and negative growth regulators on stem
cell growth and differentiation and intercellular communication
via gap junctions in a closed organ system.

One implication of this model would be that as an organism ages,
the number of stem cells would decrease, therefore the number of
potential target cells might decrease. Conversely, as we age, the
number of stem cells, which might be initiated spontaneously or induced,
would increase. Therefore, the probable additional "hits" needed for
neoplastic transformation would depend on the exposure to endogenous or
exogenous promoters.

Role of Intercellular Communication in Carcinogenesis

If the idea of cancer being a disease of stem cells which are
unable to terminally differentiate and to contact inhibit is correct,
the next question is what is (are) the normal biological process(es)
involved in controlling cell growth and regulating the differentiation
of stem cells. One of the earliest observations which helped to
distinguish normal cells from malignant cells was that normal cells
contact-inhibited (Levine et al., 1965) while cancer cells lost this
ability (Borek and Sach, 1966; Corsaro and Migeon, 1977; Abercrombie,
1979). Among several different kinds of observations (see Chang et al.,
1987), the ability to induce terminal differentiation of some neoplastic
cells in vitro by various natural differentiation factors or exogenous
chemical compounds (Huberman and Callaham, 1979; Schubert and Jacob,
1970; Yamamoto et al., 1980) lends support to the idea that initiation
has induced a partial block in the ability to terminally differentiate
(Potter, 1978).

A delicate orchestration of regulatory mechanisms exists not only
within cells, but also between cells within and between tissues. The
process of intercellular communication has evolved through the evolution
of multicellular organisms to help maintain homeostasis between stem
cells and their differentiated daughter cells, as well as to synchronize

170

activity within functional cells of a given tissue and to coordinate activity of one organ with that of other organs.

Of the several types of intercellular communication mechanisms which exist, two major ones stand out [Fig. 4]. One involves the transfer of molecular signals from cells of one cell type to another cell type via an extracellular route [i.e., with hormones, growth

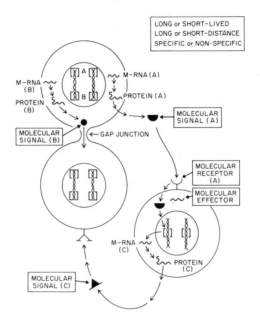

CELL–CELL COMMUNICATION

Fig. 4 Heuristic diagram illustrating two general forms of intercellular (cell-cell) communication. One involves the production and transmission of "signal" molecules over a distance through extracellular space to a target tissue. The other involves the transfer of "signal" molecules via permeable intercellular junctions between coupled cells. [From Trosko and Chang (Trosko and Chang, 1985), with permission from Scope Publ., Paris].

regulators, neurotransmitters] (Potter, 1983). The other involves the transfer of ions and relatively small molecular weight molecules via a membrane-bound protein structure, the gap junction (Pitts and Finbow, 1986).

The gap junction has been implicated in the regulation of normal cell growth and differentiation of mitotic cells and of the differentiated function of post-mitotic cells (Loewenstein, 1979). The gap junction, as a functional structure, is modulated by genetic/developmental factors in that their appearance is correlated with specific tissue development (Lo, 1985), and their inhibition by antibodies directed to the gap junction protein is correlated with abnormal development (Warner et al., 1984). Modulation of gap junctions by hormones has been correlated with the maturation of germ cells (Gilula et al., 1976; Larsen et al., 1987; Schultz, 1985). In addition, the disappearance of gap junctions during partial hepatectomy-induced regenerative stage and their reappearance after liver regeneration has been documented (Yee and Revel, 1978).

The only observation on normal presumptive human epithelial stem cells indicates that those cells do not have expressed or functional gap junctions (Chang et al., 1987). This implies, since they are normally held in check in the tissue, that they are communicating with their daughter-differentiated cells via some negative growth regulator. One of the earliest links between gap junctional communication and cancer was made by Borek et al and her co-workers (Borek et al., 1969). Over the last twenty years, many observations have suggested that the loss of gap junctions or their function is correlated with the transition of a normal cell to a cancer cell (Kanno, 1985). On the other hand, a series of observations seemed to indicate either that the loss of gap junctional communication was the consequence of malignant transformation and not the cause, or that there was no correlation at all with carcinogenesis since some cells derived from tumors were capable of gap junctional intercellular communication (Finbow and Yancey, 1981). Only recently, the demonstration of "selective communication" between cells within a transformed colony and the surrounding normal cells (Yamasaki et al., 1987; Enomoto and Yamasaki, 1984) makes it possible to explain some of these challenges to the idea that gap junctions (or the lack thereof) play a role in carcinogenesis.

Chemical Tumor Promoters, Oncogenes and Growth Factors: Modulators of Gap Junctional Intercellular Communication

In 1979, several observations provided strong evidence that gap junctions do play a major role in the tumor promotion phase of carcinogenesis. Yotti et al (Yotti et al., 1979) and Murray and Fitzgerald (Murray and Fitzgerald, 1979) showed that the powerful skin tumor promoting agent, 12-tetradecanoylphorbol-13-acetate (TPA), could inhibit gap junctional communication. Subsequently, using ultrastructural analysis, it was shown that TPA reduced the number of gap junctions seen in _vitro_ in Chinese hamsters (Yancey et al., 1982) and in _vivo_ in mouse skin (Kalimi and Sirsat, 1984). Moreover, using a wide variety of techniques and different in _vitro_ cell systems, a wide range of tumor promoting chemicals representing biological toxins, hormones, pollutants, pesticides, herbicides, drugs, food additives, heavy metals, etc., was shown to inhibit intercellular communication in a reversible manner (Trosko and Chang, in press).

More recently, several oncogenes (those genes which have a proven cancer association that appear to function primarily in the regulation of cellular proliferation and differentiation) have been shown to inhibit gap junction function, presumably by diverse molecular mechanisms (Azarnia and Loewenstein, 1984; Chang et al., 1985; Atkinson and Sheridan, 1984; Atkinson et al., 1986; El-Fouly et al., 1986; Azarnia and Loewenstein 1987).

Lastly, since chemical tumor promoters act as "growth factors" for the initiated cell and since many oncogenes either code for growth factors, growth factor receptors or mitogenic-transmembrane signalling elements (Weinberg, 1985), it seems logical to assume that growth factors, themselves, could modulate gap junction function. Epidermal growth factors and transforming growth factors, as well as bovine pituitary extract, have been shown to inhibit gap junctional communication in human keratinocytes (Madhukar et al., in press). Several growth factors have also been shown to have tumor promoting activity in _vivo_ and in _vitro_ (see Madhukar et al., in press).

Consequently, there appears to be a possible means of integrating the actions of chemical tumor promoters, oncogenes and growth factors via their shared ability to inhibit gap junctional intercellular communication (Madhukar et al., in press; Trosko et al., 1984). Normal and transient regulation of endogenous inhibitors of gap junctional communication (e.g., growth factors, cellular oncogenes, hormones) would be a powerful means to regulate cell growth and differentiation. Chronic or permanent endogenous inhibitors of intercellular communication (e.g., genetic defects overproducing endogenous hormones; mutated or over-expressed oncogenes) would, therefore, lead to homeostatic dysfunction.

Intercellular Communication and Its Implications for Risk Assessment

In the quest to determine if toxic chemicals work by genotoxic mechanisms, using less than unequivocal bioassay and STT assays, many serious interpretations are being made related to the mechanisms by which these chemicals act (Trosko, 1984; Trosko, in press). Clearly, true genotoxic chemicals are going to pose both genetic and somatic risks to humans. However, many chemicals have been falsely categorized as genotoxic, either because they "cause" cancer in the NTP bioassay or because, in one or another STT, a positive endpoint has been incorrectly interpreted as indicating they are mutagenic. In addition, the absence of any mutagenicity in STT seems to be all that is needed to issue the claim that a chemical is "safe".

Since we know chemicals can kill cells or alter gene expression (or modulate gap junctional intercellular communication), these cellular endpoints should be considered in the risk assessment of exposure to chemicals. Since both of these endpoints have been associated with threshold levels, the implications of this thorny issue cannot be overlooked.

Many tumor promoting chemicals, which are inhibitors of intercellular communication either by cytotoxic or non-cytotoxic mechanisms, have been shown to have threshold or no-effect levels (Verma and Boutwell, 1980; Goldsworthy et al., 1984; Van Duuren et al., 1973; Deml and Oesterle, 1987; Ito et al., 1986; Pereira et al., 1986; Pitot et al., 1987). They also need to be present on a regular and chronic basis (Boutwell, 1974; Pitot et al., 1981; Reddy and Fialkow, 1987). Clearly, inhibition of intercellular communication might have devastating consequences if the exposure is only once (e.g., during critical periods of development as a teratogen) or during the function of a critical organ (i.e., alcohol's effect on the brain leading to an automobile accident).

With some tumor promoting chemicals being persistent in both the environment or the body (e.g., DDT), and the demonstration that some endogenous tumor promoting chemicals can interact synergistically with endogenous chemicals (Warngard et al., 1987; Aylsworth et al., in press), one cannot automatically predict "safe" levels on the information of one chemical. In addition, genetic sensitivities (or resistance) to exogenous tumor promoters as inhibitors of intercellular communication would preclude accurate risk assessments (Wolff et al., 1987). Even differences in tissue or species response to chemical modulators on the cellular level would prevent accurate predictions of a chemical's action if it were based on only one species/cell type in vivo.

Since there seems to be multiple mechanisms by which chemicals, growth factors and oncogenes can modulate (up regulate or down regulate) gap junctional intercellular communication (Spray and Bennett, 1985; Saez et al., 1987), and since an individual is never exposed to just one chemical at a time, a given chemical, known to have the potential of modulating gap junctional communication, might have its effect either enhanced or suppressed by other genetic, developmental, sex-associated, dietary or environmental factors. Consequently, while our knowledge of this class of chemicals has provided a new perspective of the potential risk for cancer after exposure, there still are many unknown (and unknowable) factors which will prevent accurate assessment.

Acknowledgments

The authors wish to thank our co-workers, Dr. B.V. Madhukar, Dr. S.Y. Oh, Dr. D. Bombick, Dr. M. El-Fouly, Mrs. B. Lockwood, Mrs. Guixiang Zhang and Ms. H. Rupp for their intellectual support during the preparation of the manuscript. We also wish to acknowledge the excellent secretarial skills of Mrs. Judy Copeman and Mrs. Darla Conley.

References

Abercrombie, M., 1979, Contact inhibit and malignancy. Nature (London) 281:259-262.

Ames, B.N., Durston, W.E., Yamasaki, E., and Lee, F.D., 1973, Carcinogens are mutagens: A simple test system combining liver homogenates for activation and bacteria for detection. Proc. Natl. Acad. Sci. 70:2281-2285.

Atkinson, M., and Sheridan, J., 1984, Decreased junctional permeability in cells transformed by three different viral oncogenes: A quantitative video analysis. J. Cell. Biol. 99:401a.

Atkinson, M.H., Anderson, S.K., and Sheridan, J.D., 1986, Modification of gap junctions in cells transformed by a temperature - sensitive mutant of Rous sarcoma virus. J. Memb. Biol. 91:53-64.

Aylsworth, C.F., Trosko, J.E., Chang, C.C., Benjamin, K., and Lockwood, E., in press, Synergistic inhibition of metabolic cooperation by oleic acid or TPA and DDT in Chinese hamster V79 cells: Implications of a role for protein kinase C in the regulation of gap junctional intercellular communication. Cell Biol. Toxicol.

Azarnia, R., and Loewenstein, W.R., 1984, Intercellular communication and the control of growth: Alteration of junctional permeability by the src gene: A study with temperature-sensitive mutant Rous sarcoma virus. J. Memb. Biol. 82:191-205.

Azarnia, R., and Loewenstein, W.R., 1987, Polyomavirus middle T antigen down regulates junctional cell to cell communication. Molecul. Cellul. Biol. 7:946-950.

Borek, C., and Sach, L., 1966, The difference in contact inhibition of cell replication between normal cells and cells transformed by different carcinogens. Proc. Natl. Acad. Sci. U.S.A. 56:1705-1711.

Borek, C., Higashino, S., and Loewenstein, W.R., 1969, Intercellular communication and tissue growth. IV. Conductance of membrane junctions of normal and cancerous cells in culture. J. Membr. Biol. 1:274-293.

Boutwell, R.K., 1974, The function and mechanism of promoters of carcinogenesis. CRC Crit. Rev. Toxicol. 2:419-443 (1974).

Cairns, J., 1975, Mutation, selection and the natural history of cancer. Nature (London) 225:197-200.

Chang, C.C., Trosko, J.E., El-Fouly, M.H., Gibson-D'Ambrosio, R.E., and D'Ambrosio, S.M., 1987, Contact insensitivity of a subpopulation of normal human fetal kidney epithelial cells and of human carcinoma cell lines. Cancer Res. 47:1634-1645.

Chang, C.C., Trosko, J.E., Kung, H.J., Bombick, D., and Matsumura, F., 1985, Potential role of the src gene product in inhibition of gap junctional communication in NIH 3T3 cells. Proc. Natl. Acad. Sci. U.S.A. 82:5360-5364.

Chu, K.C., Brown, C.C., Tarone, R.E., and Tan, W.Y., 1987, Differentiating among proposed mechanisms for tumor promotion in mouse skin with the use of the multievent model for cancer. J. Natl. Cancer Inst. 79:789-796.

Corsaro, C.M., and Migeon, B.R., 1977, Comparison of contact-mediated communication in normal and transformed human cells in culture. Proc. Natl. Acad. Sci. 74:4476-4480.

Deml, E., and Oesterle, D., 1987, Dose-response of promotion by polychlorinated biphenyls and chloroform in rat liver foci bioassay. Arch. Toxicol. 60:209-211.

Dermietzel, R., Yancey, S.B., Traub, O., Willecki, K., and Revel, J.P., 1987, Major loss of the 28-kd protein of gap junction in proliferating hepatocytes. J. Cell Biol. 105:1925-1934.

Ehrenberg, L., Brookes, P., Druckrey, H., Lagerlof, B., Litwin, J., and Williams, G., 1973, The relation of cancer induction and genetic damages. Ambio. Spec. Rep. 3:15-16 (1973).

El-Fouly, M.H., Warren, S.T., Trosko, J.E., and Chang, C.C., 1986, Inhibition of gap junction-mediated intercellular communication in cells transfected with the human H-ras oncogene. Am. J. Human Genet. 39:A30.

Enomoto, T., and Yamasaki, H., 1984, Lack of intercellular communication between chemically transformed and surrounding non-transformed BALB/c3T3 cells. Cancer Res. 44:5200-5203.

Fialkow, P.J., 1974, The origin and development of human tumors studied with cell markers. N. Engl. J. Med. 291:26-35.

Finbow, M.E., and Yancey, S.G., 1981, The roles of intercellular junctions. in: Biochemistry of Cellular Regulation, M.J. Clemens, ed., CRC Press, Baco RAton, FL., pp. 215-249.

Foulds, L., 1975, Neoplastic Development, Vol. 1,2, Academic Press, New York.

Gilula, N.B., Fawcell, D.W., and Aoki A., 1976, The Sertoli cell occluding junctions and gap junctions in mature and developing mammalian testes. Devel. Biol. 51:142-168.

Goldsworthy, T., Campbell, H.A., and Pitot, H.C., 1984, The natural history and close-response characteristics of enzyme-altered foci in rat liver following phenobarbital and diethylnitrosumine administration. Carcinogenesis 5:67-71.

Hennings, H., Shores, R., Wenk, M.L., Spangler, E.F., Tarone, R., and Yuspa, S.H., 1983, Malignant conversion of mouse skin tumors is increased by tumor initiators and unaffected by tumor promoters. Nature 304:67-69.

Huberman, E., and Callaham, M.F., 1979, Induction of terminal differentiation in human promyelocytic leukemia cells by tumor promoting agents. Proc. Natl. Acad. Sci. U.S.A. 76:1293-1297.

Ito, N., Fukushima, S., Tamano, S., Hirose, M., and Hagiwara, A., 1986, Dose response in butylated hydroxyanisole induction of forestomach carcinogenesis in F344 rats. J. Natl. Cancer Instit. 7:1261-1265.

Jaffe, D.R., Williamson, J.R., and Bowden, G.T., 1987, Ionizing radiation enhances malignant progression of mouse skin tumors. Carcinogenesis 8:1753-1755.

Kalimi, G.H., and Sirsat, S.M., 1984, The relevance of gap junctions to stage 1 tumor promotion in mouse epidermis. Carcinogenesis 5:1671-1677.

Kanno, Y., 1985, Modulation of cell communication and carcinogenesis. Japan J. Physiol. 35:693-707.

Kawamura, H., Strickland, S.E., and Yuspa, S.H., 1985, Association of resistance to terminal differentiation with initiation of carcinogenesis in adult mouse epidermal cells. Cancer Res. 45:2748-2752.

Kerbel, R.S., Frost, P., Liteplo, R., Carlow, P.A., and Elliott, B.E., 1984, Possible epigenetic mechanisms of tumor progression:

Induction of high frequency heritable but phenotypically unstable changes in the tumorigenic and metastatic properties of tumor cell populations by 5-azacytidine treatment. J. Cell. Physiol. 3:87-97.

Larsen, W.J., Wert, S.E., and Brunner, G.D., 1987, Differential modulation of rat follicle cell gap junction populations at ovulation. Devel. Biol. 122:61-71.

Levine, E.M., Becker, Y., Boone, C.W., and Eagle, H., 1965, Contact inhibition, macromolecular synthesis, and polyribosomes in cultured human diploid fibroblasts. Proc. Natl. Acad. Sci. U.S.A. 53:350-356.

Lo, C.W., 1985, Communication compartmentation and pattern formation in development. in: Gap Junctions, M.V.L. Bennett, and D.C. Spray, eds., Cold Spring Harbor Lab., Cold Spring Harbor, New York, pp. 251-263.

Loewenstein, W.R., 1979, Junctional intercellular communication and the control of growth. Biochem. Biophys. Acta 560:1-65.

Madhukar, B.V., Oh, S.Y., Chang, C.C., Wade, M., El-Fouly, M.H., and Trosko, J.E., in press, Altered regulation of intercellular communication by epidermal growth factor, transforming growth factor-B, and peptide hormones in hormol human keratinocytes. Carcinogenesis.

Madhukar, B.V., Trosko, J.E., and Chang, C.C., in press, Chemical, oncogene and growth factor modulation of gap junctional communication in carcinogenesis. in: Cell Interactions and Gap Junctions. N. Sperelakis, and W.C. Cole, eds., CRC Press, Boca Raton, FL.

Markert, C., 1968, Neoplasia: A disease of cell differentiation. Cancer Res. 28:1908-1914.

Miller, D.R., Viaje, A., Aldaz, C.M., Conti, C.V., and Slaga, T.J., 1987, Terminal differentiation-resistant epidermal cells in mice undergoing two-stage carcinogenesis. Cancer Res. 47:1935-1940.

Moolgavkar, S.H., and Knudson, Jr., A.G., 1981, Mutation and cancer: A model for human carcinogenesis. J. Natl. Cancer Inst. 66:1037-1052.

Murray, A.W., and Fitzgerald, D.J., 1979, Tumor promoters inhibit metabolic cooperation in co-cultures of epidermal and 3T3 cells. Biochem. Biophys. Res. Commun. 91:395-401.

NaKano, S., Ueo, H., Bruce, S.A., and Ts'o, P.O.P., 1985, A contact-insensitive subpopulation in Syrian hamster cell cultures with a greater susceptibility to chemically induced neoplastic transformation. Proc. Natl. Acad. Sci. U.S.A. 82:5005-5009.

Nicolson, G.I., 1987, Tumor cell instability, diversification and progression to the metastatic phenotype: From oncogene to oncofetal expression. Cancer Res. 47:1473-1487.

O'Connell, J.F., Klein-Szanto, A.J.P., Digiovanni, D.M., Fries, J.M., and Slaga, T.J., 1986, Malignant progression of mouse skin papillomas treated with ethylnitrosourea, N-methyl-N'-nitro-N-nitrogoguanidine, or 12-0-tetradecanoylphorbol-13-acetate. Cancer Lett. 30:269-274.

Pereira, M.A., Herren-Freund, S.L., and Long, R.E., 1986, Dose-response relationship of phenobarbital promotion of diethylnitrosamine initiated tumors in rat liver. Cancer Lett. 32:305-311.

Pierce, G.B., 1980, Neoplasms, differentiation, and mutations. Am. J. Pathol. 77:103-118.

Pitot, H.C., Goldsworthy, T., and Moran, S., 1981, The natural history of carcinogenesis: Implications of experimental carcinogenesis in the genesis of human cancer. J. Supramol. Struct. Cell Biochem. 17:133-146.

Pitot, H.C., Goldsworthy, T.L., Moran, S., Kenne, W., Glauert, H.P., Maronpot, R.R., and Campbell, H.A., 1987, A method to quantitate the relative initiating and promoting potencies by hepatocarcinogenic agents in their dose-response relationships to altered hepatic foci. Carcinogenesis 8:1491-1499.

Pitts, J.D., and Finbow, M.E., 1986, The gap junction. J. Cell Sci. 4:239-261.

Potter, V.R., 1978, Phenotypic diversity in experimental hepatomas: The concept of partially blocked ontogeny. Br. J. Cancer 38:1-23.

Potter, V.R., 1981, A new protocol and its rationale for the study of initiation and promotion of carcinogenesis in rat liver. Carcinogenesis 2:3175-3179.

Potter, V.R., 1983, Cancer as a problem in intercellular communication: Regulation by growth-inhibiting factors. in: Progress in Nucleic Acid Research and Molecular Biology, Vol. 29, W.E. Cohn, ed., Academic Press, New York, pp. 161-173.

Reddy, A.L., and Fialkow, P.J., 1983, Papillomas induced by initiation-promotion differ from those induced by carcinogen alone. Nature 304:69-71.

Reddy, A.L., and Fialkow, P.J., 1987, Sequential studies of skin tumorigenesis in PGK mosaic mice: The effect of respected exposure to a carcinogen on regressed mouse skin papillomas. Carcinogenesis 8:1455-1459.

Saez, G.C., Bemmett, M.V.L., and Spray, D.C., 1987, Carbon tetrachloride at hepatotoxic levels block reversibly gap junctions between rat hepatocytes. Science 236:967-969.

Schubert, D., and Jacob, F., 1970, 5-Bromo-deoxyuridine-induced differentiation of a neuroblastoma. Proc. Natl. Acad. Sci. U.S.A. 67:247-254.

Schultz, R.M., 1985, Roles of cell to cell communication in development. Biol. Reprod. 32:27-42.

Scott, R.E., and Maercklein, P.B., 1985, An initiator of carcinogenesis selectively and stably inhibits stem cell differentiation: A concept that initiation of carcinogenesis involves multiple phases. Proc. Natl. Acad. Sci. U.S.A. 82:2995-2999.

Spray, D.C., and Bennett, M.V.L., 1985, Physiology and pharmacology of gap junctions. Ann. Rev. Physiol. 47:281-303.

Steering Committee on identification of toxic and potentially toxic chemicals for consideration by the National Toxicology Program. "Toxicity Testing - Strategies to Determine Needs and Priorities." Washington, D.C., National Academy Press (1984).

Taguchi, T., Yokoyama, M., and Kitamura, Y., 1984, Intraclonal conversion from papilloma to carcinoma in the skin of PgK-1[9]/PgK-1[6] mice treated by a complete carcinogenesis process or by an initiation-promotion regimen. Cancer Res. 44: 3779-3782.

Tennant, R.W., Margolin, B.H., Shelby, M.D., Zeiger, E., Haseman, J.K., Spalding, J., Caspary, W., Resnick, M., Stasiewicz, S., Anderson, B., and Minor, R., 1987, Prediction of chemical carcinogenicity in rodents from in vitro genetic toxicity assays. Science 236:933-941.

Trosko, J.E., 1984, A new paradigm is needed in toxicology evaluation. Environ. Mutag. 6:767-769.

Trosko, J.E., in press, A failed paradigm: Carcinogenesis is more than mutagenesis. Mutagenesis.

Trosko, J.E., in press, Towards understanding carcinogenic hazards: A crisis in paradigms. J. Amer. Coll. Toxicol.

Trosko, J.E., and Chang, C.C., 1978, Environmental carcinogenesis: An integrative model. Quart. Rev. Biol. 53:115-141.

Trosko, J.E., and Chang, C.C., 1980, An integrative hypothesis linking cancer, diabetes, and atherosclerosis: The role of mutations and epigenetic changes. Med. Hypoth. 6:455-468.

Trosko, J.E., and Chang, C.C., 1983, Potential role of intercellular communication in the rate-limiting step in carcinogenesis. in: Cancer and the Environment: Possible Mechanisms of Thresholds for

Carcinogens and Other Toxic Substances, J.A. Cimo, ed., Mary Ann Liebert, Inc., New York, pp. 5-21.

Trosko, J.E., and Chang, C.C., 1985, Implications for risk assessment of genotoxic and non-genotoxic mechanisms in carcinogenesis. in: P.V. Vouk, G.C. Butler, D.G. Hoel, and D.B. Parall, eds., Methods for Estimating Risks of Chemical Injury: Human and Non-Human Biota and Ecosystems, John Wiley and Sons, Chichester, England, pp. 181-200.

Trosko, J.E., and Chang, C.C., in press, Nongenotoxic mechanisms in carcinogenesis: Role of inhibited intercellular communication. in: Banbury Report 31: New Directions in the Qualitative and Quantitative Aspects of Carcinogen Risk Assessment. R.W. Hart, and R.B. Setlow, eds., Cold Spring Harbor Lab., Cold Spring Harbor, New York.

Trosko, J.E., Chang, C.C., Madhukar, B.V., Oh, S.Y., Bombick, D., and El-Fouly, M.H., in press, Modulation of gap junction intercellular communication by tumor promoting chemicals, oncogenes and growth factors during carcinogenesis. in: Gap Junctions, R. Johnson, and E. Hertzberg, eds., Alan R. Liss, Inc.

Trosko, J.E., Chang, C.C., and Medcalf, A., 1983, Mechanisms of tumor promotion: Potential role of intercellular communication. Cancer Invest. 1:511-526.

Trosko, J.E., Jone, C., and Chang, C.C., 1983, The role of tumor promoters on phenotypic alterations affecting intercellular communication and tumorigenesis. Ann. New York Acad. Sci. 407:316-327.

Trosko, J.E., Jone, C., and Chang, C.C., 1984, Oncogenes, inhibited intercellular communication and tumor promotion. in: Cellular Interactions by Environmental Tumor Promoters. H. Fujiki, E. Hecker, R.E. Moore, T. Sugimura, and I.B. Weinstein, eds., Japan Sci. Soc. Press, Tokyo, pp. 101-113.

Trosko, J.E., Riccardi, V.M., Chang, C.C., Warren, S., and Wade, M., 1985, Genetic predispositions to initiation or promotion phases in human carcinogenesis. in: Biomarkers, Genetics and Cancer, Anton-H. Guirgis, and N.T. Lynch, eds., VanNostrand Reinhold Co., New York, pp. 13-37.

Van Duuren, B.L., Sivak, A., Segal, A., Seidman, I., and Katz, C., 1973, Dose-response studies with a pure tumor-promoting agent, phorbol myristate acetate. Cancer Res. 33:2166-2172.

Verma, A.K., and Boutwell, R.K., 1980, Effect of dose and duration of treatment with the tumor - promotions agent, TPA, on mouse skin carcinogenesis. Carcinogenesis 1:271-276.

Warner, A.E., Guthrie, S.C., and Gilula, N.B., 1984, Antibodies to gap-junctional protein selectively disrupt junctional communication in the early amphibian embryo. Nature 311:127-131.

Warngard, L., Flodstrom, S., Ljungquist, S., and Ahlborg, U.G., 1987, Interaction between quercetin, TPA and DDT in the V79 metabolic cooperation assay. Carcinogenesis 8:1201-1205.

Weinberg, R.A., 1985, The action of oncogenes in the cytoplasm and nucleus. Science 230:770-776.

Weinstein, I.B., Gattoni-Celli, S., Kirschmeier, P., Lambert, M., Hsiao, W., Backer, J., and Jeffrey, A., 1984, Multistage carcinogenesis involves multiple genes and multiple mechanisms. J. Cellul. Physiol. 3:127-137.

Wolff, G.L., Roberts, D.W., Morrissey, R.L., Greenman, D.L., Allen, R.R., Campbell, W.L., Bergman, H., Vesnow, S., and Frith, C.H., 1987, Tumorigenic responses to Lindane in mice: Potentiation by a dominant mutation. Carcinogenesis 8:1889-1897.

Yamamoto, Y., Tomida, M., and Hozumi, M., 1980, Production by mouse spleen cells of factors stimulating differentiation of mouse myeloid leukemic cells that differ from the colony-stimulating factor. Cancer Res. 40:4804-4809.

Yamasaki, H., Hollstein, M., Mesnil, M., Martel, N., and Anguelon, A.M., 1987, Selective lack of intercellular communication between transformed and non-transformed cells as a common property of chemical and oncogene transformation of BALB/cBT3 cells. _Cancer Res_. 47:5658-5664.

Yancey, S.B., Edens, J.E., Trosko, J.E., Chang, C.C., and Revel, J.P., 1982, Decreased incidence of gap junctions between Chinese hamster V79 cells upon exposure to the gap junctions between Chinese hamster V79 cells upon exposure to the tumor promoter 12-tetradecanoyl-phorbol-13-acetate. _Exp_. _Cell_ _Res_. 139:329-340.

Yee, A., and Revel, J.P., 1978, Loss and reappearance of gap junctions in regenerating liver. _J_. _Cell_ _Biol_. 78:554-564.

Yotti, L.P., Chang, C.C., and Trosko, J.E., 1979, Elimination of metabolic cooperation in Chinese hamster cells by a tumor promoter. _Science_ 206:1089-1091.

Yuspa, S.H., and Morgan, D.L., 1981, Mouse skin cells resistant to terminal differentiation associated with initiation of carcinogenesis. _Nature_ 293:72-74.

COMPARATIVE ANALYSES OF THE TIMING AND MAGNITUDE OF GENOTOXIC AND

NONGENOTOXIC CELLULAR EFFECTS IN URINARY BLADDER CARCINOGENESIS

Leon B. Ellwein and Samuel M. Cohen

University of Nebraska Medical Center
Department of Pathology and Microbiology
Omaha, Nebraska

INTRODUCTION

Risk assessment is a complex process. It attempts to relate adverse health effects, such as cancer induction, to exposure to potentially toxic agents. The relationship between exposure and tumor incidence is studied experimentally by administering specific exposure regimens to animals followed by lifetime observation to determine tumor incidence. A pivotal issue in risk assessment centers around the estimation of risk at low exposure levels, levels significantly below those typically used in experimental toxicology studies. To quantitatively estimate risk at low exposure levels, mathematical modeling and extrapolation procedures are necessary.

Modeling directed toward the risk assessment process has proceeded on several fronts. Conceptually, this work can be categorized into three components as shown in Fig. 1. The first component deals with pharmacokinetics, where the interest is in the relationship between exposure, or administered dose, and the dose delivered to the target tissue. The second component centers around understanding cellular physiology in relating biological response in the target organ with target tissue dose. Finally, the relationship between cellular response and tumor incidence is shown under the rubric of carcinogenesis modeling. Our interest is in this latter component of modeling, where we attempt to capture the essence of the carcinogenesis process at a cellular level.

Before elaborating on the carcinogenesis component of risk assessment modeling, a few comments regarding response thresholds in the two previous components are in order. In considering the relationship between administered dose and dose delivered to the target tissue, two threshold phenomena are particularly important: one is operative at low doses and the other at high doses. For example, in the presence of detoxification mechanisms the administered dose must exceed a threshold level before the compound is delivered to the target tissue. Once the detoxification mechanism is saturated, the relationship between administered dose and dose delivered to the target tissue may follow a linear or some other more complex mathematical relationship. In a similar fashion, at high doses metabolic activation mechanisms may saturate such that the dose delivered to the target will not increase beyond a certain level even as the administered dose continues to increase. Clearly the pharmacokinetics which relate administered dose to

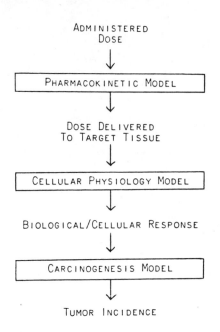

ADMINISTERED
DOSE

↓

| PHARMACOKINETIC MODEL |

↓

DOSE DELIVERED
TO TARGET TISSUE

↓

| CELLULAR PHYSIOLOGY MODEL |

↓

BIOLOGICAL/CELLULAR RESPONSE

↓

| CARCINOGENESIS MODEL |

↓

TUMOR INCIDENCE

Fig. 1. Biologically-based
risk assessment
modeling.

target tissue dose are complex, with the possibility for thresholds at the lower and upper levels of administered dose.

Modeling the relationship between delivered dose and cellular response must also be grounded in an understanding of the appropriate biological mechanisms. Intracellular treatment and/or interference with the delivered dose is critical here. Cellular metabolism and receptor interactions will influence the dose-response relationship. If the test compound influences cellular response by mechanisms similar to those operating under background conditions an additive response may be seen. On-the-other-hand if the mechanisms are different, a threshold level of delivered dose may be required before cellular response is affected. Clearly, some understanding of the biological mechanisms involved is necessary for biologically-based modeling.

Modeling of the carcinogenic process must also be based on mechanistic foundations. We build upon the two-stage theory of carcinogenesis, where in the process of becoming malignant, the progeny of a cell pass through an intermediate, initiated state, before realizing a second genetic change which transforms them into a fully malignant state.[1] The relationship between compund-induced cellular response and the ultimate appearance of a malignant tumor is modeled mathematically by accounting for these genetic events in cell progeny and for the cellular dynamics that determine the frequency of these events. The purpose of this paper is to explore the relationships between cellular response variables and tumor incidence. The changes in tumor incidence that result from variations in both the timing and magnitude of cellular response are examined. The primary benefit to be gained from sensitivity analyses such as these is insight, not the numbers associated with any one analytical scenario.

The rat urinary bladder is used as the target organ in this paper. The bladder epithelium is a simple structure with a basal or stem cell layer, an intermediate cell layer and a layer of superficial, differentiated cells. With this simple epithelium, cellular parameters are experimentally quantifiable. Although the analyses presented here are not directed toward the study of any specific compound, they were motivated by, and are based on, our previous modeling efforts using experimental data from studies of both classical genotoxic carcinogens[2,3] and non-genotoxic compounds[4]. As stated, our purpose is a general one: to develop insight into the relationships linking cellular response with tumor incidence.

CARCINOGENESIS MODEL

The biological basis of the model centers around the conceptualization of three genetically distinct cellular states: normal, initiated, and transformed. Methods for tracking the proliferation of cells within each state and the associated transitions from normal to initiated and from initiated to transformed are at the core of the mathematical implementation of this biological foundation. The target organ is represented, at any point in time, by a population of normal cells, a population of initiated cells substantially smaller than the normal cell population, and ultimately, a population of transformed cells. A cancer arises if, and when, the transformed cell population expands to some visually detectable magnitude. The important cellular events in this carcinogenic model are shown in Fig. 2. The events encompass both genetic change and nongenetic proliferative response. It is assumed that malignant cells arise only within the stem cell population, and thus, cells committed to differentiation (the intermediate cell layer in the bladder epithelium) and already differentiated cells (the superficial layer) need not be modeled.

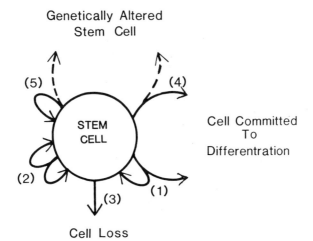

Fig. 2.   Cellular Events: 1) cell division with one stem and one committed daughter cell; 2) cell division with two stem daughter cells (cell birth); 3) cell death--no division; 4) event 1 with genetic change in one daughter stem cell; 5) event 2 with genetic change in one daughter stem cell.

In modeling these biological events over the course of time, we use a series of equal time intervals. These intervals are short enough so that it is biologically impossible for any given cell to divide more than once within one interval. Further, the events are taken to be mutually exclusive and thus no two events can occur simultaneously.

The occurrence of events 1,2,4 and 5 is driven by the mitotic rate of the cell population, represented by M_N, M_I, and M_T for the normal, initiated and transformed cell populations, respectively. These mitotic rates can be treated as probabilities if expressed in time units corresponding to the model time interval. The expected number of mitotic events in one time interval, the mitotic rate, is equivalent to the probability that a single mitotic event will occur. Another important model variable is the probability that cell birth occurs during a mitotic event. Event 2 entails the birth of an extra stem cell, both daughter cells will be stem cells rather than one stem cell and one committed cell. The probability that a cell birth occurs conditional on a mitotic event taking place pertains, as before, to normal (B_N), initiated (B_I) and transformed (B_T) cells. The unconditional probability of cell birth is represented by the product M*B. Genetic change associated with events 4 and 5 is also conditional on mitosis, the conditional probability of genetic transition during mitosis from a normal to an initiated state (P_I) or from an initiated to a transformed state (P_T). Finally, there is the probability of cell death, represented by D_N, D_I, and D_T.

Fig. 3 identifies the model outputs of primary interest, which are functions of the mathematical variables defined above. The product of the mitotic and conditional cell birth variables (M*B) and the cell death variable (D) determine the growth or regression of the cell population within each of the three states, whereas genetic transitions are determined by the product of mitotic and conditional cell transition variables (M*P). Some of the model outputs are directly relatable to data collected in animal studies. For example, the expected number of normal stem cells should parallel the developmental growth of the target organ and any exposure-related hyperplasia. The expected number of cells making the transition from the normal to the initiated state can be equated with initiated cell foci; those foci which are of some minimum size can be considered visible and correlated with experimental observation. For the transformed cell population, we are particularly interested in the probability that one or more transformed cells exist and whether any one transformed cell focus has grown to a visible size. All of these model outputs vary as a function time, as do the input variables.

MODEL VARIABLES   MODEL OUTPUTS

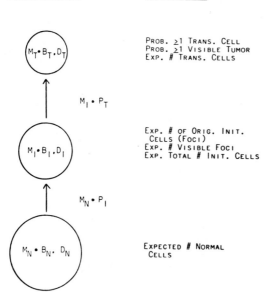

PROB. ≥ 1 TRANS. CELL
PROB. ≥ 1 VISIBLE TUMOR
EXP. # TRANS. CELLS

EXP. # OF ORIG. INIT. CELLS (FOCI)
EXP. # VISIBLE FOCI
EXP. TOTAL # INIT. CELLS

EXPECTED # NORMAL CELLS

Fig. 3. Model outputs of primary interest associated with normal, initiated, and transformed cell populations.

Several biological assumptions underlie this model. Four of these are particularly significant. First, it is assumed that the genetic alterations separating normal from transformed cells can be represented as two irreversible transitions. This does not mean, for example, that initiated cell foci cannot regress, but only that an initiated cell undergoing cell division will never produce a normal daughter cell. Another critical modeling assumption is that of independence in cell behavior. This assumption implies that the behavior of any one cell is influenced only by the biological stimulus underlying the behavior of all cells, and is not influenced directly by the behavior of other neighboring cells in the population. The third major assumption is that genetic change occurs only during mitosis and that only one of the daughter cells is affected. A fourth major assumption limits the induction of cancer to the stem cell population; therefore, for modeling purposes, we ignore the committed and differentiated cell populations.

It should be evident from the foregoing discussion that tumor induction centers around the frequency with which mitotic events take place and the likelihood of genetic change during cell division. It is the number of mitotic events, not simply elapsed time, that relates directly to tumor prevalence. Further, once an initiated cell population becomes established, mitotic events in the normal cell population are overshadowed in importance by those taking place in initiated cells.

Since each cell division is subject to some extremely small, but non-zero, probability of mutation or other genetic change (P_I and P_T), cancers occur spontaneously. Exposure to nongenotoxic compounds increase cancer incidence, not by increasing the conditional probability of genetic change, but by increasing the number of mitotic events, i.e., the number of opportunities for spontaneous genetic change. For nongenotoxic compounds, these spontaneous genetic alterations are the mechanism by which initiation and malignant transformation take place. The resulting effect is no different than one which occurs by increasing the conditional probability of genetic change instead of the number of mitotic events. The influence of any compound on cancer induction must be viewed as a combination of both genotoxic and nongenotoxic proliferative effects. Terminology classifying compounds as co-carcinogens, initiators, promoters, completers, etc. has no direct interpretation in this framework and, indeed, can be confusing.

This carcinogenesis model is based on the same underlying biological framework as that presented by Moolgavkar and Knudson;[5] however, our mathematical implementation is entirely different. We use a discrete-time approach in contrast to their continuous-time implementation and use a recursive method of solution rather than attempting to solve closed-formed equations. As a result, we are not faced with simplifying the dynamics of the biological model to ensure computational tractability. The price we pay for this modeling realism is the sacrifice of traditional methods of statistical inference in estimating experimentally unobservable model variables.

ANALYSES

Although the mathematical relationship between the probability of a visible tumor and the mitotic, birth, death, and transition probabilities of the normal, initiated, and transformed cell populations is complex,[2] an intuitive understanding of this and other relationships can be fostered by examining the results from a series of simulations designed for this purpose. Using the rat urinary bladder as the target organ, we first contrast the relative influence of biological change during the early developmental period of the organ with that which takes place during the post-weaning, two-year adult period. Under normal conditions, the proliferative response associated with bladder formation gradually slows until it is relatively quiescent during adulthood. Spontaneous bladder tumors are uncommon in most experimental species.

Table 1 provides baseline cellular response values for a simplified two period model. The specific values shown are based on information gained during the course of considerable modeling analyses directed toward examination of the effects of both genotoxic and nongenotoxic compounds in Fischer and Sprague-Dawley rats. The dynamism of the development period is greatly simplified by the use of "average" values for mitotic rates and conditional birth probabilities. For our purpose in sensitivity analysis, this simplification serves to facilitate comprehension without significant loss of reality.

Table 1. Baseline Cellular Response Probabilities in the Rat Bladder

Development Period (30 Days)

	Mitosis	Birth	Death	Transistion
Normal Cells	.333	.500	0.0	5.0×10^{-6}
Initiated Cells	.333	.500	0.0	5.0×10^{-6}
Transformed Cells	.333	1.000	0.0	5.0×10^{-6}

Adult Period (720 Days)

	Mitosis	Birth	Death	Transistion
Normal Cells	.005	.010	0.0	5.0×10^{-6}
Initiated Cells	.005	.010	0.0	5.0×10^{-6}
Transformed Cells	.100	1.000	0.0	

Table 2 shows values for some of the output variables of interest in the baseline scenario. As can be seen, one-third of the cell divisions take place by the time of weaning, even though this represents only four percent of the animal's lifespan. We see that the typical bladder is expected to have one initiated cell focus at this time, comprising four or five cells. (Although not shown, at birth there is a .20 probability that one initiated cell will already be present.) By the end of the two year adult period, the normal bladder is expected to have three initiated cell foci. The probability of one or more malignant cells is 10^{-3} (not shown) and the probability of a visible bladder tumor is 10^{-4}. Obviously, this represents a very low spontaneous tumor rate.

We begin the sensitivity analyses by examining first the influence of cellular proliferation during the adult period. Cellular proliferation is induced by increasing both mitotic rates and conditional birth probabilities for initiated cells, but increasing only the former for normal cells (to preclude an unrealistic growth in bladder size). As shown in Fig. 4, if cellular response variables corresponding to mitotic rates and conditional birth probabilities are increased 20- to 40-fold over baseline values (producing 200- to 800-fold increases in their product) for durations that range from six months to the entire 24 month adult period, we see a widely varying tumor response. For example, doubling cellular response (M*B) from

Table 2. Outcomes Associated with Baseline Cellular Response in the Rat Bladder

Time	Accum. Normal Cell Div.	Exp. # Norm. Cell Transit.	Exp. # Init. Cells	Prob. Visible Tumor
Weaning	2.0×10^5	1.0	4.3	–
$\frac{1}{2}$ year	2.8×10^5	1.4	4.8	3.5×10^{-5}
1 year	3.7×10^5	1.9	5.3	5.5×10^{-5}
$1\frac{1}{2}$ years	4.7×10^5	2.3	5.8	7.8×10^{-5}
2 years	5.6×10^5	2.8	6.3	1.0×10^{-4}

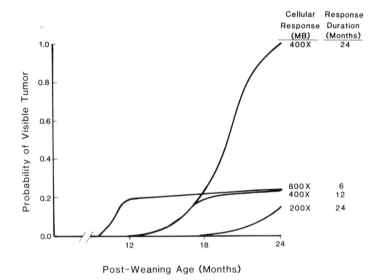

Fig. 4. Nonlinear relationship between post-weaning proliferative effects and bladder tumors.

200 to 400 times over baseline while halving the response duration from 24 to 12 months produces different results, illustrating the fallacy of linear thinking. Over the near term, increasing the magnitude of the cellular response has a greater effect than increasing its duration. This is due primarily to the relative importance of cellular proliferation that occurs early versus that which occurs toward the end of the adult period. Cellular response at the latter part of the adult period is of lesser influence because of the reduced time remaining for initiated cells which are generated during this latter period to make the transition to the transformed state and for the new transformed cells to proliferate in number to a visible tumor. (If the analysis period is increased beyond 24 months, however, the 200x curve will cross the 400x and 800x curves before leveling off.)

Fig. 4 also illustrates the existence of a latency period before tumors are seen and the eventual leveling off of tumor occurrence once cellular response drops to baseline.

The relationship between the probability of a visible tumor by two years and the magnitude of the enhancement of cellular response during the entire two year adult period is shown in Fig. 5 (represented by the curve labeled $M_I B_I$ adult). As in Fig. 4, we see that once the cellular response is increased on the order of 400-fold, tumor prevalence reaches 100 percent. Fig. 5 illustrates the greater sensitivity associated with increasing cellular response during the development period (the first thirty days). Once cellular response is increased five- to six-fold during this short, but early, thirty day period, tumors are expected in all animals. This seemingly disproportionate importance of the development period of the bladder is due to its early position in the time sequence, the fact that it contains one-third of all mitotic events, and its cellular dynamics are 100-fold greater than the adult period under normal conditions.

Fig. 5 provides a comparison of nongenotoxic cellular response with a strictly genotoxic response. The genetic transition probabilities P_I and P_T require substantial increases over the spontaneous baseline levels before comparable effects on tumor incidence are seen. These probabilities must be increased on the order of 10,000- to 100,000-fold before tumor prevalence reaches 100 percent. The relative importance of influencing P_I versus P_T during development and adult periods is illustrated.

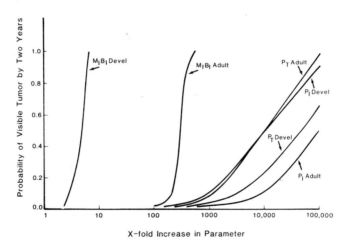

Fig. 5. Comparative influence of proliferative and genotoxic response on bladder tumors.

If P_I is influenced, there is an obvious advantage to increasing it during the development period. The rationale for this is that initiated cells which come into existence during the development period have two years of time over which to become transformed. If the initiated cell population is not established until well into the adult period, there is significantly less time remaining for transformation. On-the-other-hand, in influencing P_T, there is an advantage to be gained by waiting until the adult period. An increased P_T during the development period, when initiated cells are not in existence until the end, is not as effective as increasing P_T after the time of weaning, when initiated cells are present at the outset. The difference in influence between P_I and P_T centers around the existence of spontaneously produced initiated cells at the time of weaning. If initiated cells did not exist at weaning, the effects of increasing P_I versus P_T would be equivalent.

Of greatest interest for risk assessment purposes is the relationship between tumor incidence and both nongenotoxic and genotoxic response, but at levels typified by low exposures. Subsequent analyses focus on examining further the lower portions of the curves in Fig. 5, corresponding to small increases in cellular response over baseline and the associated small increases in tumor risk.

In Fig. 6, mitotic rates of both normal and initiated cells are increased as much as 12-fold over baseline levels. The conditional birth probability has not been changed, only the mitotic rate. (The impact on tumor incidence is maximized by increasing only M in achieving some target increase in the M*B product.) As before, increasing cellular response during the development period has a relatively dramatic effect on increasing the probability of tumor, again demonstrating the importance of cell prolif-eration during this early, dynamic time period. Influencing mitotic rates during the adult period is represented by the remaining three curves. Increasing the mitotic rate during the first year as compared to the second year of the adult period has a differential effect on tumor production.

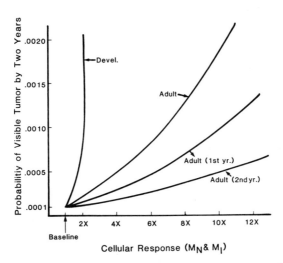

Fig. 6. Relationships between mitotic response and bladder tumors.

Fig. 7 is a comparable analysis focusing on genetic response. In this figure, the conditional transition probabilities, P_I and P_T, are increased up to 12-fold over baseline values. As before, the relative advantage of increasing P_I during the development period and P_T during the adult period is shown, along with the comparative advantage of changing both P_I and P_T in the development period compared to changing both in the adult period.

Fig. 8 demonstrates a genetic response combined with a delayed cell proliferative response. This scenario might represent a circumstance where an agent is administered with genotoxic effects at very low exposure levels

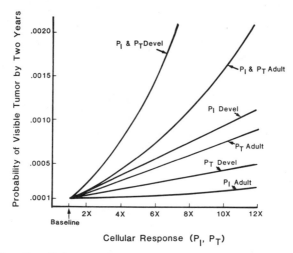

Fig. 7. Relationship between genotoxic response and bladder tumor.

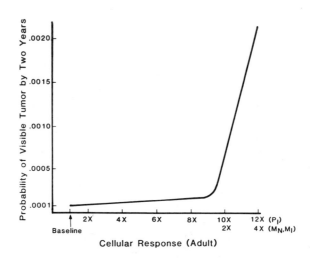

Fig. 8. Genotoxic response with threshold mitotic response.

and cell proliferative effects at higher levels. In the scenario shown, increases in mitotic rates come into play only after the point at which genotoxic effects have already produced a 10-fold increase in the transition probability P_I. This is more than merely a superpositioning of the P_I adult curve from Fig. 7 with the adult mitotic response curve from Fig. 6. Once the mitotic response comes into play, a synergism between genetic and proliferative effects is seen which goes beyond a simple additive relationship. This scenario, and the resulting hockey stick shaped tumor curve, might be representative of a number of genotoxic agents. It demonstrates the importance of considering dose-related cell proliferative effects even in analyzing agents identified a priori as being genotoxic. Without an understanding of the potential for synergistic effects between genotoxic response and nongenotoxic response, observations such as this in experimental situations would be difficult to explain.

DISCUSSION

Bioassays currently focus on measuring the ultimate response end point, tumor incidence. To produce statistically significant increases in tumor incidence, unrealistically high doses of the test compound are generally required. At so-called maximum tolerated doses, mechanistic distortions affecting the integrity of the biological test system can be expected. Thus, information gained using these severely stressed physiological systems may not be completely relevant for establishing quantitative relationships between tumor incidence and exposure at low doses. By measuring response at the cellular level, the doses used in testing can be substantially reduced. Compounds which produce a statistically significant increase in tumor incidence at high doses can be expected to produce significant increases in genotoxic and/or nongenotoxic cellular response at much lower doses. As noted in the foregoing analyses, any measurable increase in cellular response will lead to an increase in tumor risk.

Modeling the carcinogenic process gives us the basis for establishing analytically the relationships between cellular response and tumor incidence. Animal experimentation can be directed towards determination of doses below which cellular response is not observed. Thus, experimentation could focus on the question of whether thresholds exist, thresholds that pertain to cellular response in the target tissue. This experimentation will require development of new laboratory methods for quantifying both DNA and proliferative effects. Currently, these measurements entail a great deal of effort and cost. The objective of new technology should be to detect increases in cellular response no more than two-fold over baseline levels. At these levels the associated increase in tumor response is expected to be far below that detectable in the traditional bioassay.

With current technology it is not possible, at least in the urinary bladder, to identify the initiated cell population. Whether the initiated cell population is stimulated to a greater extent than normal cells upon exposure to nongenotoxic or genotoxic agents is subject to speculation. If the influence on initiated cells is significantly greater than that on normal cells, this heightened cellular response may go undetected. This differential effect can be extremely important, however; increasing the mitotic rate of initiated cells is more influential in producing a tumor than increasing the mitotic rate of normal cells, just as influencing P_T during the adult period was shown to produce a greater tumor risk than influencing P_I. If initiated cells are selectively receptive to a proliferative influence, cellular response measurements based on normal cell behavior will underestimate the true risk. It is expected that analyses using other target organs, such as the liver will only reinforce these results. Since the differential behavior of initiated cells and normal cells is extremely important, it is necessary that the mechanism for specification within the model be comparable. In the liver, observations of cell foci identified as initiated cells provide an opportunity to examine differences between normal and initiated cell behavior.

The preceding results have demonstrated the necessity of incorporating the entire lifetime of an animal in model analyses. As part of starting conditions, we must specify the distribution of cells among the normal, initiated, and transformed states. Since we have no basis for doing this, all cells are assumed to be normal at the start. It is safe to make this assumption only at the beginning of target organ development. As evidence of the importance of this, we noted that the differential influence of P_I compared to P_T was due entirely to the existence of spontaneously initiated cells by the time of weaning.

In closing it should be noted that, as with all modeling and analytical exercises, we do not fully capture the qualities of the real world. Indeed no complex reality, biological or other, can be captured analytically in its entirety. Our purpose in studying an abstraction of reality is to improve upon the perspective that exists in minds of people and, thereby, improve upon the relevance of yet-to-be designed experimental studies and their interpretation.

ACKNOWLEDGMENTS

This work was supported by the International Life Sciences Institute -- Nutrition Foundation. The authors are grateful for the assistance of Ms. Cheryl Kibler in preparation of the manuscript.

REFERENCES

1. T.J. Slaga, Mechanisms Involved in Two-stage Carcinogenesis in Mouse Skin, in: "Mechanisms of Tumor Promotion," Vol. II, T.J. Slaga, ed., CRC Press, Boca Raton (1984).
2. R.E. Greenfield, L.B. Ellwein, and S.M. Cohen, A General Probabilistic Model of Carcinogenesis: Analysis of Experimental Urinary Bladder Cancer, Carcinogenesis 5:437 (1984).
3. R. Hasegawa, S.M. Cohen, M. St. John, M. Cano and L.B. Ellwein, Effect of Dose on the Induction of Urothelial Proliferation by N-[4-(5-nitro-2-furyl)-2-thiazolyl]formamide and it Relationship to Bladder Carcinogenesis in the Rat, Carcinogenesis 7:633 (1986).
4. L.B. Ellwein and S.M. Cohen, A Cellular Dynamics Model of Experimental Bladder Cancer: Analysis of the Effect of Sodium Saccharin in the Rat, Risk Analysis 8:215 (1988).
5. S. H. Moolgavkar and A.G. Knudson, Jr., Mutation and Cancer: A Model for Human Carcinogenesis, Journal of the National Cancer Institute 66:1037 (1981).

ALTERATIONS IN GENE EXPRESSION IN MOUSE HEPATOCARCINOGENESIS

Tommaso A. Dragani, Giacomo Manenti, Marina R.M. Sacchi, Bruno Colombo and Giuseppe Della Porta

Division of Experimental Oncology A, Istituto Nazionale Tumori, Milan, Italy

ABSTRACT

Alteration in gene expression is one of several molecular changes observed in cancer. The great relevance on cell phenotype of quantitative alterations in the levels of particular mRNAs is well documented. To isolate genes under-expressed in mouse liver tumors compared to normal adult liver, we have screened a normal adult liver cDNA library with RNA probes prepared from a normal adult liver and from a hepatocellular carcinoma. Three different clones showed the common feature to be expressed at relatively high levels in normal adult liver and to be undetectable or expressed at 10-50-fold lower levels, in liver carcinomas and in 14-day-old normal liver. Therefore, these clones should represent genes regulated during liver development. Preliminary nucleotide sequence analysis of a 3' terminal region of one clone indicated that the clone may be identical to mouse major urinary protein. The characterization of the other two clones is in progress.

INTRODUCTION

In the past decade our understanding of the molecular origins of cancer has changed greatly. Much of the progress derived from the identification of the oncogenes. These genes are normal cellular genes,

_____

Abbreviations AFB1, aflatoxin B1; CD, choline-deficient diet; CDE, choline-deficient diet containing ethionine; DAB, p-dimethylaminoazobenzene; DEN, diethylnitrosoamine; HO-DHE, 1'-hydroxy-2',3'-dehydroestragole; 3'-Me-DAB, 3'-methyl-4-dimethylaminoazobenzene; MUP, major urinary protein; N-HO-AAF, N-hydroxy-2-acetylaminofluorene; PB, phenobarbital; TPA, 12-O-tetradecanoyl phorbol-13-acetate; PDGF, platelet-derived growth factor; VC, vinyl carbamate.

involved in important cell functions. Their activation, through different mechanisms, may lead to malignant transformation (Bishop, 1987). At present, more than 30 distinct oncogenes are known. The cellular functions of the protein products are not yet clear for the majority of oncogenes, both in normal and in cancer cells.

Activation of oncogenes may occur by different mechanisms: point mutation, insertional mutagenesis, chromosomal translocation, gene amplification. The activation of a single oncogene has been proved to be insufficient for malignant transformation of a normal diploid cell (Land et al., 1983). It is now widely recognized that multiple molecular alterations are necessary to convert a normal cell into a fully tumorigenic cell. The requirement for multiple, independently activated genes may explain multistep carcinogenesis. The multistep carcinogenesis has been well studied in laboratory animals, and it has been demonstrated also for human cancer (Farber, 1984).

Recently, a new category of genes involved in some tumors has been discovered. These genes are named 'antioncogenes' or 'tumor-suppressor genes'. Their functions appear different from those of the oncogenes. They appear involved in negative growth-regulatory pathways, and their loss of function, creating a predisposition to malignant transformation, may represent one event in the multistage carcinogenesis process (Klein, 1987).

Activation of cellular oncogenes by a single point mutation in their coding sequence has been observed in different cases. The ras gene family (H-ras, K-ras and N-ras) has been most frequently involved, both in human and rodent tumors (Barbacid, 1987). The activated ras genes were detected by the NIH/3T3 transfection assay or by modifications of this technique.

Another form of activation of oncogenes is an altered expression of a structural normal gene. The altered expression may be caused by different mechanisms, including insertional mutagenesis, chromosomal translocation, gene amplification. Examples exist in the literature for each of these mechanisms (Alitalo and Schwab, 1986; Bishop, 1987; Klein, 1987; Ymer et al., 1985). In all cases where they have been studied, the amplified oncogenes have been found abundantly expressed at the RNA level. Therefore, gene amplification may mean increased expression of specific genes (Alitalo and Schwab, 1986).

In different human tumors amplification of specific oncogenes has been associated with a poor prognosis and with more malignant characteristics of the tumor. In particular, amplification of N-myc in neuroblastomas is strongly correlated with advanced clinical stages, i.e., stages III and IV (Seeger et al., 1985). Analysis of progression-free survival in patients with neuroblastomas revealed that amplification of N-myc was associated with the worst prognosis.

Similar results were obtained in human breast cancer for amplification of the HER-2 gene (also named neu or erbB-2). A significant correlation was found between HER-2 amplification and both disease-free survival and overall survival in lymphonode-positive patients with breast cancer. Greater HER-2 copy number were associated with a worst prognosis (Slamon et al., 1987).

Taken together, these results suggest that amplification of N-myc in neuroblastomas and of HER-2 in mammary carcinomas, may have a determinant role in the progression of these two tumors. New data indicate that amplification of both N-myc and HER-2 genes correspond to an over-expression of these genes (Alitalo et al., 1987; Berger et al., 1988). The biochemical activity of their over-expressed protein products most probably accounts for the role of N-myc and HER-2 genes in neuroblastomas and mammary carcinomas, respectively.

However, gene amplification may represent only one of different possible mechanisms that can modify gene expression in tumors. Irrespectively of the responsible mechanism, altered expression of specific genes appears to be very important in the pathogenesis of tumors, and it deserves further studies.

ACTIVATED ONCOGENES IN RODENT LIVER TUMORS

Point mutation

Recently, activated oncogenes of the ras family have been found by transfection assays in a high percentage of mouse liver tumors. The results have been obtained in different laboratories, with tumors induced by different carcinogens or even spontaneously arisen (Reynolds et al., 1987; Stowers et al., 1988; Wiseman et al., 1988). Up to 40% of adenomas and up to 80% of carcinomas were positive in the trasfection assay (Table 1). Further analysis demonstrated that the activated oncogene was Ha-ras in the great majority of the cases.

It should be noted that all the analysed tumors derived from B6C3 mice, a hybrid with high genetical susceptibility to hepatocarcinogenesis (Becker, 1982; Della Porta et al., 1987; Dragani et al., 1987; Ward et al., 1979). Therefore, we do not know whether or not similar results may be obtained with liver tumors originated in murine strains genetically resistant to hepatocarcinogenesis.

Interestingly, in rat liver tumors a quite different pattern of oncogene activation has been found by the transfection assay (Table 2). A high frequency of activated unknown oncogenes has been reported in a single experiment using AFB1-induced liver carcinomas (McMahon et al., 1986). However, the transforming activity of these tumors were not examined for stability upon secondary and tertiary transfections into NIH/3T3. Therefore, the results obtained with AFB1-induced rat liver tumors cannot be considered as conclusive. On the other hand, three other different laboratories failed to detect a significant percentage of rat liver tumors as positive in transfection assays (Farber et al., 1984; Ishikawa et al., 1985; Stowers et al., 1988). The biological

Table 1. Activated oncogenes detected in hepatocellular tumors of B6C3 mice

Treatment	Tumor type	Transfection frequency	Activated oncogene			
			H-ras	K-ras	raf	Unknown
Vehicle [a]	Adenoma	3/10	3	–	–	–
	Carcinoma	14/17	12	–	1	1
Furan [a]	Adenoma	9/19	7	2	–	–
	Carcinoma	4/10	3	–	1	–
Furfural [a]	Adenoma	2/3	2	–	–	–
	Carcinoma	11/13	7	1	–	3
N-HO-AAF [b]	Hepatoma	7/7	7	–	–	–
VC [b]	Hepatoma	7/7	7	–	–	–
HO-DHE [b]	Hepatoma	11/11	10	1	–	–
DEN [c]	Adenoma	8/22	8	–	–	–
	Carcinoma	6/11	6	–	–	–
Total	Adenoma	22/54 (41%)	20	2	–	–
	Carcinoma + Hepatoma	60/76 (79%)	52	2	2	4

[a] from Reynolds et al., 1987; [b] from Wiseman et al., 1986; [c] from Stowers et al., 1988.

significance of this clear difference at molecular level, between B6C3 mice and rat liver tumors, in the presence of activated ras oncogenes need further studies to be clarified.

Over-expression

To study gene expression at RNA level two methods are currently available:
1) study of expression of already cloned genes (probes available)
2) study of genes to be cloned on the basis of their characteristics of expression.

In the first case, we have a certain number of reports in which the expression of cellular oncogenes has been investigated in rodent liver

Table 2. Activated oncogenes detected in hepatocellular tumors of F344 rats

Treatment	Tumor type	Transfection frequency	Activated oncogene		
			H-ras	K-ras	Unknown
AFB1 [a]	Carcinoma	10/11	-	2	8
DEN [b]	Carcinoma	1/24	-	-	1
	Neoplastic nodule	0/4	-	-	-
DEN [c]	Carcinoma	0/20	-	-	-
2-amino-3-methylimidazo [4,5-f] quinoline [d]	Carcinoma	1/5	1	-	-
Total		12/64 (19%)	1	2	9

[a] from McMahon et al., 1986; [b] from Stowers et al., 1988; [c] from Farber, 1984; [d] from Ishikawa et al., 1985.

tumors. The oncogenes most widely studied are those of the ras family and the c-myc gene.

Table 3 shows the results obtained from different laboratories. They include analysis of expression made in tumor tissue, in tumor cell lines and in samples containing mixed tumor tissue and normal tissue.

In the majority of cases an increased expression of ras genes, as well as of c-myc gene was found. The results obtained with the tumor tissue showed a modest increase or no changes in expression of Ha-ras gene, and a considerable increase of c-myc RNA levels in most of the rat liver tumors (Hsieh et al., 1987; Makino et al., 1984). Interestingly, in rat liver tumors, transcripts homologous to the src oncogene were detected at unchanged levels compared to normal liver (Yaswen et al., 1985), and c-raf oncogene transcripts were seen at decreased levels (Hsieh et al., 1987).

Studies on oncogene expression in mouse liver tumors, however, are much more limited. We found in mouse liver tumors a slightly increased expression of Ha-ras gene, i.e., about 1.5- to 2-fold higher levels in tumors than in normal liver. On the other hand, c-myc gene was strongly induced in mouse liver tumors, compared to the normal liver (Dragani et al., 1986). In the same mouse liver tumor samples, other sequences, not related to oncogenes, but to specific families of endogenous retroviral

Table 3. Altered expression of cellular oncogenes in rat liver tumors

Strain	Treatment	No. of samples	Oncogenes			
			H-ras	K-ras	N-ras	c-myc
Sprague-Dawley [a]	3'-Me-DAB	6*	+			++
		4**	+			++
Sprague-Dawley [b]	DEN	3*	+	+	+	+
		4***	++	++	++	+
		1**	++	++	++	+
F344 [c]	3'-Me-DAB	5***	++			+
		4**	+	+		+
Sprague-Dawley [d]	CDE, CD	8***	=+	++		++
Sprague-Dawley [e]	DEN + PB	16*	=			++

*Tumor tissue, **Tumor cell line, ***Mixed tumor and normal tissue.
[a] Makino et al., 1984; [b] Corcos et al., 1984; [c] Cote et al., 1985; [d] Yaswen et al., 1985; [e] Hsieh et al., 1987.

genes were also over-expressed. Sequences related to Mo-MuLV and IAP were over-expressed in liver tumors. VL30 related RNA levels were increased in 4 tumors, but they were not substantially changed in the other 8 tumors. Mouse mammary tumor virus related sequences were absent both in normal liver and in tumor liver RNAs (Dragani et al., 1986).

It is important to note that our results and the results from other laboratories (Yaswen et al., 1985; Hsieh et al., 1987) indicate that mouse, as well as rat liver tumors, are associated with abnormalities in the expression of specific genes, but not with alteration in the overall pattern of gene expression.

DIFFERENTIAL SCREENING OF cDNA LIBRARIES

The second approach to study gene expression is represented in Table 4, in which a method to clone specific genes whose expression is modulated in different situations is shown. This method is named 'differential' or 'plus-minus' screening of cDNA libraries.

First, it is necessary to construct or to have available the cDNA library of interest. Filter replicas are then prepared from each plate. The filter replicas represent the exact copy of the plate, and they contain the DNA of the different recombinant phages bound to nitrocellulose. The filter replicas are then hybridized with RNA or

Table 4. Differential or 'plus-minus' screening of cDNA libraries

---

- Construction of a cDNA library
- Replica filters
- Labelling of mRNA (or cDNA) with ^{32}P
- Hybridization
   - driver of the reaction: filter-bound DNA
   - hybridization signal of each clone is proportional
   - to the relative abundance of the homologous mRNA
   - in the labelled mRNA population
- Identification and isolation of clones displaying differential ibridization signals
- Secondary and tertiary screenings
- Isolation of single clones displaying differential hybridization signals

---

cDNA probes synthetized from different RNA populations. The driver of hybridization reactions is the filter-bound DNA, present in large excess with respect to the homologous species in solution. The hybridization signal displayed by each clone is, therefore, proportional to the relative abundance of the omologous RNA in the labelled RNA population.

Differential expression is reflected by differences in the signal intensities displayed by specific clones. This technique allows the identification of individual clones displaying a differential hybridization signal. Once identified, the clones of interest are then isolated not pure, but mixed with other clones from the agar plate. A secondary, and perhaps a tertiary screening, at lower plaque densities than the first one, are necessary to purify the clones of interest.

The differential screening allowed to isolate specific genes expressed at levels as low as 0.05%. For the identification of genes expressed at levels lower than 0.05% other methodologies, such as the use of subtraction libraries and subtraction probes are more adequate (Davis, 1986). A number of genes, whose expression is changed in different situations, have been isolated by the differential screening. For example, this kind of screening has been used to identify sequences induced in response to various factors, including serum, PDGF, interferon, and TPA (Lau et al., 1985; Cochran et al., 1983; Friedman et al., 1984; Johnson et al., 1987).

With regard to genes over-expressed or under-expressed in experimental rodent tumors we can consider the results of three published studies. Yamamoto et al. (1983) screened 4,000 colonies of cDNA libraries from rat ascitic hepatoma cell lines. They isolated 160 clones displaying differential hybridization signal and characterized 31 clones, of which 14 contained repetitive sequences. The expression of these clones was increased in ascitic hepatoma cells, compared to normal rat liver. No information was available on the nucleotide sequence of the cloned genes. The same group reported in 1985 the nucleotide sequence of one clone insert (Endo et al., 1987). They found a complete homology between their clone and the gene of rat glyceraldehyde-3-phosphate dehydrogenase, an enzyme of glycolysis. Corral et al. (1986) followed a similar approach and characterized 3 clones showing a stronger hybridization signal with rat liver carcinomas than with normal rat liver. The authors did not report the nucleotide sequence of the cloned genes. Melber et al. (1986) reported the isolation, from mouse skin carcinoma cDNA libraries, of 6 clones over-expressed in mouse skin papillomas and carcinomas compared to normal skin. Information on nucleotide sequence of the isolated clones were not given.

Molecular cloning of genes under-expressed in mouse liver tumors

In our laboratory we have screened a normal adult mouse liver cDNA library to identify genes under-expressed in liver tumors compared to normal liver. This approach was chosen because we think that the identification of genes under-expressed in tumors may help in understanding some mechanisms of the carcinogenesis process.

In fact, genes may be under-expressed in tumors, compared to normal tissue, due to:
1) structural alterations of the genes in tumor tissue (e.g. deletions, translocations, loss of alleles, etc.)
2) depletion of trans acting factors in tumor cells
3) changes of differentiative functions in tumor cells

In all these cases, the study of genes under-expressed in tumors may lead to insights in the molecular alterations occurring in tumors and, in addition, the isolated genes may prove to be useful as tumor markers, that could be used in short- or medium-term carcinogenesis experiments (Bannash, 1986).

Fig. 1 shows an example of differential screening we performed using a normal liver cDNA library. The probes used were prepared from normal liver RNA and tumor liver RNA.

There were different plaques with different hybridization signals. For each plaque the signal was proportional to the relative abundance of the homologous RNA in the probe population. Some clones, indicated by the arrows, showed a much stronger signal when hybridized with normal liver RNA than with tumor liver RNA. Interestingly, most of the plaques displayed identical hybridization signals with both normal liver RNA and tumor liver RNA probes. Therefore, the majority of sequences expressed in normal adult liver does not change their RNA levels in liver tumors.

We constructed a cDNA library from a normal adult C3Hf male liver, using the vector lambda gt10. We obtained 10^6 recombinants. Therefore, the library contained also low abundant RNA species. The mean length of the inserts was not very high, about 0.5 kb, because we did not make the size selection of cDNAs before ligation with the phage arms.

First, we screened 3,600 plaques with probes from normal liver and from a spontaneous C3H hepatocellular carcinoma. We isolated 20 plaques displaying a hybridization signal stronger with normal liver RNA probe than with the tumor liver RNA probe. A subsequent screening was done with 4,000 plaques using RNA probes from normal liver and from DAB-induced hepatocellular carcinoma. We identified and isolated 35 clones with a hybridization signal stronger with normal liver than with tumor liver probes. In both cases we performed secondary screening at low plaque densities to purify the clones of interest. Several clones proved to be identical. Some clones showed similar response to both normal liver RNA and tumor RNA. 3 clones appeared more interesting and they were further characterized.

A clone, named al-1, contained a 600 bp insert. Clone al-1 was present at a relatively high abundance, since it was identical with 17 out of 20 and with 19 out of 35 clones isolated in the first and in the second screening, respectively.

Northern blot analysis, of 14-day-old liver (lane 1), adult livers (lanes 2 and 3), spontaneous hepatocellular carcinoma (lane 4) and DAB-induced hepatocellular carcinoma (lane 5) showed that clone al-1 displayed a strong signal with normal mouse liver RNA, but a very weak signal with tumor RNA, and no signal with 14-day-old liver RNA. The clone recognized a single transcript of about 1 kb (Fig. 2).

Clone al-2 detected in normal adult liver 3 transcripts of 4 kb, 3 kb and 1.1 kb. Transcripts of 4 and 3 kb were 3-4-fold more abundant in normal liver than in 14-day-old liver and in liver tumors. 1.1 kb RNA was detected only in normal liver. We do not know whether the shorter molecular weight transcripts represent splicing products of the 4 kb

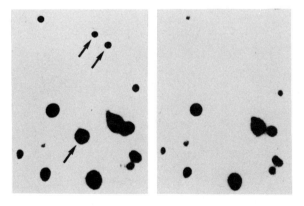

Fig. 1. Differential hybridization of mouse normal liver cDNA library. Duplicate filters were hybridized to ^{32}P-labelled RNA probes synthesized from (left) normal mouse liver or (right) mouse hepatocellular carcinoma. Arrows indicate clones displaying differential hybridization signals.

transcript, or whether they derived from different transcriptional starting points of the al-2 gene.

Clone al-3 showed a pattern of expression similar to clone al-1. (Fig. 3). The single 1 kb transcript displayed a strong signal with normal liver RNA and a very weak signal with 14-day-old liver and liver tumors. Clone al-3 was different from clone al-1, as judged by absence of cross-hybridization between the two clones.

Clone al-4 displayed differential hybridization signal during the differential screenings, but the Northern blot analysis showed that the clone is transcribed at similar levels in 14-day-old liver, in normal adult livers, and in liver carcinomas (Fig. 3). This clone, however, represented a good control, since it demonstrated that similar amounts of RNA were loaded in the different lanes. Therefore, the differences in the signal intensities observed using the other clones as probes were really due to different levels of transcripts.

Taken together, these results indicated that all the 3 clones we isolated represent, presumably, genes which are developmentally regulated in mouse liver. The decreased expression of these genes in liver tumors most likely represent loss of differentiated functions.

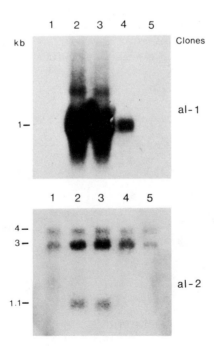

Fig. 2. Northern blot analysis of mouse normal liver cDNA clones. Lane 1, 14-day-old liver; Lanes 2 and 3, normal adult liver; Lane 4, spontaneous hepatocellular carcinoma; Lane 5, DAB-induced hepatocellular carcinoma.

We subcloned the 3 clones in the plasmid vector Bluescript, and we are carrying out the nucleotide sequence analysis. We have sequenced 121 nucleotides in the 3'-terminal region of clone al-1. This nucleotide sequence was screened for related sequences contained in the GenBank. Our sequence matched exactly, except for 2 gaps, with the 3'-terminal region of mouse MUP gene (Shahan et al., 1987) (Fig. 4).

MUP belongs to a multigene family of about 30 to 40 genes per aploid genome, which are clustered on mouse chromosome 4. MUP genes are expressed in liver, lacrimal glands, mammary glands and salivary glands, where they are subjected to different developmental and hormonal controls. MUP genes expressed in male liver are regulated by testosterone, growth hormone, and thyroid hormone (Held et al., 1987). To our knowledge a decreased MUP expression in liver tumors has not yet been reported. The decreased MUP expression we found in murine liver tumors may represent a loss of hormone responsivity of the tumor tissue.

Nucleotide sequence of about 200 bases of al-3 gene also matched with the MUP sequence, although without a complete homology (data not shown). To explain the lack of cross-hybridization between clone al-1 and clone al-3 we think that clone al-3 may represent a portion of the same MUP gene not contained in the al-1 clone, or, alternatively, al-3 may represent a different MUP-like gene, containing regions of homology with the MUP sequence. We are carrying out experiments to clarify this point.

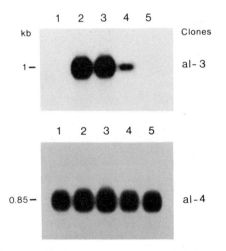

Fig. 3. Northern blot analysis of mouse normal liver cDNA clones. Lane 1, 14-day-old liver; Lanes 2 and 3, normal adult liver; Lane 4, spontaneous hepatocellular carcinoma; Lane 5, DAB-induced hepatocellular carcinoma.

The next step in our project is the characterization of the role of the isolated genes in mouse hepatocarcinogenesis. To this aim we are planning to use antibodies against their protein products, in immunoperoxidase techniques. The use of immunoperoxidase technique on histological slides containing small and large liver nodules may allow the assessment of:
1) whether or not the decreased expression of these genes occur at early or late stages of mouse hepatocarcinogenesis
2) whether or not the cloned genes may represent good tumor markers for mouse hepatocarcinogenesis.

CONCLUSIONS

In conclusion, the differential screening represents a powerful technique to isolate genes whose expression is altered in tumors compared to the normal tissue. This tecnique is not very easy to carry out and it may lead to the isolation of already known genes. However, we think that it may also allow the identification and isolation of genes playing an important role in tumor development.

The available murine model of hepatocarcinogenesis and the modern methodologies of molecular biology can allow us to study the genes involved in the different stages of the carcinogenesis process, from the early neoplastic nodules, to the hepatocellular adenomas and carcinomas. Once genes presumably involved in the pathogenesis of mouse liver tumors have been isolated, the murine model will allow us also to compare spontaneously occurring liver tumors in genetically susceptible strains, with chemically-induced liver tumors.

In perspective, we should be able to understand whether or not the carcinogen-induced genetic lesions in specific genes are identical to the lesions observed in spontaneous liver tumors. Therefore, the possible relevance of newly identified genes may be evaluated in detail

```
               .         .        .         .        .
al-1      TGTTACCTAGGATACCTCATTCAAGAATC.AAGACTTCTTTAAATTTTTC
MUP  804  --------------------.---------A---------------------  852

                    .                  .           .
al-1      TTTGATATACCCATGACAATTTTTCATGAATTTCTTCCTCTTCCTGTTCA
MUP  853  -------------------------------------------------  902

                 .         .
al-1      ATAAATGATTACCCTTGCACTT
MUP  903  --------------------- 924
```

Fig. 4. Partial nucleotide sequence of clone al-1 compared to MUP sequence. Conserved bases are indicated by dashes, dots indicate the introduction of gaps for alignment.

in murine hepatocarcinogenesis. In addition, a comparison could also be done between results obtained in murine liver tumors and results that could be obtained in liver tumors of other species, for example rats, hamsters and also humans, using the newly isolated genes in hybridization reactions performed at relaxed stringency conditions.

ACKNOWLEDGEMENTS

The authors wish to thank Mrs. Stefania Falvella and Mrs. Teresa Radice for their valuable technical assistance. This investigation was supported by a grant from the Consiglio Nazionale delle Ricerche (Finalized Project "Oncology") Rome, Italy, and by Associazione Italiana Ricerca sul Cancro.

REFERENCES

Alitalo K., Koskinen P., Makela T.P., Saksela K., Sistonen L., Winqvist R. (1987) myc Oncogenes: activation and amplification. Biochim. Biophys. Acta, 907: 1-32.

Alitalo K., Schwab M. (1986) Oncogene amplification in tumor cells. Adv. Cancer Res., 47: 235-281.

Bannasch P. (1986) Preneoplastic lesions as end points in carcinogenicity testing. I. Hepatic preneoplasia. Carcinogenesis, 7: 689-695.

Barbacid M. (1987) ras Genes. Ann. Rev. Biochem., 56: 779-827.

Becker F.F. (1982) Morphological classification of mouse liver tumors based on biological characteristics. Cancer Res., 42: 3918-3923.

Berger M.S., Locher G.W., Saurer S., Gullick W.J., Waterfield M.D., Groner B., Hynes N.E. (1988) Correlation of c-erbB-2 gene amplification and protein expression in human breast carcinoma with nodal status and nuclear grading. Cancer Res., 48: 1238-1243.

Bishop M.J. (1987) The molecular genetics of cancer. Science, 235: 305-310.

Cochran B.H., Reffel A.C., Stiles C.D. (1983) Molecular cloning of gene sequences regulated by platelet-derived growth factor. Cell, 33: 939-947.

Corcos D., Defer N., Raymondjean M., Paris B., Corral M., Tichonicky L., Kruh J. (1984) Correlated increase of the expression of the c-ras genes in chemically induced hepatocarcinomas. Bioch. Biophys. Res. Comm., 122: 259-264.

Corral M., Defer N., Paris B., Raymondjean M., Corcos D., Tichonicky L., et al. (1986) Isolation and characterization of complementary DNA clones for genes overexpressed in chemically induced rat hepatomas. Cancer Res., 46: 5119-5124.

Cote G.J., Lastra B.A., Cook J.R., Huang D.-P., Chiu J.-F. (1985) Oncogene expression in rat hepatomas and during hepatocarcinogenesis. Cancer Lett., 26: 121-127.

Davis M.M. (1986) Subtractive cDNA hybridization and the T-cell receptor genes. in: "Handbook of Experimental Immunology. Vol. 2: Cellular Immunology", D.M. Weir ed., Ch. 76. Blackwell Sci. Publ., Oxford.

Della Porta G., Dragani T.A., Manenti G. (1987) Two-stage liver carcinogenesis in the mouse. Toxicol. Pathology, 15: 229-233.

Dragani T.A., Manenti G., Della Porta G., Gattoni-Celli S., Weinstein I.B. (1986) Expression of retroviral sequences and oncogenes in murine hepatocellular tumors. Cancer Res., 46: 1915-1919.

Dragani T.A., Manenti G., Della Porta G. (1987) Genetic susceptibility to murine hepatocarcinogenesis is associated with high growth rate of NDEA-initiated hepatocytes. J. Cancer Res. Clin. Oncol., 113: 223-229.

Endo H., Fujiyoshi T., Maehara Y., Shikata I., Nogae I. (1987) Conserved sequences abundantly expressed in tumor cells. in: "Molecular Biology and Differentiation of Cancer Cells (Oncogenes, Growth Factors, Receptors)", K. Lapis, S. Eckhardt eds., pp. 21-26. Akademiai Kiado', Budapest.

Farber E. (1984) Cellular biochemistry of the stepwise development of cancer with chemicals: G.H.A. Clowes Memorial Lecture. Cancer Res., 44: 5463-5474.

Friedman R.L., Manly S.P., McMahon M., Kerr I.M., Stark G.R. (1984) Transcriptional and posttranscriptional regulation of interferon-induced gene expression in human cells. Cell, 38: 745-755.

Held W.A., Gallagher J.F., Hohman C.M., Kuhn N.J., Sampsell B.M., Hughes R.G. (1987) Identification and characterization of functional genes encoding the mouse major urinary proteins. Mol. Cell. Biol., 7: 3705-3712.

Hsieh L.L., Hsiao W.-L., Peraino C., Maronpot R.R., Weinstein I.B. (1987) Expression of retroviral sequences and oncogenes in rat liver tumors induced by diethylnitrosamine. Cancer Res., 47: 3421-3424.

Ishikawa F., Takaku F., Nagao M., Hayashi K., Takayama S., Sugimura T. (1985) Activated oncogenes on a rat hepatocellular carcinoma induced by 2-amino-3-methylimidazo 4,5-f quinoline. Gann, 76: 425-428.

Johnson M.D., Housey G.M., Kirschmeier P.T., Weinstein I.B. (1987) Molecular cloning of gene sequences regulated by tumor promoters and mitogens through protein kinase C. Mol. Cell. Biology, 7: 2821-2829.

Klein G. (1987) The approaching era of the tumor suppressor genes. Science, 238: 1539-1545.

Land H., Parada L.F., Weinberg R.A. (1983) Cellular oncogenes and multistep carcinogenesis. Science, 222: 771-778.

Lau L.F., Nathans D. (1985) Identification of a set of genes expressed during the G0/G1 transition of cultured mouse cells. EMBO J., 4: 3145-3151.

Makino R., Hayashi K., Sato S., Sugimura T. (1984) Expression of the c-Ha-ras and c-myc genes in rat liver tumors. Bioch. Biophys. Res. Comm., 119: 1096-1102.

McMahon G., Hanson L., Lee J.-J., Wogan G.N. (1986) Identification of an activated c-Ki-ras oncogene in rat liver tumors induced by aflatoxin B1. Proc. Natl. Acad. Sci. USA, 83: 9418-9422.

Melber K., Krieg P., Fustenberger G., Marks F. (1986) Molecular cloning of sequences activated during multi-stage carcinogenesis in mouse skin. Carcinogenesis, 7: 317-322.

Reynolds S.H., Stowers S.J., Patterson R.M., Maronpot R.R., Aaronson S.A., Anderson M.W. (1987) Activated oncogenes in B6C3F1 mouse liver tumors: implications for risk assessment. Science, 237: 1309–1316.

Seeger R.C., Brodeur G.M., Sather H., Dalton A., Siegel S.E., Wong K.Y., Hammond D. (1985) Association of multiple copies of the N-myc oncogene with rapid progression of neuroblastomas. N. Engl. J. Med., 313: 1111–1116.

Shahan K., Gilmartin M., Derman E. (1987) Nucleotide sequences of liver, lachrymal, and submaxillary gland mouse major urinary protein mRNAs: mosaic structure and construction of panels of gene-specific synthetic oligonucleotide probes. Mol. Cell. Biol. 7: 1938–1946.

Slamon D.J., Clark G.M., Wong S.G., Levin W.J., Ullrich A., McGuire W.L. (1987) Human breast cancer: correlation of relapse and survival with amplification of the HER-2/neu oncogene. Science, 235: 177–182.

Stowers S.J., Wiseman R.W., Ward J.M., Miller E.C., Miller J.A., Anderson M.W., Eva A. (1988) Detection of activated proto-oncogenes in N-nitrosodiethylamine-induced liver tumors: a comparison between B6C3F1 mice and Fisher 344 rats. Carcinogenesis, 9: 271–276.

Ward J.M., Goodman D.G., Squire R.A., Chu K.C., Linhart M.S. (1979) Neoplastic and nonneoplastic lesions in aging (C57BL/6NxC3H/HeN)F1 (B6C3F1) mice. J. Natl. Cancer Inst., 63: 849–854.

Wiseman R.W., Stowers S.J., Miller E.C., Anderson M.W., Miller J.A. (1986) Activating mutations of the c-Ha-ras protooncogene in chemically induced hepatomas of the male B6C3 F1 mouse. Proc. Natl. Acad. Sci. USA, 83: 5825–5829.

Yamamoto M., Maehara Y., Takahashi K., Endo H. (1983) Cloning of sequences expressed specifically in tumors of rat. Proc. Natl. Acad. Sci. USA, 80: 7524–7527.

Yaswen P., Goyette M., Shank P.R., Fausto N. (1985) Expression of c-Ki-ras, c-Ha-ras, and c-myc in specific cell types during hepatocarcinogenesis. Mol. Cell. Biol., 5: 780–786.

Ymer S., Tucker W.O.J., Sanderson C.J., Hapel A.J., Campbell H.D., Young I.G. (1985) Constitutive synthesis of interleukin-3 by the leukaemia cell line WEHI-3B is due to retroviral insertion near the gene. Nature, 317: 255–258.

MEDIUM-TERM BIOASSAY MODELS FOR ENVIRONMENTAL CARCINOGENS — TWO-STEP LIVER AND MULTI-ORGAN CARCINOGENESIS PROTOCOLS

Nobuyuki Ito, Hiroyuki Tsuda, Ryohei Hasegawa,
Masae Tatematsu, Katsumi Imaida and Makoto Asamoto

First Department of Pathology, Nagoya City University
Medical School, Mizuho-cho, Mizuho-ku, Nagoya 467, Japan

INTRODUCTION

Epidemiological studies have made it increasingly clear that the variation in individual cancer rates in different regions of the world is a direct reflection of the presence or absence of exogenous, causal factors (Wynder and Gori, 1977; Doll, 1978). The investigation of possible nutritional and other environmentally derived influences in animal experiments has further established that a vast array of compounds are capable of playing a role in tumorigenesis, and it is now recognized that detection and appropriate regulation of these compounds are of prime importance for the management of neoplasia in man. Moreover, since it is now evident that neoplastic development is a multistep process, this question is complicated by the problem of different stages at which exogenous factors could interact (Foulds, 1969; Berenblum, 1974; Wynder, 1983). Until recently 2-year long-term _in vivo_ testing using rats, mice or hamsters has been considered to be the most reliable method for the prediction of carcinogenic potential in man (NCI, 1976; IARC, 1980). However, to be internationally accepted these long-term tests must satisfy costly regulatory guidelines for appropriate facilities, long duration (2 years), maintenance of animals, sufficiently large numbers of rodents and careful histopathological examination. Therefore the vast number of compounds which have been introduced into our environment in recent years is far beyond our capacity to assess using such comprehensive carcinogenicity tests in each case.

For the purpose of performing mass screening of compounds, _in vitro_ short-term screening assays using gene mutation, including the _Salmonella_ /microsome assay (Ames' test), chromosomal aberration and various other test systems have been developed (Ames, 1975; Ishidate et al., 1981; IARC, 1982; IARC, 1986). Using these methods, a variety of compounds were shown to be genotoxic with apparently good correlation to their known carcinogenicity (Rinkus et al., 1979; Haworth et al., 1983; Kier et al., 1986).

Recently, however, as the number of compounds tested increased, it became clear that genotoxicity results did not always show direct correlation to carcinogenicity (ICPMC, 1984; Kier et al., 1986; Zeiger, 1987) (see Table 1). Thus, although the tests are very rapid and

Table 1.   Example list of carcinogens negative in the Salmonella assay

Chemical	Principal site of tumor induction	Chemical	Principal site of tumor induction
Acetamide	liver	Diethylstilbestrol	mammary gland
Aldrin	liver	1,2-Dimethylhydrazine	large intestine
3-Amino-1H-1,2,4-triazole	thyroid	Ethyl carbamate	liver
Auramine	liver	Safrole	liver
Butylated hydroxyanisole	forestomach	Sodium saccharin	urinary bladder
Carbon tetrachloride	liver	Thioacetamide	liver
Cycasin	liver	Trypan blue	liver
DDT	liver		

inexpensive, the existence of discrepancies indicates that in vivo testing is indeed necessary. This paper is primarily concerned with efforts in our laboratory to develop suitable medium term systems.

BACKGROUND

Sequential Analysis of Neoplastic Development

Since the development of the concepts of initiation and promotion, as originally proposed on the basis of research into skin carcinogenesis, subsequent investigations have demonstrated their applicability to a large number of other organ or tissue models, including the alimentary tract, thyroid, respiratory tract, kidney, mammary gland, urinary bladder, and liver (reviewed by Berenblum, 1974; Pitot and Sirica, 1980). This last organ is of particular importance, since a number of attributes combine to make it a model system for the investigation of carcinogenesis. Ease of induction of neoplasms, large size, and relative homogeneity have, for example, contributed to the use of the liver for the vast majority of investigations into changes in biochemical parameters during carcinogenesis, although interpretation of such data is complicated both by consideration of zoning of hepatocyte populations (Rappaport, 1979) and by the focal nature of neoplastic development (Foulds, 1975).

Histogenesis of Hepatocellular Neoplasias

For similar reasons, the histopathology of liver lesion development has also been best studied although it is important to remember that similar sequences have been established for all organs investigated. The earliest recognizable foci of altered hepatocytes in the liver after carcinogen application are distinguishable from background parenchyma on the grounds of morphology (Farber, 1980; Williams, 1980; Bannasch, 1986) and changed enzyme phenotype (Kitagawa, 1971; Pugh and Goldfarb, 1978; Butler et al., 1981) and demonstrate a quantitative dependency on the dose of carcinogen given (Moore et al., 1982; Vesselinovitch and Mihailovich, 1983; Tamano et al., 1983; Scherer, 1984).

A sequence of development from small foci of cells, usually characterized by excessive storage of glycogen but sometimes presenting as basophilic populations, to nodular lesions comprising mixtures of basophilic, clear, and acidophilic cells to the final basophilic tumors has been established (Bannasch et al., 1980; Institute of Laboratory Animal Resources, 1980). This sequence is accompanied by a correlated change in the pattern of enzymes involved in carbohydrate metabolism (Hacker et al., 1982) and an increase in proliferation rate, which appears independent of further carcinogen administration (Bannasch et al., 1982). Investigation of the growth kinetics of cells making up enzyme-altered foci has consistently revealed increases, as compared to the rate of tritiated incorporation into "normal" background hepatocytes both in vivo and in vitro (Rabes et al., 1972). The increase in conformity of expression of different enzyme markers evident in larger and more advanced lesions (Ogawa et al., 1980; Moore et al., 1983) has, moreover, been demonstrated tb correlate positively with an increased proliferation rate (Pugh and Goldfarb, 1978).

In our experience of the liver, the most promising positive marker enzymes appear to be glutathione S-transferase placental form (GST-P) and glucose-6-phosphate dehydrogenase (G6PDH) (Hacker et al., 1982; Sato et al., 1984; Tatematsu et al., 1985). Use of immunohistochemically demonstrated GST-P has practical advantages because of the ease of staining which enables rapid processing of large numbers of specimens and clear contrast recognition allowing the use of a semi-automatic image analysis system. An overview of analogous lesions involved in tumor development in a range of organs and our knowledge of the best marker enzymes in each case is given in Table 2.

Table 2. Markers of preneoplastic lesions in different organs

Organ	Phenotypic expression		Preneoplastic change
	Histology	Marker enzyme	
Nasal cavity	Dysplasia	?	PN hyperplasia
Lung	Hyperplasia	GST-P	Adenomatous hyperplasia
Esophagus	Dysplasia	?	Dysplastic epithelium
Forestomach	Dysplasia	?	PN hyperplasia
Glandular stomach	Dysplastic tubules	Pg 1 (-)	Adenomatous hyperplasia
Intestine	Dysplastic tubules	?	Adenomatous hyperplasia
Liver	Foci	GST-P, γ-GT, G6PDH	Hyperplastic nodule
Pancreas	Duct hyperplasia	GST-P	Dysplastic epithelium
Kidney	Dysplastic tubules	GST-A, G6PDH	Dysplastic epithelium
Urinary bladder	Dysplasia	G6PDH, SDH	PN hyperplasia
Mammary gland	Duct hyperplasia	?	HAN
Prostate	Hyperplasia	?	Dysplastic epithelium

PN hyperplasia : Papillary or nodular hyperplasia
HAN : Hyperplastic alveolar nodule

DEVELOPMENT OF ASSAY MODELS

1) Two-step Liver Medium-term Assay Protocol

The importance of liver cell proliferation for enhancement of carcinogenesis in both the initiation (Craddock, 1974; Pitot et al., 1978; Tsuda et al., 1980) and promotion (Solt and Farber, 1976; Hasegawa et al., 1982) stages in two-step models has been stressed. Recently, several medium-term duration assay systems for liver carcinogens and promoters have been developed, utilizing the initiation-promotion concept (Peraino et al., 1975; Pitot et al., 1980; Williams, 1982; Goldsworthy, 1986; Preat et al., 1986; Bannasch, 1986).

Since the introduction of the two-step liver model for rapid induction of lesions with 2-acetylaminofluorene (2-AAF) as a potent promoting agent (Farber et al., 1976; Solt and Farber, 1976), our attention has been focused on the development of a short-term assay system, preferably not only for liver but also for non-liver carcinogens, with a suitably short duration but sufficient effects to allow demonstration of significance. For example, when rats were treated with diethylnitrosamine (DEN) or 2-AAF for the initiation step followed by administration of various test compounds combined with partial hepatectomy, an increased number and area of preneoplastic focal lesions distinguished as hyperplastic nodules (HN) or γ-glutamyl transpeptidase (γ-GT) positive foci was noted with good correlation to known potency to promote hepatocarcinogenesis in long-term studies (Ito et al., 1980, 1982; Tatematsu et al., 1983)

More recent studies in our laboratory indicated that immunohistochemically demonstrated GST-P positive staining of foci showed good conformity to γ-GT positivity with the advantage of far less background hepatocyte staining (Sato et al., 1984; Tatematsu et al., 1985). Therefore, we introduced GST-P staining for the novel end-point marker lesions of the assay method (see Fig. 1). It should be noted that ∿60% of the environmental carcinogens which were rated to have "sufficient evidence" of capacity to cause cancer in man listed in IARC (IARC, 1982) proved to be hepatocarcinogens. Therefore theoretically more than half of all environmental carcinogens could be screened by liver assay systems.

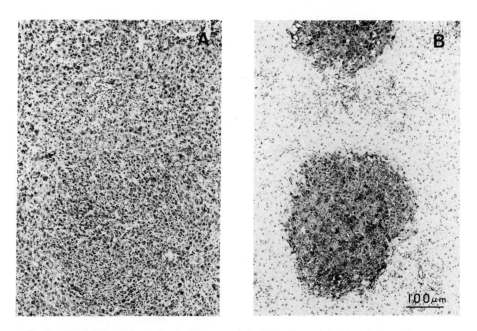

Fig. 1. Serial liver sections after performance of the DEN-PH model, A) H & E, B) immuno-histochemical staining for GST-P.

a) DEN-PH model

Materials and methods   Male F344 rats (Charles River Japan Inc., Atsugi, Japan) weighing ∿160 g at the commencement were maintained on basal diet (Oriental M, Oriental Yeast Co., Tokyo, Japan) ad libitum and housed in plastic cages in an air-conditioned room at 24°C. The animals in each experiment were divided into three groups. Group 1 was given a single i.p. injection of DEN (200 mg/kg) dissolved in 0.9% NaCl to initiate hepatocarcinogenesis. After 2 weeks on basal diet, they received one of the test compounds in the basal diet (D), drinking water (W), or by i.p. or i.v. injection at different concentrations. Animals were subjected to two-thirds partial hepatectomy (PH) at week 3 to maximize any interaction between proliferation and the effects of the compounds tested (Hasegawa et al., 1986). Group 2 was given DEN and PH in the same manner as for group 1 without administration of any test compounds. Group 3 animals were injected with 0.9% NaCl instead of DEN solution and then subjected to administration of test compound and PH. Rats in each group were killed for examination at week 8 (10 to 25 rats each group) (Fig. 2). The doses of test compounds were chosen on the basis of preliminary investigations as permitting >70% survival of rats after PH performed during the administration, or from chronic toxicity data when available.

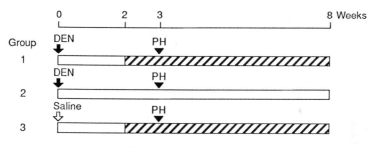

Animals : F344 male rats, 6-weeks-old
↓ : DEN (diethylnitrosamine), 200 mg/kg, i.p.
▼ : PH (2/3 partial hepatectomy)
▨ : 136 different test compounds

Fig. 2.   DEN-PH model protocol.

Table 3.   Positive rates for 136 compounds of different categories (%)

Test compound	Genotoxicity			Total
	+	−	Unknown	
Liver carcinogen	14 / 15 (93) *	13 / 15 (87) **	0 / 0	27 / 30 (90)
Non-liver carcinogen	1 / 14 (7)	1 / 6 (17)	0 / 1 (0)	2 / 21 (10)
Non-carcinogen	0 / 6 (0)	0 / 19 (0)	0 / 2 (0)	0 / 27 (0)
Unknown	1 / 8 (13)	7 / 28 (25)	4 / 22 (18)	12 / 58 (21)

* Diaminodiphenylmethane (DDPM) was negative

** Clofibrate and di(2-ethylhexyl)phthalate (DEHP) were negative

213

Table 4. Association between positive results, genotoxicity and site of carcinogenicity

Compound	Geno-Toxicity	Carcino-genicity	Principal site of tumor induction
Aromatic amines and azodye			
2-Acetylaminofluorene (2-AAF)	+	+	liver, bladder, Zymbal gland
2-Amino-3-methylimidazo[4,5-f]quinoline (IQ)	+	+	liver, forestomach, intestines
3'-Methyl-4-dimethylaminozobenzene (3'-Me-DAB)	+	+	liver
Nitrosamines			
Dibutylnitrosamine (DBN)	+	+	liver, bladder, esophagus, forestomach
Diethylnitrosamine (DEN)	+	+	liver
Dimethylnitrosamine (DMN)	+	+	liver, kidney
N-Ethyl-N-hydroxyethylnitrosamine (EHEN)	+	+	liver, kidney
Polycyclic aromatic hydrocarbons			
Benzo[a]pyrene	+	+	lung, application site, liver?
Aflatoxin B$_1$	+	+	liver
Sterigmatocystin	+	+	liver
Hormones and endogenous metabolites			
Cholic acid	−	−	
Diethylstilbestrol	−	+	mammary, pituitary, liver?
17-α-Ethinyl estradiol	−	+	liver, mammary, pituitary
Orotic acid	−		
Taurine	−		
Malonic acid	−		
Pesticides			
Aldrin	−	+	liver
Captafol	+	+	liver, heart
Carbazole	+	+	liver, forestomach
Chlorodane	−	+	liver
Dieldrin	−	+	liver
Disulfiram	−		
α-Hexachlorocyclohexane (α-HCH)	−	+	liver
Phenytoin	−	−	
Tetramethylthiuram disulfide (Thiram)	+	−	
Drugs and dyes			
Aminopyrine	−		
Auramine	−	+	liver
Barbital	−	+	liver
Dipyrone (Sulpyrin)	+	+	liver
Ethenzamide	−	+	liver
HC Blue 1	+	+	liver
Phenobarbital	−	+	liver
Miscellaneous chemicals			
D,L-Ethionine	−	+	liver
Monoaldehyde bis(diethylacetate) (MABD)	−		
Safrole	+	+	liver
Sodium benzoate	−		
Sodium nitrate	−		
Sodium propionate	−		
Thioacetamide	−	+	liver
Urethane	−	+	liver, lung
Quinoline	+	+	liver

Immediately upon sacrifice, the livers were excised and sections 2-3 mm thick were cut with a razor blade. Four slices, one each from the right posterior and caudate lobes and two from the right anterior lobe, were fixed in ice-cold acetone for immunohistochemical examination of GST-P. Anti-GST-P antibody was raised as described previously (Satoh et al., 1985). The avidin-biotin-peroxidase complex (ABC) method described by Hsu et al. (1981) was used to determine the location of GST-P binding in the liver (Vectastain ABC Kit, PK 4001, Vector Laboratories Inc.,

Burlingame, CA). As a negative control for the specificity of anti-GST-P antibody binding, pre-immune rabbit serum was used instead of antiserum.

The numbers and areas of GST-P positive foci or areas of >0.2 mm in diameter were measured using a color video image processor (VIP-21C, Olympus-Ikegami Tsushin Co., Tokyo, Japan) as described previously (Ito et al., 1980; Tatematsu et al., 1983). The results were assessed by comparing the values of foci between group 1 (DEN-test compounds) and group 2 (DEN alone), while group 3 served for the assay of potential to induce GST-P positive foci without prior DEN. Statistical analysis was carried out using the Student's t-test and scoring of the results was made on the basis of the P value for the difference between groups 1 and 2: an increase at P < 0.05 in either number or area of foci was regarded as positive.

Results   The results for different classes of chemicals which were tested for enhancement of the induction of GST-P positive foci are summarized in Table 3. Most liver carcinogens gave positive results (27 out of 30, 90%) whereas positivity for non-liver carcinogens was low (2 out of 21, 10%). It should be noted that 13 out of 15 (87%) non-genotoxic liver carcinogens gave positive results. GST-P positive foci were also induced in group 3 rats given potent hepatocarcinogens such as 2-AAF, DEN, dimethylnitrosamine, 3'-methyl-4-dimethylaminoazobenzene (3'-Me-DAB) aflatoxin B1, 2-amino-3-methylimidazo[4,5-f]quinoline and thioacetamide. However these values were far less than for group 1. No false-positive results were recorded because none of the test chemicals without carcinogenic activity (27 compounds) enhanced the induction of GST-P positive foci.

Table 5.   Compounds showing inhibitory effects

Compound	Geno-toxicity	Carcinogenicity (site)	Note
Antioxidant			
Butylated hydroxyanisole (BHA)	−	+ (forestomach)	
Caffeic acid	−		
Catechol	−		
Esculin	−		
Eugenol	−	−	
Ferulic acid			
Gallic acid	−		
p-Methoxyphenol			
Sesamol			
tert-Butylhydroquinone (TBHQ)	−		
α-Tocopherol	−	−	
Peroxisome proliferator			
Clofibrate	−	+ (liver)	peroxidation product
Di(2-ethylhexyl)phthalate (DEHP)	−	+ (liver)	peroxidation product
Drugs, pesticides and others			
Acetaminophen	−	−	anti-pyretic drug
Diphenyl	−		pesticide
Ethyl alcohol	−	−	
2-(2-furyl)-3(5-nitro-2-furyl)acrylamide (AF-2)	+	+ (forestomach)	food additive
Harman	+		
Indomethacin	−		anti-inflammatory drug
Linolic acid hydroperoxide A	+		peroxidation product
Linolic acid hydroperoxide B			peroxidation product
Methyltestosterone			sex hormone
o-Aminophenol	−		acetaminophen derivative

Forty one chemicals which enhanced development of GST-P positive foci calculated from the groups 1 and 2 quantitative values of each experimental series are presented in Table 4 along with data for known genotoxicity and carcinogenicity in long term in vivo experiments. A number of chemicals, in contrast, were shown to have inhibitory effects, the majority of these being antioxidants (see Table 5).

Summary   The described experimental protocol was found to be of advantage for rapid screening of the large number of environmental chemicals which may possess the potential to induce liver cancer in man. Although the results with non-hepatocarcinogens were less than satisfactory, it was concluded that the system could nevertheless be of practical use because ∿60% of the environmental carcinogens which were rated to have "sufficient evidence" of capacity to cause cancer in man listed in the IARC (1982) proved to be hepatocarcinogens.

b) DEN-Galactosamine-PH model

Since results with non-liver carcinogens in DEN-PH model were far from satisfying, we attempted to develop a model which might also detect some of these compounds by alteration of our liver system. To this end, since treatment with D-galactosamine is well known to cause liver damage and hepatocellular proliferation (Keppler et al., 1968; Decker et al., 1972; Tsuda et al., 1987) an investigation of its effects on GST-P positive foci development in our medium-term bioassay system was performed (Ito et al., 1988).

Materials and methods   A total of 410 6-week-old male F344 rats (Charles River Japan Inc.) were used. Rats were divided into 3 groups. The animals in Groups 1 and 2 were given a single i.p. injection of 200 mg of DEN per kg body weight in saline. Animals in Group 3 received saline i.p. in place of carcinogen. After 2 weeks on basal diet, all groups received a single i.p. injection of D-galactosamine (Wako Pure Chemical Industries, Osaka, Japan) at a dose of 300 mg/kg. At the same time, treatment with test chemicals mixed in the basal diet (Oriental M, Oriental Yeast Co.) or the drinking water was commenced (Fig. 3). The doses of test chemicals used were the same as in the DEN-PH model. In group 3, which served as the control, basal diet and tap water were given continuously for 8 weeks after the exposure to DEN. All groups underwent PH at week 5, and rats were sacrificed at the end of week 8 for assessment of liver lesion development. The liver was similarly

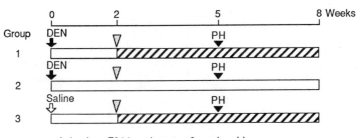

Animals : F344 male rats, 6-weeks-old
↓ : DEN (diethylnitrosamine), 200 mg/kg, i.p.
▽ : D-Galactosamine, 300 mg/kg 5 ml saline, i.p.
▼ : PH (2/3 partial hepatectomy)
▧ : Test compounds

Fig. 3. DEN-Galactosamine-PH model protocol.

processed for immunohistochemical staining of GST-P and quantitatively analyzed as in the DEN-PH model.

Results   The results are summarized in Table 6. Hepatocarcinogens such as 2-AAF, 3'-Me-DAB, DL-ethionine (ethionine), and phenobarbital (PB) all showed positive results, as in the DEN-PH bioassay system. The false negative compound 4,4'-diaminodiphenylmethane (DDPM) in the DEN-PH model moreover gave a positive result. Furthermore, non-liver carcinogens such as N-butyl-N-(4-hydroxybutyl)nitrosamine (BBN), 3-methylcholanthrene (3-MC) and 7,12-dimethylbenz(a)anthracene (DMBA) also gave positive results, in clear contrast to the data from the previous assay system. N-Methyl-N'-nitro-N-nitrosoguanidine (MNNG) was, however, negative in both cases. In confirmation of earlier results, butylated hydroxyanisole (BHA) demonstrated an inhibitory effect on the induction of GST-P foci (Table 7).

Summary   The present results clearly demonstrated that a single necrogenic treatment with D-galactosamine at the commencement of test chemical administration increases the sensitivity of our medium-term bioassay system to carcinogens which do not normally induce liver tumors.

Table 6.   Positive rates for 15 compounds of different categories in the DEN-Galactosamine-PH model (%)

Test compound	Genotoxicity			Total
	+	−	Unknown	
Liver carcinogen	4 / 4 (100)	1 / 2 (50) [a]	0 / 0	5 / 6 (83)
Non-liver carcinogen	4 / 5 (80) [b]	0 / 1 (0)	0 / 0	4 / 6 (67)
Non-carcinogen	0 / 0	0 / 3 (0)	0 / 0	0 / 3 (0)

[a] Clofibrate was negative.
[b] N-Methyl-N'-nitro-N-nitrosoguanidine (MNNG) was negative.

Table 7.   Numbers and total areas of GST-P positive foci in livers of rats using the DEN-Galactosamine-PH model

Test chemical	Dose (%)	Route [a]	No. of rats	GST-P positive foci		Previous results [b]
				No./cm²	Area (mm²/cm²)	
2-AAF	0.01	D	19	51.7 ± 14.6 ***	55.2 ± 12.4 ***	+
3'-Me-DAB	0.06	D	17	58.8 ± 12.6 ***	37.9 ± 15.7 ***	+
Ethionine	0.25	D	11	32.2 ± 8.1 ***	4.1 ± 1.5 ***	+
Phenobarbital	0.05	D	7	17.0 ± 6.9 ***	1.3 ± 0.4 ***	+
Clofibrate	0.03	D	10	3.3 ± 1.5	0.2 ± 0.1	−
DDPM	0.1	D	9	9.1 ± 4.9 *	0.7 ± 0.5 *	−
Benzo[a]pyrene	0.02	D	18	7.9 ± 2.5 ***	0.5 ± 0.2 ***	+
BHA	1	D	18	1.6 ± 1.0 ***	0.1 ± 0.1 ***	−
BBN	0.1	W	18	5.6 ± 2.4 *	0.3 ± 0.2 *	−
3-MC	0.02	D	17	16.5 ± 5.1 ***	1.3 ± 0.2 ***	−
MNNG	0.005	W	18	5.0 ± 2.6	0.3 ± 0.2	−
DMBA	0.01	D	18	8.0 ± 6.0 **	0.5 ± 0.4 **	N. E.
Control 1	—	—	20	4.1 ± 1.5	0.2 ± 0.1	
Control 2	—	—	10	4.9 ± 2.3	0.3 ± 0.1	

[a] D, in diet; W, in drinking water
[b] DEN-PH model, N.E., not examined

c) Comparison of dose-dependence in the medium-term liver assay
model with results of long-term carcinogenicity testing

The experiment was carried out to examine whether results with medium-term assay model using preneoplastic hepatocyte lesion as an end-point marker might parallel the induction of hepatocellular carcinomas in the long-term (Osigo et al., 1985).

Materials and methods   In the medium-term experiment, rats were subjected to feeding of 2-AAF (0.0008, 0.004, 0.02%), 3'-Me-DAB (0.0024, 0.012, 0.06%) or ethionine (0.01, 0.05, 0.25%) mixed in the basal diet during weeks 2 to 8 of the same regimen as for the DEN-PH model. The long-term experiment was carried out by 104 weeks continuous feeding of the 3 compounds at 3 doses as in the medium-term experiment without prior initiation with DEN (Fig. 4). Rats becoming moribund due to development of tumors, mainly in the liver, were immediately sacrificed and examined histopathologically. Immunohistochemical staining of GST-P and quantitative analysis of preneoplastic lesions were performed on liver sections from medium-term experiment rats as described above.

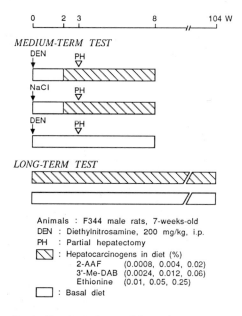

Fig. 4.   Experimental protocol for comparative medium-
and long-term test studies.

Results   In the medium-term assay, induction GST-P positive foci and nodules by 2-AAF and 3'-Me-DAB was clearly dose-dependent. In contrast, ethionine showed enhancing effects on development of GST-P positive foci and nodules only in the group given the highest dose level. Similarly, in the long-term experiment, induction of hepatocellular carcinomas by 2-AAF and 3'-Me-DAB was clearly dose-dependent, whereas liver neoplasms were only induced by the highest dose level of ethionine. These results indicate that the degree of induction of GST-P positive foci and nodules in the short-term in vivo test for liver carcinogens clearly corresponds to the incidences of hepatocellular carcinomas as revealed by a long-term in vivo assay (Fig. 5).

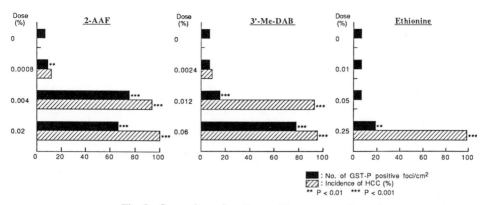

Fig. 5. Comparison of medium and long-term results.

Summary   It is concluded that results from the current medium-term assay model (DEN-PH model) utilizing quantitative analysis of GST-P positive hepatocyte foci are representative of findings after long-term carcinogenicity testing.

d) *Assessment of three-dimensional GST-P positive focus quantitative values*

The applicability of mathematical formulae for the calculation of numbers of foci per volume was examined by graphic three-dimensional reconstruction of the shape of individual GST-P positive foci.

Materials and methods   GST-P positive foci were induced by the DEN-PH protocol. As test chemicals, liver carcinogens of different potency, N-ethyl-N-hydroxyethylnitrosamine (EHEN, 0.05% in drinking water), dibutylnitrosamine (DBN, 0.1% in drinking water), aldrin (0.005% in diet), and PB (0.05% in diet), and an inhibitory agent, BHA (2% in diet) were used. The acetone-fixed and paraffin embedded liver was serially sectioned (3-4 μm thick) and immunohistochemically stained with GST-P at 10 to 15 μm steps (every 3-4 sections) for up to 150 sections. Numbers and areas of GST-P positive foci were measured as in the assay study. Number of GST-P positive foci was calculated using Fullman's formula (Fullman, 1953) which introduced to liver models by Campbell et al. (1982) and Enzmann's formula (Enzmann et al., 1987).

Several GST-P positive foci or nodules were selected and three-dimensionally reconstructed using a computer graphic system (Spicca Computer System-TRI, Vippon Avionics Co., Ltd., Tokyo, Japan).

Results   Numbers of GST-P positive foci/cm² and calculated numbers of foci/liver for each of the compounds are compared in Fig. 6. It is clear that promoting potential of EHEN, DEN, aldrin and PB or inhibition by BHA are equally expressed either as numbers of foci per cm² or per liver irrespective of which formula was employed. Stereological reconstitution demonstrated that the shape of GST-P positive foci was not always spherical but rather that many demonstrated irregular branching forms.

The results thus clearly indicated that both two- and three-dimensionally expressed quantitative values adequately represent the modifying potential of test chemicals and since calculation of three-dimensional values is based on the partially false assumption that foci are spherical, the use of two-dimensional data is validated.

Summary   Quantitative values for GST-P positive foci in our medium-term assay system gave the same result whether expressed per unit area or volume. Indeed, irregularity of the three-dimensional shape of foci suggests that, given the assumptions underlying the presently available transformation formulae, assessment of focus development from two-dimensional data may be more accurate.

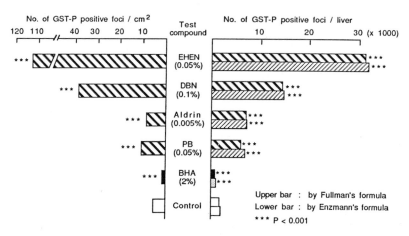

Fig. 6.   Three dimensional estimation of GST-P positive foci development by mathematical correction of data gained from two dimensional sections

2) Multi-organ Carcinogenesis Protocol

Since the two-step liver assay model is based on the induction of preneoplastic hepatocyte lesions, it primarily provides information as to whether a test compound is carcinogenic for the liver (DEN-PH model) although additional of the galactosamine step did allow detection of some carcinogens not normally active in this organ (DEN-Galactosamine-PH model). For the purpose of developing an alternative assay approach to detection of carcinogenicity in a variety of target organs we have investigated two different medium-term assay systems using multi-organ wide-spectrum initiation.

a) MNU model

N-Methyl-N-nitrosourea (NMU) is well known to induce neoplastic lesions in many different organs (IARC, 1974; Imaida et al., 1984; Tsuda et al., 1984) and thus was chosen as a wide-spectrum initiator.

Materials and methods   A total of 150 F344 male rats were divided into three groups. Groups 1 and 2 were initially given 8 doses of MNU (20 mg/kg, i.p.) within a 4-week period (total 160 mg/kg). Then group 1 rats were administered 3,2'-dimethyl-4-aminobiphenyl (DMAB, 50 mg/kg, once weekly, s.c.) or placed on basal diet (D) or drinking water (W) containing DBN (0.05%, W), dihydroxy-di-N-propylnitrosamine (DHPN, 0.1%, W), diethylstilbestrol (DES, 2.5 ppm, D), sodium o-phenylphenate (S-OPP,

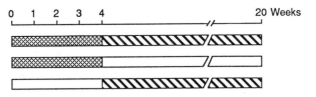

Animals : F344 male rats, 6-weeks-old
▨ : MNU (20 mg/kg i.p.) twice a week
▧ : Test compounds

Fig. 7. MNU model protocol.

2%, D) or captafol (0.15%, D). Group 2 (control) rats were given basal diet without supplement after MNU (20 to 25 rats each). Group 3 rats were initially given vehicle without MNU (citrate buffer at pH 6) and then administered one of the above 6 compounds (15 rats each). All animals were killed at week 16 and all major organs were histologically examined for development of preneoplastic and neoplastic lesions (Fig. 7).

    Results   In the liver, all 6 compounds in Group 1 significantly increased the values (number or area/cm^2 or both) of GST-P positive foci as compared to control group 2, DBN being associated with the highest values. Similarly incidences of thyroid tumors in the DHPN and S-OPP groups, lung tumors in the DHPN group, esophageal tumors in DBN and DHPN groups, forestomach hyperplasias in all except the DMAB group and urinary bladder hyperplasia/tumors in DMAB, DBN, DHPN, S-OPP and captafol groups were significantly increased as compared to control group values. Thus it was clearly shown that after initiation with MNU, the various carcinogens promoted the induction of preneoplastic and neoplastic lesions in their respective target organs. However due to earlier development of malignant lymphoma/leukemia, 10-20% of rats died before the termination of experiment. Results for the liver, small intestine, esophagus, forestomach, kidney and urinary bladder lesions are shown in Table 8.

Table 8.   Summary of MNU model results

	DMAB	DBN	DHPN	DES	S-OPP	Captafol
Thyroid	→	→	↑	→	↑	→
Lung	→	→	↑	→	→	→
Liver	↑	↑	↑	↑	↑	↑
Pancreas	↑	→	→	→	→	→
Esophagus	→	↑	↑	→	→	→
Forestomach	→	↑	↑	↑	↑	↑
Small intestine	↑	→	↑	→	→	→
Kidney (pelvis)	→	→	→	→	↑	→
Urinary bladder	↑	↑	↑	→	↑	↑
Judgement	+	+	+	+	+	+

↑ : Enhancement, → : No change

221

Summary   Using MNU as a wide-spectrum initiating agent, organotropic carcinogenicity of test compounds could be detected in as short as 20 weeks.

b) Combined initiators: model-I (DEN-MNU-DHPN protocol)

Consecutive application of three different carcinogens was used to cause wide-spectrum initiation. In addition to DEN and MNU which were also used in the previous experiments, DHPN was utilized as one of the initiators. Known sites of tumor induction of DHPN are the lung, thyroid and kidney (Hiasa et al., 1985; Shirai et al., 1988).

Materials and methods   A total of 65 male F344 rats were divided into 3 groups. Groups 1 and 2 were treated sequentially with DEN (100 mg/kg, i.p., single dose at commencement), MNU (20 mg/kg, i.p., 4 doses at days 2, 5, 8 and 11), and DHPN (0.1% in drinking water, during weeks 3 and 4). After this initiating procedure, groups 1 and 3 were fed known carcinogens as the test compound, PB at 0.05% in the diet or DBN at 0.005% in the drinking water. Group 2 rats were given basal diet and tap water after the initiation treatment and served as controls. Group 3 received vehicles without carcinogens during the initiation period. All animals were sacrificed at week 18 (Fig. 8). The main organs were excised and fixed in buffered formalin, then hematoxylin and eosin-stained sections were examined for histopathological lesion development. Liver fixed in ice-cold acetone was also used for the quantitative assessment of immunohistochemically stained GST-P positive foci. Statistical analysis was performed as for the two-step liver protocol.

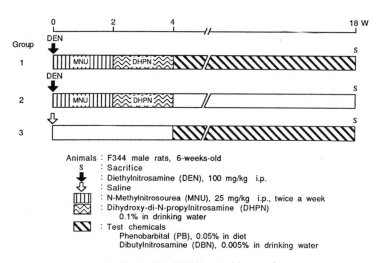

Fig. 8.   Combined initiators model protocol.

Results   The numbers and the areas of GST-P positive foci in the liver were significantly increased by the PB treatment as compared to group 2 values (Table 9). The incidences of thyroid hyperplasia and adenoma in PB-treated animals were also significantly higher than those of controls (87%, $P < 0.01$ and 47%, $P < 0.01$, respectively, Table 10). In group 1, the incidence of lung adenoma was significantly increased by DBN treatment (47%, $P < 0.05$), as were those of hyperplasia and papilloma of the esophagus (47%, $P < 0.01$, and 80%, $P < 0.001$, respectively) and forestomach hyperplasia (27%, $P < 0.05$, Table 10).

Table 9. The numbers and areas of GST-P positive foci in the rat livers in DEN-MNU-DHPN model

Group	Initiation	Test chemical	No. of rats	GST-P positive foci [a] No. / cm^2	Area (mm^2/ cm^2)
1	DEN + MNU + DHPN	PB	15	5.26 ± 1.76 **	0.29 ± 0.12 **
1	DEN + MNU + DHPN	DBN	15	0.19 ± 0.52	0.02 ± 0.02
2	DEN + MNU + DHPN	control	15	0.47 ± 0.46	0.05 ± 0.09
2	—	PB	10	0	0
3	—	DBN	10	0	0

[a] Mean ± SD.
** Statistically different from respective control group at $P < 0.01$.

Table 10. Incidences of neoplastic lesions in rats in DEN-MNU-DHPN model

Group	Test chemical	No. of rats	Lung (%) Hyperplasia	Adenoma	Thyroid (%) Hyperplasia	Adenoma	Esophagus (%) Hyperplasia	Adenoma	Forestomach (%) Hyperplasia	Adenoma
1	PB	15	14 (93)	4 (27)	13 (87)**	7 (47)**	0 (0)	1 (7)	0 (0)	0 (0)
1	DBN	15	15 (100)	7 (47)*	4 (27)	2 (13)	7 (47)**	12 (80)***	4 (27)*	3 (20)
2	control	15	15 (100)	1 (7)	4 (27)	0 (0)	0 (0)	0 (0)	0 (0)	0 (0)
2	PB	10	1 (10)	0 (0)	0 (0)	0 (0)	0 (0)	0 (0)	0 (0)	0 (0)
3	DBN	10	1 (10)	0 (0)	0 (0)	0 (0)	0 (0)	0 (0)	0 (0)	0 (0)

* Statistically different from control group at $P < 0.05$.
** Statistically different from control group at $P < 0.01$.
*** Statistically different from control group at $P < 0.001$.

Summary   The results of the present experiment demonstrated enhancing effects of PB in the liver and thyroid gland, and of DBN in the lung, esophagus and forestomach. Thus induction of preneoplastic and neoplastic lesions was clearly enhanced by feeding of carcinogens given after the DEN-MNU-DHPN protocol in the respective organotropic sites.

c) Combined initiators: model-II (DHPN-EHEN-DMAB protocol)

Consecutive application of three different carcinogens was again used to cause wide-spectrum initiation. Known sites of tumor induction are as follows: DHPN, the lung, thyroid and kidney (Hiasa et al. 1985; Shirai et al., 1988); EHEN, the kidney, liver and esophagus (Tsuda et al., 1983,); DMAB, the colon, small intestine, prostate, urinary bladder (Shirai, et al., 1986).

Materials and methods   A total of 275 F344 male rats were divided into 3 groups. Groups 1 and 2 were consecutively treated with the 3 different carcinogens, DHPN (1000 mg/kg, i.p., 2 doses in week 1), EHEN (1500 mg/kg, i.g., 2 doses in week 2) and DMAB (75 mg/kg, s.c., 2 doses in week 3) for initiation. One week later group 1 rats were given D or W containing 2-AAF (0.01%, D), 3'-Me-DAB (0.06%, D), ethionine (0.25%, D), PB (0.05%, D) as hepatocarcinogens, 3-MC (0.02%, D), DMBA (0.01, D), BBN (0.01, D), as non-hepatocarcinogens or DDPM (0.1%, D) as an equivocal chemical for 12 weeks (15 rats each). Group 2 rats (controls) were given vehicles for the initiating carcinogens then fed the respective test chemicals (5 rats each). All major organs were carefully examined as in the MNU model (Fig. 9).

<u>Results</u>   Values for GST-P positive foci in the liver were significantly increased in the groups treated with 3-MC, DMBA, DDPM, 2-AAF, 3'-Me-DAB, PB and ethionine. In the lung, data (No./cm²) for hyperplasias/adenomas demonstrated significant enhancement in rats given 3-MC. In the thyroid, the incidence of carcinomas was significantly elevated by DDPM while PB only promoted the development of hyperplasias. In the urinary bladder, incidences of papillary/nodular (PN) hyperplasias and transitional cell carcinomas were significantly increased in rats treated with BBN, whereas induction of simple hyperplasias was promoted by BHA, 2-AAF, 3'-Me-DAB and ethionine (Table 11).

<u>Summary</u>   After multiple organ, wide-spectrum initiation using a DHPN-EHEN-DMAB protocol, various non-liver as well as liver carcinogens enhanced preneoplastic and neoplastic lesions in their respective target organs. In addition, their organotropic inhibitory potential was also demonstrated. The model appears more suitable than that using MNU alone because of better survival.

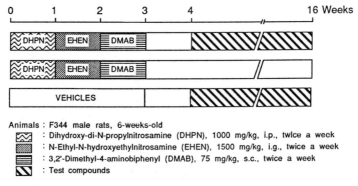

Animals : F344 male rats, 6-weeks-old
- : Dihydroxy-di-N-propylnitrosamine (DHPN), 1000 mg/kg, i.p., twice a week
- : N-Ethyl-N-hydroxyethylnitrosamine (EHEN), 1500 mg/kg, i.g., twice a week
- : 3,2'-Dimethyl-4-aminobiphenyl (DMAB), 75 mg/kg, s.c., twice a week
- : Test compounds

Fig. 9.   Combined initiators model protocol.

Table 11.   Summary of combined initiator model results

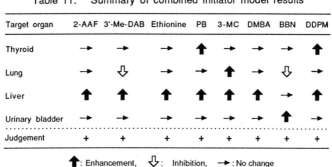

Target organ	2-AAF	3'-Me-DAB	Ethionine	PB	3-MC	DMBA	BBN	DDPM
Thyroid	→	→	→	↑	→	→	→	↑
Lung	→	⇩	→	→	↑	→	⇩	→
Liver	↑	↑	↑	↑	↑	↑	→	↑
Urinary bladder	→	→	→	→	→	→	↑	→
Judgement	+	+	+	+	+	+	+	+

↑: Enhancement,   ⇩: Inhibition,   →: No change

DISCUSSION

The results obtained using the presently described experimental protocols showed positive association with carcinogenicity, mainly to the liver, without obvious correlation to the results of <u>Salmonella</u> genotoxicity testing. As summarized in Tables 3 and 4, 15 genotoxic as well as 14 non-genotoxic carcinogens were successfully detected as positive compounds.

It is especially noteworthy that in the 2-step medium-term liver protocols 27 of 30 (90%) hepatocarcinogens gave a positive result, irrespective of their mutagenicity, leaving only three compounds, DDPM, di(2-ethylhexyl)phthalate and clofibrate, as false negatives (Reddy et al., 1979; Kluwe et al., 1982; Lamb et al., 1986). As expected, positive results for non-liver carcinogens were not as clear as for hepatocarcinogens since only two non-hepatocarcinogens were associated with increased lesion development. Most important is the fact that none of the compounds currently considered as non-carcinogens proved positive. In other words, the bioassay system did not generate false-positive results, an essential advantage for practical use.

D-Galactosamine causes periportal necrosis in liver parenchyma (Keppler et al., 1968; Decker et al., 1972), thus stimulating hepatocellular proliferation. Indeed, it was earlier shown that D-galactosamine at the present dose is almost as effective as partial hepatectomy for generation of nodular lesions in a modification of the Solt-Farber model (Tsuda et al., 1987). In the present system, a combination of D-galactosamine and partial hepateactomy treatments was applied to give proliferative stimuli at both the commencement of and during test chemical administration. As a result, the numbers and areas of preneoplastic lesions were increased relative to the previous results from the same bioassay system without D-galactosamine. A clear advantage was thereby achieved, since the non-hepatocarcinogens, BBN, 3-MC and DMBA, and the hepatocarcinogen, DDPM, which was previously a false-negative, all gave positive responses (Ito, et al., 1988).

Thus, even though MNNG remained a false-negative (and even in this case a slight increase was observed) the addition of a D-galactosamine step to the bioassay system gave a clear improvement in sensitivity. The enhancing effects of D-galacatosamine may be related to altered enzyme activity in the hepatocytes which metabolize non-liver carcinogens to proximate form (Daikuhara et al., 1979). However, the shift towards increased susceptibility of the liver to what are normally regarded as non-hepatocarcinogens is also presumably directly related to the proliferative effects, which acted to enhance promotion by test compounds.

As is evident from Table 5, the liver assay system also possesses the advantage that detection of inhibitory agents for hepatocarcino-genesis is possible. For example, a number of antioxidants (11 out of 22 inhibitory agents), mostly naturally occurring, brought about a reduction of GST-P positive foci induction (Thamavit et al., 1985). BHA, ethoxyquin and α-tocophenrol were previously reported as inhibitory agents for liver or colon carcinogenesis in long-term experiments (Cook et al., 1980; Tsuda et al., 1984). However, since some antioxidant species such as BHA and sodium ascorbate are also carcinogenic or exert promoting effects in other organs (Imaida et al., 1983, 1984), investigation using protocols based on wide-spectrum initiating protocols or some appropriate modification of the method are necessary to clarify their potential as environmental hazards.

Furthermore, even though the DEN-Galactosamine-PH model could be utilized for the detection of non-liver carcinogens, it does not provide information on the site of tumor induction. For this purpose the presently described wide-spectrum initiation protocols appear of advantage. Initiation procedures that induce lesions in multiple organs apparently sensitize the animals for detection of subsequent enhancing and/or modifying effects of test chemicals. The present data clearly indicate that administration of different wide-spectrum carcinogens has potential for development of medium-term bioassay systems for environmental carcinogens to supplement those already established for the liver (Ito et al., 1988).

In conclusion it is proposed that the presently described experimental protocols have advantages for rapid screening of the large number of environmental chemicals which may possess hazardous potential in man. These include shorter experimental periods and therefore costs than long-term in vivo carcinogenicity studies and in some cases better accuracy than in vitro short-term screening results. Moreover not only carcinogenic potency of chemicals but also possible target organs may be determined. Thus these systems should find wide application in surveying and establishing dose-dependence of modifying and inhibitory factors and conditions in environmental carcinogenesis and therefore play an important role in regulatory risk assessment.

AKNOWLEDGEMENTS

The research documented in this review was supported in parts by grants-in-aid for Cancer Research from the Ministry of Education, Science, and Culture, and from the Ministry of Health and Welfare of Japan, by a grant-in-aid from the Ministry of Health and Welfare for the Comprehensive 10 Year Strategy for Cancer Control, Japan and by grants from the Society for Promotion of Pathology of Nagoya and Experimental Pathological Research Association, Nagoya.

REFERENCES

Ames, B. N., McCann, J., and Yamasaki, E., 1975, Methods for detecting carcinogens and mutagens with the Salmonella/mammalian microsome mutagenicity test, Mutat. Res., 32:347.

Bannasch, P., Mayer, D., and Hacker, H. J., 1980, Hepatocellular glycogenesis and hepatocarcinogenesis, Biochim. Acta., 605:217.

Bannasch, P., Moore, M. A., Klimek, F., and Zerban, H., 1982, Biological markers of preneoplastic foci and neoplastic nodules in rodent liver, Toxicol. Pathol., 10:19.

Bannasch, P., 1986, Preneoplastic lesions as end points in carcinogenicity testing. I. Hepatic neoplasia, Carcinogenesis, 7:689.

Berenblum, I., 1974, "Carcinogenesis as a Biological Problem," North-Holland Publ., Amsterdam.

Butler, W. H., Hempsall, V., and Stewart, M. G., 1981, Histochemical studies on the early proliferating lesions induced in the rat liver by aflatoxin, J. Pathol., 133:325.

Campbell, H. A., Pitot, H. C., Potter, V. R., and Laishes, B. A., 1982, Application of quantitative stereology to the evaluation of enzyme-altered foci in rat liver, Cancer Res., 42:465.

Cook, M. G., and McNamara, P., 1980, Effect of dietary vitamin E on dimethylhydrazine-induced colonic tumors in mice, Cancer Res., 40:1329.

Craddock, V. M., and Frei, J. V., 1974, Induction of liver cell adenoma in the rat by a single treatment with N-methyl-N-nitrosourea given at various times after partial hepatectomy, Br. J. Cancer, 30:503.

Daikuhara, Y., Tamada, F., Takigawa, M., Takeda, Y., and Mori, Y., 1979, Changes in polyamine metabolism of rat liver after administration of

D-galactosamine, Gastroloenterology, 77:123.

Decker, K., and Keppler, D., 1972, Galactosamine induced liver injury, in: "Progress in Liver Disease," H. Popper, and S. Fenton, ed., Grune & Stratton, New York and London.

Doll, R., 1978, Strategy for detection of cancer hazards to man, Nature, 265:589.

Enzmann, M., Edler, L., and Bannasch, P., 1987, Simple elementary method for the quantification of focal liver lesions induced by carcinogens, Carcinogenesis, 8:231.

Farber, E., Parker, S., and Gruenstein, M., 1976, The resistance of putative premalignant liver cell populations, hyperplastic nodules, to the acute cytotoxic effects of some hepatocarcinogens, Cancer Res., 36:3879.

Farber, E., 1980, The sequential analysis of liver cancer induction, Biochim. Biophys. Acta, 605:149.

Foulds, L., 1969, "Neoplastic Development," 1, Academic Press, New York.

Foulds, L., 1975, "Neoplastic Development," 2, Academic Press, New York.

Fullman, R.L., 1953, Measurement of particle sizes in opaque bodies, Trans. AIME, 197:447.

Goldsworthy, T. L., Hanigan, M., and Pitot, H. C., 1986, Models of hepatocarcinogenesis in the rat -- contrast and comparisons, CRC Crit Rev. Toxicol., 17:61.

Hacker, H.-J., Moore, M. A., Mayer, D., and Bannasch, P., 1982, Correlative histochemistry of some enzymes of carbohydrate metabolism in preneoplastic and neoplastic lesions in the rat liver, Carcinogenesis, 3:1265.

Hasegawa, R., Tatematsu, M., Tsuda, H., Shirai, T., Hagiwara, A., and Ito, N., 1982, Induction of hyperplastic liver nodules in hepatectomized rats treated with 3'-methyl-4-dimethylaminoazobenzene, benzo(a)pyrene or phenobarbital before or after exposure to N-2-fluorenylacetamide, Gann, 73:264.

Hasegawa, R., Tsuda, H., Shirai, T., Kurata, Y., Masuda, A., and Ito, N., 1986, Effect of timing of partial hepatectomy on the induction of preneoplastic liver foci in rats given hepatocarcinogens, Cancer Lett., 32:15.

Haworth, S., Lawlor, T., Morlelmans, K., Spesk, W., and Zeiger, E., 1983, Salmonella mutagenicity test results for 250 chemicals, Environ. Mutagen., Suppl. 1:3.

Hiasa, Y., Kitahori, Y., Konishi, N., Shimoyama, T., and Lin, J.-C., 1985, Sex differential and dose dependence of phenobarbital promoting activity in N-bis(2-hydroxypropyl)nitrosamine-initated thyroid tumorigenesis in rats, Cancer Res., 45:4087.

Hsu, S. M., Raine, L., and Fanger, H., 1981, Use of avidin-biotin-peroxidase complex (ABC) in immunoperoxidase techniques: A comparison between ABC and unlabeled antibody (PAP) procedures, J. Histochem. Cytochem., 29:577.

IARC, 1974, IARC Monograph on the Evaluation of Carcinogenic Risk of Chemicals to Man, vol. 17, Lyon, France.

IARC, 1980, Long-term and Short-term Screening Assays for Carcinogens. A Critical Appraisal, IARC Monographs, Suppl. 2 IARC Scientific Publications, Lyon.

IARC, 1982, IARC Monograph on the Evaluation of the Carcinogenic Risk of Chemicals to Humans, Suppl. 4, IARC Lyon.

IARC, 1986, Long-term and Short-term Assays for Carcinogens: A Critical Appraisal, IARC Scientific Publications, No. 83, Lyon.

ICPMC Publication No. 9, 1984, Report of ICPMC task group 5 on the differentiation between genotoxic and non-genotoxic carcinogens, Mutat. Res., 133:1.

Imaida, K., Fukushima, S., Shirai, T., Ohtani, M., Nakanishi, K., and Ito, N., 1983, Promoting activities of butylated hydroxyanisole and butylated hydroxytoluene on 2-stage urinary bladder carcinogenesis and inhibition of γ-glutamyltranspeptidase-positive foci development in the liver of rats, Carcinogenesis, 4:895.

Imaida, K., Fukushima, S., Shirai, T., Masui, T., Ogiso, T., and Ito, N., 1984, Promoting activities of butylated hydroxyanisole, butylated hydroxytoluene and sodium L-ascorbate on forestomach and urinary bladder carcinogenesis initiated with methylnitrosourea in F344 male rats, Gann, 75:769.

Institute of Laboratory Animal Resources, 1980, Histologic typing of liver tumors of the rat, J. Natl. Cancer Inst., 64:179.

Ishidate, M., Jr, Sofuni, T., and Yoshikawa, K., 1981, Chromosomal aberration test in vitro as a primary screening tool for environmental mutagens and/or carcinogens, in: "Mutation, Promotion and Transformation in vitro, Gann Monograph," N. Inui, T. Kuroki, M. A. Yamada, and C. Heidelberger, eds., Japanese Scientific Society Press, Tokyo.

Ito, N., Tatematsu, M., Nakanishi, K., Hasegawa, R., Takano, T., Imaida, K., and Ogiso, T., 1980, The effects of various chemicals on the development of a hyperplastic liver nodules in hepatectomized rats treated with N-nitrosodiethylamine or N-2-fluorenylacetamide, Gann, 71:832.

Ito, N., Tsuda, H., Hasegawa, R., and Imaida, K., 1982, Sequential observation of pathomorphologic alterations in preneoplastic lesions during the promoting stage for hepatocarcinogenesis and the development of short-term test system for hepatopromoters and hepatocarcinogens, Toxicol. Pathol., 10:37.

Ito, N., Tsuda, H., Tatemastu, M., Inoue, T., Tagawa, Y., Aoki, T., Uwagawa, S., Ogiso, T., Masui, T., Imaida, K., Fukushima, S., and Asamoto, M., 1988, Enhancing effect of various hepatocarcinogens on induction of preneoplastic glutathione S-transferase-P form positive foci in rats -- An approach for a new medium-term bioassay system, Carcinogenesis, 9:387.

Ito, N., Imaida, K., de Camargo, J.L.V., Takahashi, S., Asamoto, M., and Tsuda, H., 1988, A new medium-term bioassay system for detection of environmental carcinogens using diethylnitrosamine-initiated rat liver followed by D-galactosamine treatment and partial hepatectomy, Jpn. J. Cancer Res. (Gann), 79:573.

Keppler, D., Lesch, R., Reutter, W., and Decker, K., 1968, Experimental hepatitis induced by D-galactosamine, Exp. Mol. Pathol., 9:279.

Kier, L. W., Brusick, D. J., Auletta, A. E., Von Halle, E. S., Brown, M. M., Simmon, V. F., Dunkel, V., McCann, J., Mortelmans, K., Prival, M., Rao, T. K., and Ray, V., 1986, The salmonella typhimurium/mammalian microsomal assay. A report on the U. S. Environmental Protection Agency Gene-Tox Program, Mutat. Res., 168:69.

Kitagawa, T., 1971, Histochemical analysis of hyperplastic lesions and hepatomas of the liver of rats fed 2-fluorenylacetamide, Gann, 62:207.

Kluwe, W. M., Haseman, J. K., Douglas, J. F., and Huff, J. E., 1982, The carcinogenicity of dietary di(2-ethylhexyl)phthalate (DEHP) in Fischer 344 rats and B6C3F1 mice, J. Toxicol. Environ. Health., 10:797.

Lamb, J. C., Huff, J. E., Haseman, J. K., Murth, A. S. K., and Lilga, H., 1986, Carcinogenesis studies of 4,4'-methylenedianiline dihydrochloride given in drinking water to F344/N rats and B6C3F$_1$ mice, J. Toxicolg. Environ. Health, 18:325.

Moore, M. A., Mayer, D., and Bannasch, P., 1982, Sequential appearance of putative preneoplastic populations induced in the rat liver by stop experiments with N-nitrosomorpholine, Carcinogenesis, 3:1429.

Moore, M. A., Hacker, H.-J., Kunz, H. W., and Bannasch, P., 1983,

Enhancement of NNM-induced carcinogenesis in the rat liver by phenobarbital: a combined morphological and enzyme histochemical approach, Carcinogenesis, 4:473.

NCI, 1976, Guidelines for carcinogen bioassay in samll rodents, National Cancer Institute Carcinogenesis Technical Report Series, NCI, USA.

Ogawa, K., Solt, D. B., and Farber, E., 1980, Phenotypic diversity as an early property of putative preneoplastic hepatocyte populations in liver carcinogenesis, Cancer Res.,40:725.

Ogiso, T., Tatematsu, M., Tamano, S., Tsuda, H., and Ito, N., 1985, Comparative effects of carcinogens on the induction of placental glutathione S-transferase-positive liver nodules in a short-term assay and of hepatocellular carcinomas in a long-term assay, Toxicol. Pathol., 13:257.

Peraino, C., Fry, R., Staffeldt, E., and Christopher, J. P., 1975, Comparative enhancing effect of phenobarbital, diphenylhydantoin, and dichlorodiphenyltrichloroethane on 2-acetylaminofluorene induced hepatic tumorigenesis in the rat, Cancer Res., 35:2884.

Pitot, H. C., Barsness, L., Goldsworthy, T., and Kitagawa, T., 1978, Biochemical characterization of stages of hepatocarcinogenesis after a single dose of diethylnitrosamine, Nature (Lond.), 271:456.

Pitot, H. C., Goldsworthy, T., Campbell, H. A., and Poland, A., 1980, Quantitative evaluation of the promotion by 2,3,7,8-tetra-chlorodibenzo-p-dioxin of hepatocarcinogenesis from diethylnitrosamine, Cancer Res., 40:3616.

Pitot, H. C., and Sirica, A. E., 1980, The stages of initiation and promotion in hepatocarcinogenesis, Biochim. Biophys. Acta, 605:191.

Preat, V., de Gerlache, J., Lans, M., Taper, H., and Roberfroid, M., 1986, Comparative analysis of the effects of phenobarbital dichlorodiphenyltrichloroethane, butylated hydroxytoluene and nafenopin on rat hepatocarcinogenesis, Carcinogenesis, 7:1025.

Pugh, T. D., and Goldfarb, S., 1978, Quantitative histochemical and autoradiographic studies of hepatocarcinogenesis in rats fed 2-acetylaminofluorene followed by phenobarbital, Cancer Res., 38:4450.

Rabes, H. M., Scholze, P. and Jantsch, B., 1972, Growth kinetics of diethylnitrosamine-induced enzyme-deficient "preoplastic" liver cell populations in vivo and in vitro, Cancer Res., 32:2577.

Rappaport, A. M., 1979, Physioanatomical basis of toxic liver injury, in: "Toxic Injury of the Liver, Part A," E. Farber, and M. M. Fischer, eds., Marcel Dekker, New York.

Reddy, J. K., and Qureshi, S. A., 1979, Tumorigenicity of the hypolipidaemic peroxisome proliferator ethyl-α-p-chlorophenoxyisobutyrate (clofibrate) in rats, Br. J. Cancer, 40:476.

Rinkus, S., and Legator, M. S., 1979, Chemical characterization of 465 known or suspected carcinogens and their correlation with mutagenic activity in the Salmonella typhimurium system, Cancer Res., 39:3289.

Sato, K., Kitahara, A., Satoh, K., Ishikawa, T., Tatematsu, M., and Ito, N., 1984, The placental form of gluathione S-transferase as a new marker protein for preneoplasia in rat chemical hepatocarcinogenesis, Gann, 75:199.

Satoh, K., Kitahara, A., Soma, Y., Inaba, Y., Hayama, I., and Sato, K, 1985, Purification, induction and distribution of placental glutathione transferase: a new marker enzyme for preoplastic cells in the rat chemical carcinogenesis, Proc. Natl. Acad. Sci. USA, 82:3964.

Scherer, E., 1984, Neoplastic progression in experimental hepatocarcinogenesis, Biochim. Biophys. Acta, 738:219.

Shirai, T., Fukushima, S., Ikawa, E., Tagawa, Y., and Ito, N., 1986, Induction of prostate carcinoma in situ at high incidence in F344 rats by a combination of 3,2'-dimethyl-4-aminobiphenyl and ethinyl estradiol, Cancer Res., 46:6423.

Shirai, T., Masuda, A., Imaida, K., Ogiso, T., and Ito, N., 1988, Effects of phenobarbital and carbazole on carcinogenesis of the lung, thyroid, kidney, and bladder of rats pretreated with N-bis(2-hydroxypropyl)nitrosamine, Jpn. J. Cancer Res. (Gann), 79:460.

Solt, D., and Farber. E., 1976, New principle for the analysis of chemical carcinogenesis, Nature (London), 262:701.

Tamano, S., Tsuda, H., Fukushima, S., Masui, T., Hosoda, K., and Ito, N., 1983, Dose and sex dependent effects of 2-acetylaminofluorene, 3'-methyl-4-dimethylaminoazobenzene and DL-ethionine in induction of γ-glutamyltranspeptidase-positive liver cell foci in rats, Cancer Lett., 20:313.

Tatematsu, M., Hasegawa, R., Imaida, K., Tsuda, H., and Ito, N., 1983, Survey of various chemicals for initiating and promoting activities in a short-term in vivo system based on generation of hyperplastic liver nodules in rats, Carcinogenesis, 4:381.

Tatematsu, M., Mera, Y., Ito, N., Satoh, K., and Sato, K., 1985, Relative merits of immunohistochemical demonstrations of placental, A, B and C forms of glutathione S-transferase and histochemical demonstration of γ-glutamyl transferase as markers of altered foci during liver carcinogenesis in rats, Carcinogenesis, 6:1621.

Thamavit, W., Tatematsu, M., Ogiso, T., Mera, Y., Tsuda, H., and Ito, N., 1985, Dose-dependent effects of butylated hydroxyanisole, butylated hydroxytoluene and ethoxyquin in induction of foci of rat liver cells containing the placental form of glutathione S-transferase, Cancer Lett., 27:295.

Tsuda, H., Lee, G., and Farber, E., 1980, Induction of resistant hepatocytes as a new principle for a possible short-term in vivo test for carcinogens, Cancer Res., 40:1157.

Tsuda, H., Sakata, T., Tamano, S., Okumura, M., and Ito, N., 1983, Sequential observations on the appearance of neoplastic lesions in the liver and kidney after treatment with N-ethyl-N-hydroxyethylnitrosamine followed by partial hepatectomy and unilateral nephrectomy, Carcinogenesis, 4:523.

Tsuda, H., Sakata, T., Shirai, T., Kurata, Y., Tamano, S., and Ito, N., 1984, Modification of N-methyl-N-nitrosurea initiated carcinogenesis in the rat by subsequent treatment with antioxidants, phenobarbital and ethinyl estradiol, Cancer Lett., 24:19.

Tsuda, H., Masui, T., Ikawa, E., Imaida, K., and Ito, N., 1987, Compared promoting potential of D-galactosamine, carbon tetrachloride and partial hepatectomy in rapid induction of preneoplastic liver lesions in the rat, Cancer Lett., 37:163.

Vesselinovitch, S. D., and Mihailovich, M., 1983, Kinetics of diethylnitrosamine hepatocarcinogenesis in the infant mouse, Cancer Res., 43:4253.

Williams, G. M., 1980, The pathogenesis of rat liver cancer caused by chemical carcinogens, Biochim. Biophys. Acta, 605:167.

Williams, G. M., 1982, Phenotypic properties of preneoplastic rat liver lesions and applications to detection of carcinogens and tumor promoters, Toxicol. Pathol., 10:3.

Wynder, E. L., and Gori, G. B., 1977, Contribution of the environment to cancer incidence: An epidemiologic exercise, J. Natl. Cancer Inst., 58:825.

Wynder, E. L., 1983, Tumor enhancers: underestimated factors in the epidemiology of life style-associated cancers, Environ. Health Perspect., 50:15.

Zeiger, E., 1987, Carcinogenesis of mutagens: Predictive capability of the Salmonella mutagenesis assay for rodent carcinogenicity, Cancer Res., 47:1287.

THE USE OF ALDH INDUCTION AS A CARCINOGENIC RISK MARKER

IN COMPARISON WITH TYPICAL IN VITRO MUTAGENICITY SYSTEM

V. Vasiliou, K. Athanasiou and M. Marselos

Department of Pharmacology, Medical School, University of

Ioannina, P.O. Box 1186, GR 451 10 - Ioannina, Greece

INTRODUCTION

Several aldehyde-oxidizing isozymes, the aldehyde dehydrogenases (ALDHs), are distributed in the mitochondrial, the microsomal and the cytosolic fraction of the rat liver (Deitrich, 1966; Tottmar et al., 1973). Previous studies have described the induction of two cytosolic aldehyde dehydrogenases by a variety of xenobiotics (Deitrich, 1971; Deitrich et al., 1977). Phenobarbital induces a specific ALDH (PB-ALDH) in certain genetically defined rat strains (Deitrich, 1971; Marselos, 1976). In addition, another cytosolic ALDH (T-ALDH) is induced by 2,3,7,8-tetrachlorodibenzo-p-dioxin (TCDD) and certain carcinogenic polycyclic aromatic hydrocarbons (P.A.Hs) in all rat strains tested (Marselos and Hänninen, 1974; Deitrich et al., 1978; Marselos et al., 1979). This isozyme is induced also in cultures of human hepatocytes, after in vitro exposure to 3-methylcholanthrene (Marselos et al., 1987).

The inducible isozymes (PB-ALDH and T-ALDH) are two distinct proteins, which differ in terms of substrate preference, use of coenzyme, sensitivity of inhibitors, physicochemical and immunochemical properties (Deitrich et al., 1977; Marselos et al., 1979; Lindahl and Evces, 1984; Simpson et al., 1985). Conventionally, the measurment of the PB-ALDH activity is carried out with propionaldehyde and NAD, whereas benzaldehyde and NADP are routinely used for the T-ALDH activity.

A great deal of interest has been focused on the T-ALDH isozyme, because of its apparent similarity to a tumor-associated ALDH detected in rat hepatomas induced by various protocols of chemical carcinogenesis. Several studies suggest that the tumor-specific ALDH and the T-ALDH share common properties to such an extent, that they should be considered identical (Lindahl et al., 1978; Lindahl, 1980; Lindahl and Evces, 1984).

In the present study we have examined the possible expression of T-ALDH activity in the rat liver, after treatment with different classes of chemical carcinogens. In addition, the mutagenicity of the same compounds has been determined by the Ames/Salmonella test. The latter is the most widely used test for mutagenicity (Maron and Ames, 1983) and has been also used to demonstrate a probable correlation between mutagenicity and carcinogenicity, both qualitatively and quantitavely (Bartsch et al., 1980).

MATERIALS AND METHODS

Chemicals   All chemicals used were reagent grade. Pyrazole was obtained
from Fluka (W. Germany), propionaldehyde and benzaldehyde from Ferak (W.
Germany), butadiene epoxide, ethylene dibromide, 4-dimethyl-aminoazobenzene
and 2-propionolactone from Aldrich (USA). The nitroso-compounds were obtained
from Serva (France). All the other chemicals were obtained from Sigma (USA).

Treatment of the animals   Male albino rats (weighing 200-250 g) of the
Wistar/Af/Han/Mol/Kuo/Io strain were used, originating from the Animal Center
of the University of Kuopio (Finland). These animals have been inbred as two
separate groups, according to their phenotype to respond to phenobarbital,
as far as the induction of ALDH is concerned (Marselos, 1976). In the present
study we used only animals non-responsive to phenobarbital treatment. The rats
were kept in plastic cages (Makrolon) with beddind of wood (Populus sp.)
and had free access to tap water and pelleted chow (Elviz, Greece). All
compounds were tested in groups of six animals and were given intraperitonealy
for four days, at the following daily doses: polycyclic aromatic hydrocarbons,
80 mg/kg, in olive oil (Minerva, Greece); aromatic amines, 80 mg/kg, in olive
oil; aliphatic nitrosoamines, 10 mg/kg, in saline; 4-dimethylaminoazobenzene,
10 mg/kg, in olive oil; nitrosamides and nitrosoureas, 40 mg/kg, in saline;
butadiene epoxide, 10 mg/kg, in saline; 2-propionolactone, 40 mg/kg, in
saline; ethylene dibromide 20 mg/kg in olive oil. Control groups of six
animals were given the respective vehicle. All animals were killed 24 hours
after the last injection.

Preparation of the cytosolic fraction   The rats were killed with
decapitation and the livers were homogenized in three volumes of ice-cold
0.25 M sucrose solution. The homogenate was first spun at 10.000 X g for
30 min. An equal volume of 0.024 M CaCl2 in 0.25 M sucrose was added to the
supernatant. The diluted supernatant was stirred and left to stand on ice
for 10 min. The microsomal fraction was sedimented by centrifugation at
10.000 X g for 30 min (Kamath et al., 1971). The soluble fraction was used
for the assays.

Aldehyde dehydrogenase was measured at $37^{\circ}C$, by following the reduction
of NAD(P)H at 340 nm in a Hitachi 100-80A spectrophotometer. The reaction
cuvette contained sodium pyrophosphate buffer (0.075 M, pH 8.0) 1 mM
pyrazole (to inhibit the alcohol dehydrogenase), 1 mM NAD and 5 mM
propionaldehyde (P/NAD activity). For measuring the B/NADP activity, the
substrate was benzaldehyde (5 mM) and the coenzyme was NADP (2.5 mM). In
either enzyme assay, the reaction was started by adding the substrate after
a 5 min pre-incubation. A blanc was run without the substrate (Marselos and
Michalopoulos, 1986).

Protein determination was carried out with the biuret method (Gornall
et al., 1949). Bovine serum albumin was used as the standard.

Ames/Salmonella assay   The two Salmonella typhimurium histidine
auxotroph strains TA 98 and TA 100 were obtained from Dr. B.N. Ames for use
in the plate incorpotation test. The rat liver homogenate (S9) and S9 mix
were prepared according to the method of Ames et al. (1975) after induction
by Aroclor 1254. Various concentrations of each carcinogen dissolved in 0.1
ml DMSO, 0.5 ml 0.1 M sodium phosphate buffer (pH 7.4), or 0.5 ml S9 mix,
0.1 ml overnight cultured bacterial suspension and 2 ml soft top agar
(0.7% Difco Nobel agar, 0.6% NaCl, 0.1 μmole biotin, 0.1 μmole histidine),
were added in sequence to a test tube. The contents were mixed and poured
onto a minimal agar plate. After 2 days incubation at $37^{\circ}C$ his-revertant
colonies were counted.

Statistical analysis of the results was performed with Student's t-test.

RESULTS

The doses of the different compounds administered to the animals (see Materials and Methods) did not produce gross signs of toxicity such as unwashed fur, haemorrhage, decreased notility or hypothermia.

Polycyclic aromatic hydrocarbons When ALDH was measured as P/NAD, a 2- and 4-fold increase in the activity was detected in the dimethylbenzanthacene and benzanthracene groups (Table 1). Benzopyrene produced a 30-fold increase and 3-methylcholanthrene a 40-fold increase in ALDH activity.

When ALDH measured as B/NADP only traces of activity could be detected in the control animals. The activities in the dimethylbenzanthracene, benzanthracene, benzopyrene and 3-methylcholanthrene treated animals were 30, 60, 380 and 460 times higher, compared to the respective controls.

Aromatic amines The P/NAD enzyme activity showed a 2-fold increase in the 2-naphylamine treated animals, while the B/NADP activity had a 7-fold and a 30-fold increase after treatment with 2-acetylaminofluorene and 2-naptylamine (Table 1). On the contrary, 1-naphtylamine did not affect the enzyme activities.

Nitrosoamines The ALDH activities were unchanged after treatment with dimethylnitrosoamine and diethylnitrosoamine.

The azo dye 4-dimethylaminoazobenzene produced a 15-fold increase only in the B/NADP activity.

Direct acting carcinogens From the direct-acting carcinogenic compounds tested (see Table 1) only the boutadiene epoxide produced a 7-fold increase in the B/NADP activity.

Mutagenicity of the compounds As it can be seen in tables 3 and 4, from the various non-direct acting carcinogens, the highest mutagenecity was seen by benzopyrene and acetylaminofluorene which for a dose of 10μg/plate induced a mutagenicity 20 and 17 times higher compared to the control levels. Diethylnitrosamine did not increase the mutagenicity, while the rest of them induced intermediate mutagenicity levels. From the direct carcinogens, N-methyl-nitrosoguanidine showed extremely high levels of mutagenicity in TA 100 Salmonella strain, while the highest dose of N-methyl-N-nitroso-urethane only doubled the TA 98 his revertant level compared to the controls (Table 2).

DISCUSSION

Environmental and biological monitoring are two complementary approaches for evaluanting human exposure to genotoxic agents. Biological monitoring relies on two groups of tests: those based on determination of the substances or their biotransformation products in various biological media and those based on detection and, possibly, quantification of those biological changes that result from reaction of the organism to exposures (Berlin et al.,

1984). Assays of specific enzyme activities of an organism after the exposure to environmental carcinogens might be a usefull biological marker.

It has ben previously reported that the rat liver cytosolic T-ALDH can be acutely induced by benzanthracene, benzpyrene, 3-methylcholanthrene (Törrönen et al., 1981) and TCDD (Deitrich et al., 1978). Induction of ALDH has also been found in cultures of human hepatoma cell lines (HepG2) and normal human hepatocyte cultures after application of 3-methylcholanthrene (Marselos et al., 1987). In addition, rat hepatomas induced by various protocols of chemical carcinogenesis exhibit higher ALDH activities than the normal liver (Feinstein and Cameron, 1975; Allen and Lindahl 1982; Jones et al., 1987).

In the present study we have shown for the first time that the carcinogens dimethylbenzanthracene, dimethylaminoazobenzene, 2-napthylamine, butadiene epoxide and acetylaminofluorene can also induce the rat liver T-ALDH. These findings probably suggest that other families of carcinogens additionally to P.A.Hs, such as aromatic amines or azo dyes, can increase the enzyme activity after acute treatment.

The mechanism of T-ALDH induction is not fully understood. Even with large doses of 3-methylcholanthrene, given to rat in vivo (Törrönen et al., 1981) or applied to hepatocyte cultures in vitro (Marselos et al., 1986) a lag time of at least three days is necessary, before the induction of the enzyme activity becomes evident. These observations suggest that the eventual effect of the inducer on the ALDH activity is mediated through an active metabolite. This hypothesis is further supported by the fact that the direct-acting carcinogens tested by us did not affect the enzyme activity. Nevertheless the well-known strong hepatocarcinogens dimethyl- and diethylnitrosamine, which need metabolic activation (Lijinsky and Reuber, 1981) did not show any increase of the ALDH activity. On the contrary rat hepatic tumors induced by diethylnitrosamine have elevated ALDH activity (Wischusen et al., 1982). However, the role of this increase in the process of hepatocarcinogenesis is still unknown.

The ALDH activity was also found to be unchanged compared to the respective controls, when the rats were treated with the noncarcinogenic aromatic amine 1-napthylamine.

According to the present data, it could be said that the inducers of the T- ALDH have the following characteristics: a) they are carcinogenic b) they need metabolic activation and c) they have aromatic ring(s) in their molecule.

Törrönen et al., (1980; 1981) have previously suggested that the induction of rat liver cytosolic T-ALDH activity reflects the carcinogenic potency of the compounds admistered to animals. Our results further confirm and extend this view. When the enzyme activity is compared to another biological parameter, namely the mutagenicity of the xenobiotics used, a close correlation can be seen after administration of indirect carcinogens (Table 5). Since the mutagenicity of a compound reflects its carcinogenic potency to a substantially high degree (Ames and Hooper, 1983), it could be concluded that the model of ALDH induction might be used as a marker of the exposure to certain indirect carcinogens. The hypothesis that this might be the case also with other groups of carcinogens is now under investigation by us.

Acknowledgements   This work supported by a grant from the Greek Ministry of Research and Technology.

234

Table 1. Effects of treatment with chemical carcinogens (for 4 days) on the rat liver cytosolic ALDH[α]

Daily dosage (mg/kg)		Enzyme activity nmol NAD(P)H / min / mgr protein	
		P/NAD	B/NADP
Olive oil (48)		7.2±1.2	1.2±0.3
Benzanthracene (6)	80	29.4±3.3*	73.6±9.6*
Dimethylbenzanthracene (6)	80	14.8±1.0*	33.2±5.9*
Benzopyrene (6)	80	239.0±30.4*	453.7±50.0*
Methylcholanthrene (6)	80	280.7±40.2*	552.5±55.4*
Acethylamidofluorene (6)	80	11.8±2.3	8.2±0.5*
2-Napthylamine (6)	80	15.7±1.6*	36.4±6.1*
1-Napthylamine (6)	80	6.9±2.2	1.0±0.2
2-Dimethylaminoazobenzene (6)	10	10.0±0.7	19.0±1.9*
Saline (48)		7.4±1.8	1.1±0.4
Dimethylnitrosamine (6)	10	7.5±0.8	0.8±0.2
Diethylnitrosoamine (6)	10	6.4±0.8	1.3±0.4
N-Methyl-N'-nitrosoguamidine (6)	80	7.6±0.8	1.4±0.1
N-Methylnitrosourethane (6)	80	7.8±1.3	0.9±0.6
N-Methylnitrosourea (6)	80	10.4±0.2	1.4±0.1
Ethylene dibromide (6)	20	9.0±1.0	1.1±0.2
Butadiene epoxide (6)	10	10.2±1.0	8.5±1.7*
β-propionolactone (6)	40	7.6±0.3	0.9±0.4

α The values are means ±S.D. and the number of animals in each group is given in parentheses. Statistical symbol* $p < 0.001$ (Student's t-test)

Table 2. Mutagenicity of various direct acting carcinogens for S. typhimurium.

Carcinogen	Dose (μg/plate)	Revertants/plate[α] TA 98		TA 100	
		−S9	+S9	−S9	+S9
Ethylene	0	15.3±3.7	20.6±4.1	115.0±7.0	128.3±17.0
Dibromide	50	18.0±2.8	20.3±3.2	121.6±4.5	129.6±17.2
	100	14.3±3.0	22.3±5.5	96.3±14.0	118.3±7.0
	500	16.0±1.0	27.3±3.0	170.0±8.5	176.3±12.5
	1000	13.3±2.0	14.3±1.5	171.0±14.1	163.6±22.7
N-Methyl-	0	18.0±1.7	15.0±4.0	106.0±4.5	133.6±7.6
N'-nitro-	0.3	22.3±5.5	45.3±12.3	188.6±27.4	261.6±17.0
soguani-	1.0	15.0±3.6	38.6±11.9	1816.3±221.3	350.6±15.5
dine	3	39.6±9.2	60.0±6.5	2345.0±302.4	1037.6±71.4
	10	56.0±12.1	77.0±17.0	—	—
N-Methyl-	0	16.6±1.1	19.3±4.1	97.3±8.5	126.0±8.7
nitroso-	10	15.0±3.6	13.6±2.3	101.3±2.0	124.3±13.6
urethane	50	28.0±6.0	15.6±1.5	104.3±9.7	106.0±7.8
	100	31.0±7.5	19.0±2.6	107.3±5.5	120.6±6.1
	500	33.3±8.3	21.3±3.7	98.6±9.0	120.6±6.1

(continued)

Table 2 (Continued)

	Dose	-S9	+S9	-S9	+S9
N-Methyl-nitroso-urea	0	15.3±4.0	22.0±6.0	112.6±9.2	123.0±13.5
	5	15.3±2.0	28.3±6.0	169.3±8.7	160.0±13.1
	10	17.6±3.7	26.0±3.0	264.3±32.5	228.6±16.1
	50	16.0±2.0	15.6±4.1	354.6±43.3	335.3±43.7
	100	18.6±4.1	24.6±8.0	625.3±37.2	608.0±25.5
Butadiene Epoxide	0	15.3±3.7	20.6±4.1	102.6±8.0	128.3±17.0
	2.5	16.3±0.5	16.3±2.0	118.0±6.2	123.0±14.0
	5	17.6±1.5	19.3±3.7	144.3±6.6	148.0±6.2
	10	17.3±4.1	22.3±3.7	196.0±12.4	173.0±11.5
	50	14.6±4.0	24.0±5.2	307.6±41.0	245.0±10.1
β-Propio-lactone	0	15.3±3.7	20.6±4.1	115.0±7.0	128.3±17.0
	2.5	18.3±3.5	15.3±1.1	145.0±8.5	152.0±12.0
	10	11.3±2.5	17.6±4.0	204.6±20.0	196.0±28.2
	30	24.3±5.8	16.6±4.0	612.0±20.7	506.0±17.7
	100	19.6±4.0	18.3±3.2	854.0±50.4	796.6±26.1

α Data given the mean values of three plates ±SD

Table 3. Mutagenicity of various non-direct acting carcinogens for S. Typhimurium

Carcinogen	Dose (μg/plate)	Revertants/plate[α]			
		TA 98		TA 100	
		-S9	+S9	-S9	+S9
Benzanthra-cene	0	17.0±1.0	20.6±2.0	101.3±3.0	123.0±13.1
	2.5	15.6±2.8	25.5±4.9	100.3±6.8	147.6±30.0
	10	16.6±5.5	32.0±6.0	109.3±9.4	177.0±14.1
	33	20.3±3.2	39.3±6.4	103.3±14.7	215.6±18.7
	100	15.0±6.1	48.3±4.0	115.3±5.8	337.0±38.1
Dimethyl-benzanthra-cene	0	15.0±3.6	28.3±4.0	98.3±7.1	123.3±12.5
	2.5	15.6±1.5	40.3±7.6	101.3±8.0	157.6±5.0
	5	17.3±4.7	69.6±15.9	111.0±9.5	170.0±32.6
	10	15.3±3.2	126.3±12.1	116.6±5.5	224.0±27.0
	20	22.3±3.5	175.6±24.1	108.3±13.3	320.0±28.6
Benz-pyrene	0	17.0±1.0	21.0±2.8	101.3±3.1	123.0±13.1
	1	19.0±3.0	66.0±6.5	109.3±7.5	207.0±13.5
	2.5	13.0±1.0	194.0±6.2	98.3±12.5	482.0±39.4
	5.0	16.3±2.0	270.3±26.5	112.0±10.0	605.0±39.8
	10	12.3±0.5	410.0±31.8	121.0±7.8	693.3±48.9
Methyl-cholanthrene	0	18.3±3.2	19.0±4.2	113.3±9.0	140.6±14.7
	2.5	17.3±6.1	43.6±6.8	113.0±15.7	180.0±17.5
	10	12.0±3.6	81.0±16.0	127.6±10.0	193.3±38.2
	33	15.3±2.0	127.6±9.2	136.6±8.0	244.6±18.5
	100	15.3±2.0	166.0±13.8	185.3±12.0	391.0±10.4

(continued)

Table 3 (Continued)

Dimethyl-	0	15.3±3.7	26.6±5.0	92.3±12.3	135.3±6.5
aminoazo-	2.5	16.3±0.5	30.3±7.3	130.3±4.5	149.0±9.5
benzene	10	19.0±3.6	30.3±4.7	97.0±4.3	157.3±12.6
	33	13.0±9.8	56.3±6.6	111.3±7.3	203.0±21.6
	100	20.3±4.7	66.3±11.5	96.3±18.1	247.0±15.1

α Data give the mean values of three plates ±SD

Table 4. Mutagenicity of various non-direct acting carcinogens for S. Typhimurium

Carcinogen	Dose (μg/plate)	Revertants/plate[α]			
		TA 98		TA 100	
		-S9	+S9	-S9	+S9
Acetyl-	0	17.0±1.0	20.6±2.0	121.3±5.5	123.0±13.1
amino-	1	22.3±2.5	86.0±4.0	110.6±5.6	138.0±14.4
fluorene	2.5	18.0±2.6	177.6±11.5	96.0±9.1	180.3±11.0
	5	15.3±2.5	272.6±26.6	109.6±13.0	203.3±20.5
	10	22.0±2.0	344.0±15.0	117.3±10.5	344.3±15.6
1-Napthyl-	0	12.3±2.8	29.6±4.9	98.0±7.0	133.3±10.9
amine	10	17.6±6.1	30.3±3.2	119.0±6.0	161.3±2.0
	30	16.1±4.4	41.0±7.2	99.3±6.5	232.6±32.7
	100	15.6±4.7	26.6±3.2	107.0±13.0	355.3±46.7
	300	16.0±5.0	30.6±7.7	96.0±5.2	412.3±43.3
2-Napthyl-	0	12.0±1.7	29.6±6.6	92.3±8.3	130.3±21.0
amine	2.5	16.3±5.5	37.0±5.5	94.6±11.3	178.6±14.5
	5	19.0±4.3	58.6±6.6	113.6±10.1	298.3±32.8
	10	12.6±4.0	112.3±12.8	108.6±10.5	535.3±59.6
	30	17.3±4.5	187.6±39.6	117.0±7.0	773.6±65.0
Dimethyl-	0	15.6±2.5	24.0±2.0	90.3±5.5	129.3±7.0
nitrosa-	100	20.0±2.6	27.6±5.1	104.6±10.2	178.0±34.7
mine	250	15.0±3.6	23.6±5.6	99.6±12.6	348.6±30.5
	500	16.6±2.5	17.3±2.0	99.0±19.6	456.0±50.0
	1000	20.6±6.1	26.6±8.0	88.3±10.9	871.6±78.6
Diethyl-	0	15.6±2.5	24.0±2.0	90.3±5.5	129.3±7.0
nitrosa-	50	13.3±3.2	28.3±6.0	100.3±7.6	135.3±8.6
mine	100	16.5±0.7	26.3±3.7	95.0±4.0	124.3±13.6
	300	13.6±2.5	26.6±5.0	104.0±12.1	125.3±20.2
	1000	16.6±5.5	31.0±3.6	111.6±7.2	141.3±14.4

α Data give the mean values of three plates ±SD

Table 5. Comparison of ALDH in induction and mutagenicity of the inducers.

Carcinogen	ALDH induction		Ames test	
	P/NAD	B/NADP	TA 98	TA 100
Benzanthracene	+	++	−	+
Dimethylbenzanthracene	+	++	+	+
Benzopyrene	+++	+++	+++	+++
Methylcholanthrene	+++	+++	+++	+++
Acetylaminofluorene	−	+	+++	+++
1-Napthylamine	−	−	−	+
2-Naphtylamine	+	++	+++	+++
Dimethylaminoazobenzene	−	++	+	+
Dimethylnitrosamine	−	−	−	−
Diethylnitrosoamine	−	−	−	−
N-Methyl-N'-nitrosoguanidine	−	−	−	+++
N-Methylnitrosourethane	−	−	−	−
N-Methylnitrosourea	−	−	+	++
Butadiene epoxide	−	+	+	+
Ethylene dibromide	−	−	−	+++
β-propionolactone	−	−	−	+++

REFERENCES

Allen, B., and Lindahl, R., 1982, Sequential 2-acetylaminofluorene-
    phenobarbital exposure induces a cytosolic aldehyde dehydrogenase during
    rat hepatocarcinogenesis, Carcinogenesis, 3:533.

Ames, B.N., McCann J. and Vamasaki E., 1975, Methods for detecting
    carcinogens and mutagens with the Salmonella/mammalian-microsome
    mutagenicity test, Mutation Res., 31:347.

Ames, B.N. and Hooper, K., 1978, Does carcinogenic potency correlate with
    mutagenic potency in the Ames assay? Areply, Nature (London), 271:19.

Berlin, A., Draper, M., Hemminki, K., and Vainio, H., 1984, Monitoring human
    exposure to carcinogenic and mutagenic agents, IARC Scientific Publication
    No. 59, Lyon.

Deitrich, R.A., 1966, Tissue and subcellular distribution of mammalian
    aldehyde-oxidizing capacity, Biochem. Pharmacol., 15:1911.

Deitrich, R.A., 1971, Genetic aspects of increase in rat liver aldehyde
    dehydrogenase induced by phenobarbital, Science 173:334.

Deitrich, R.A., Bludeau, P., Stock, T., and Roper, M., 1977, Induction of
    different rat liver supernatant aldehyde dehydrogenase by phenobarbital
    and tetrachlorodibenzo-p-dioxin, J. Biol. Chem., 252:6169.

Deitrich, R.A., Bludeau, P., Roper, M., and Schmuck, J., 1978, Induction of
    aldehyde dehydrogenase, Biochem. Pharmacol., 27:2343.

Feinstein, R.N., and Cameron, E.C., 1972, Aldehyde dehydrogenase activity in rat hepatomas, Biochem. Biophys. Res. Commun., 48:1140.

Gornall, A.G., Bardawill, C.J., and David, M.M., 1949, Determination of serum proteins by means of the biuret reaction, J. Biol. Chem., 177:751.

Jones, J.D.E., Evces, S., and Lindahl, R., 1984, Expression of tumor-associated aldehyde dehydrogenase during rat hepatocarcinogenesis using the resistant hepatocyte model, Carcinogenesis, 5:1679.

Kamath, S.A., Kummerow, F.A., and Narayan K.N., 1971, A simple procedure for the isolation of rat liver microsomes, FEBS Lett., 17:90.

Lijinsky, W., and Reurer, M.D., 1981, Comparative carcinogenicity of some alifatic nitrosoamines in Ficher rats, Cancer Lett. 14:297.

Lindahl, R., Roper, M., and Deitrich, R.A., 1978, Rat liver aldehyde dehydrogenase-immunochemical idendity of 2,3,7,8-tetrachlorodibenzo-p-dioxin-inducible normal liver and 2-acetylaminofluorene-inducible hepatoma isozymes, Biochem. Pharmacol., 27:2463.

Lindahl, R., 1980, Differentiation of normal and inducible rat liver aldehyde dehydrogenase by disulfiram inhibition in vitro, Biochem. Pharmacol., 29:3026.

Lindahl, R., and Evces, S., 1984, Rat liver aldehyde dehydrogenase. II. Isolation and characterization of four inducible isozymes, J. Biol. Chem. 259:11991.

Maron, M.M., and Ames B.N., 1983, Revised methods for the mutagenicity test, Mutation Res., 113:173.

Marselos, M., and Hänninen, O., 1974, Enhancement of D-glucuronolactone and aldehyde dehydrogenase activity in the rat liver by inducers of drug metabolism, Biochem. Pharmacol., 24:1457.

Marselos, M., 1976, Genetic variation of drug metabolizing enzymes in the Wistar rat, Acta Pharmacol. et Toxicol., 39:186.

Marselos, M., Törrönen, R., Koivula, T., and Koivusalo, M., 1979, Comparison of phenobarbital - and carcinogen - induced aldehyde dehydrogenase in the rat, Biochim. Biophys. Acta, 583:110.

Marselos, M., and Michalopoulos, G., 1986, Phenobarbital enhances the aldehyde dehydrogenase activity of rat hepatocyte in vitro and in vivo, Acta Pharmacol. et Toxicol., 59:405.

Marselos, M., Strom, S., and Michalopoulos, G., 1987, Effect of phenobarbital and 3-methylcholanthrene on aldehyde dehydrogenase activity in cultures of HepG2 and normal human hepatocytes, Chem. Biol. Interactions, 62:75.

Simpson, V.J., Baker, R., and Deitrich, R.A., 1985, Inducible aldehyde dehydrogenase from rat liver cytosol, Toxicol. Appl. Pharmacol., 79:193.

Törrönen, R., Nousiainen, U., and Marselos, M., 1980, Induction of liver aldehyde dehydrogenase activity-An indicator of chemical exposure? Abstract, Int. Congress on Toxicology, July 6-11, Brussels.

Törrönen, R., Nousiainen, U., and Hänninen, O., 1981. Induction of aldehyde dehydrogenase by polycyclic aromatic hydrocarbons in rats, Chem. Biol. Interactions, 36:33.

Tottmar, S.O.C., Pettersson, H., and Kiessling, K.H., 1973, The
    subcellular distribution and properties of aldehyde dehydrogenase in rat
    liver, Biochem. J., 135:577.

Wischusen, S., Evces, S., and Lindahl, R., 1982, Changes in aldehyde
    dehydrogenase phenotype during the promotion phase of rat
    hepatocarcinogenesis, Proc. Am. Assoc. Cancer Res., 23:59.

EXPRESSION OF INDUCIBLE CYTOCHROME P-450 mRNAs

DURING PROMOTION OF EXPERIMENTAL CHEMICAL HEPATOCARCINOGENESIS

Maria Celeste Lechner
Laboratory of Biochemistry
Instituto Gulbenkian de Ciencia
Oeiras, Portugal

INTRODUCTION

The transformation of normal into neoplastic cells produced in a given tissue under the action of a carcinogenic chemical, develops as a sequential process through successive stages which are determined by different biochemical mechanisms. This concept initially elaborated on the basis of the observation of experimental skin carcinogenesis has been confirmed to apply to all kinds of living tissues[1-3].

The first stage or initiation, considered as a somatic mutation, resulting from the genotoxic action of the carcinogen, starts to be reasonably understood. It comprises several events which are the biotransformation of the pre-carcinogens followed by the covalent binding of the active metabolite or ultimate carcinogen to the DNA. The DNA adducts which are formed can be eliminated by the DNA repair systems in the cell but, if not correctly restored they may lead to a mutation. The genetic lesion thus produced may however remain latent, under the physiological control of the organism.

At this stage further stimuli are needed for the lesion to be revealed, such as an aggression by the same carcinogenic chemical or by other exogenous or endogenous agents, the tumor promoters. These promoters are believed to act essentially at an epigenetic level since they are not proven to be active mutagens or carcinogens by themselves. Tumor promotion is indeed poorly understood, and there is not even a clear definition of it, since carcinogenic promoters, acting after a true carcinogen, may increase the number of tumors or shorten the latency period, which obviously correspond to more than one single mechanism. Besides, the mechanisms displayed are complex, comprising different stages which may differ from one promoter to another as well as from tissue to tissue.

The biological effects of chemicals straightly depend on their biotransformation. Cytochrome P450 (P450) mediated mono-oxygenases play a central role in the pharmacodynamic phase of chemical induced carcinogenic processes since they are the main enzyme systems acting on the biotransformation of lipophilic xenobiotics. The existence of a wide superfamily of P450 apoproteins coded by at least 10 different gene families[4] explains their polymorphism, as well as the substrate and position differential stereospecificity underlying the dual role played by these enzy-

matic systems, now in the inactivation, now in the potentiation of xenobiotic genotoxicity through the transient generation of electrophylic
metabolites.

Considering the key role of P450 in drug metabolism, their inducibility by both initiators and promoters of chemical carcinogenesis and the
effect of mono-oxygenase inducers on both the generation of genetic alterations and the proliferation of phenotype altered hepatocyte foci[5], we
undertook a comparative study of the modulation of several P450 mRNA
during promotion of hepatocarcinogenic process by PB in parallel with the
study of liver developmental marker mRNAs.

Our observations suggest that P450 apoproteins are under strong epigenetic regulation. Besides, a net unbalance of PB inducible P450 forms
belonging to sub-families IIB, IIC and IIIA is generated in the liver of
animals undergoing a carcinogenic process which could be related to the
increased risk for tumor progression.

GENETIC SUSCEPTIBILITY OF INDIVIDUALS TO CHEMICAL CARCINOGENESIS DEPENDS ON DIFFERENTIAL ACTIVITIES OF CRITICAL GENES

The manifestation of the complex multistep chemical carcinogenesis
process depends upon the conjugation of exogenous and endogenous factors.
The genetic susceptibility of each individual may widely vary, since a
genetic control can be exercised at virtually every stage of chemical
carcinogenesis determining its rate of progression.

The first step in chemical carcinogenesis depends on the exposure,
uptake and distribution of the carcinogenic agent within the organism.
Although the uptake is primarily related to the level of exposure, the
transport and distribution among the different organs or within the cells
of a given tissue is determined in many cases by the presence of specific
receptor molecules in the cytoplasm[6-7], which can subsequently act as
trans-acting factors regulating the expression of target genes[8].There are
important genetic differences in receptor concentration resulting from
the relative activities of the genes coding for the receptor proteins in
each organism or cell type[9].

Importance of the pharmacodynamics of chemical carcinogens

Carcinogens as well as pre-carcinogens undergo biotransformation to
their elimination from the organism. The metabolic pathways leading to
the production of excretable polar end-products are very complex depending on several enzyme systems which catalyze a sequence of reactions. In
most cases these constitute a biphasic process, the presence and relative
concentrations of oxidative enzymes (phase I) and conjugation systems
(phase II) in each organism and in each tissue being also genetically
determined.

Cytochrome P450 mediated mono-oxygenases, the enzyme systems responsible for most of the phase I detoxication reactions of a great majority
of apolar xenobiotics are particularly important since in some cases they
give rise to metabolites which are more toxic and carcinogenic than the
parent compound, the pre-carcinogen[10].

These agents, or their electrophylic metabolites, the ultimate carcinogens, can be detoxified and eliminated from the organism but they can instead bind to macromolecules, either without appreciable damage to the cell or bind to critical target molecules such as the genomic DNA and cromosomal proteins. The balance of the different enzymes and other intervening proteins, determines in each case the risk of chemically induced mutation resulting in the initiation of a carcinogenic process.

Tumor promotion, instead can be considered as the proliferation of an abnormal genotype, originating transformation into the tumor phenotype. Cellular promotion will depend on both the quiescence and death of the tumor cells and the immune system that can recognize and remove them from the body or not.

It is evident that at virtually every stage, the chemical induced carcinogenic process is under genetic control since it depends on the presence of specific proteins, receptors, enzymes or even antibodies, all them final products of active genes of the target cells aggressed by the chemical carcinogen.

P450 MONO-OXYGENASES AND CHEMICAL CARCINOGENESIS

Liver P450 mono-oxygenases are inducible enzymes, responding to chemical aggression of the organism, which constitute a typical example of enzyme adaptation in somatic cells.

At present 67 different P450 mRNA or protein sequences have been characterized, from eight eukaryotic species and one prokaryote[11].

A large number of the P450 entities which have been so far identified are expressed in mammalian liver.

The hepatocyte responds to chemical injury by overproducing different forms of P450. Depending on the identity and balance of P450 forms in presence, a xenobiotic may be inactivated through oxidation inside the cell, detoxified and eliminated from the organism or transiently transformed into active electrophylic intermediates, capable of damaging critical cellular targets.

In the P450 superfamily, each form shows a different substrate and position specificity towards the different xenobiotic molecules, being induced at different extents by different substrates.

The presence and the relative activity of individual P450 enzyme forms in the liver in a given species strikingly depend on the animal's age, sex and exposure to xenobiotics[12], being a major factor determining the risk of chemical carcinogenesis.

The role of P450IA, inducible by the polycyclic aromatic hydrocarbons- inducers Type II - in the generation of 7,8-diol-epoxides, as well as the relationship between susceptibility of different animal strains or tissues to PAH initiated tumors and the activity of Ah genetic locus controlling P450IA gene expression, has been widely documented[13].

PHENOBARBITAL AS AN INDUCER OF SPECIFIC P450 FORMS AND A LIVER TUMOR PROMOTER

Phenobarbital (PB) a prototype the mono-oxygenase of inducers type I stimulates the expression of structurally, genetically and enzymatically distinct forms of P450, catalyzing the hydroxylation of many carcinogen and pre-carcinogen molecules in a way that they often improve detoxication[14-15]. However PB has been recognized as a strong promoter of experimental hepatocarcinogenesis. When given to rats previously fed with AAF or DEN, PB promotes the development of differentiated hepatocarcinomas[16-17], leading to the manifestation of a higher number of islands in a shorter time period than in the absence of PB treatment. This effect has been attributed to the well known liver hypertrophic properties of PB.

A better understanding of the promoter effect of PB on pre-initiated liver cells needs a good knowledge of the molecular mechanisms underlying the modulation of gene expression operated by this drug, which are not comparable to the mechanisms triggered by other inducers of the P450 mono- oxygenases such as PAH's and steroid hormones. Conversely to inducers type II, PB does not bind to any specific receptor molecule, neither does it interact with DNA in a way that its positive gene regulatory action can be understood.

Phenobarbital significantly changes the relative abundance of different polysomal mRNA classes in rat liver

The pleiotropic action of PB on the liver, results in a marked cell hypertrophy due to an intense proliferation of the endoplasmic reticulum membranes which is associated to the induction of specific forms of P450 such as P450 IIB1,2, de novo induced by the barbiturate and several other forms of P450 sub family IIC, as well as family IIIA, (steroid inducible)[11] both constitutively expressed and responsive to PB stimulation .

Although increased transcription of specific genes has been demonstrated to occur in the liver under PB treatment[18] important changes in the post-transcriptional metabolism of mRNA have been described, supporting the view that epigenetic phenomena can be responsible for the overall modification in the cell homeostasis and the shift of the liver phenotype operated by this xenobiotic[19-20].

In order to further investigate the different levels, and the possible mechanisms involved in the modulation of gene expression by PB in the liver, we have constructed a library of recombinant bacterial plasmids containing DNA copies of the active mRNA, isolated from PB treated rat liver polysomes, which has been compared to an identically prepared cDNA library from untreated control rat liver polysomal mRNA.

One thousand clones from each library, control (C) and PB, have been hybridized in situ with [32 P]cDNA probes from the homologous and from the heterologous rat liver poly(A)-rich RNA.

In the experimental conditions used, employing a large excess of cDNA, the extent of [32P] label hybridized to each clone is a function of the relative abundance of the complementary poly(A)-rich mRNA species in the RNA population represented in the corresponding [32P] cDNA probe[21].

This global analysis revealed that although a large similarity exists in the pattern of gene expression in both control and PB-treated rat liver, a significant change (P=0.01) on the relative abundance of different polysomal mRNA classes is produced by the xenobiotic as deduced from the statistical analysis of the results.

The similarities and differences in the relative abundance of the cloned mRNA sequences in the liver of C and PB treated (16h, 80mg/kg b.wt,i.g.) young adult male rats, were evaluated by comparing the in situ hybridization signals of each replica plate with the homologous and the heterologous [32P] cDNA probe.

The semi-quantitative analysis of the changes in abundance of speci-fic mRNA sequences represented in each library, at concentrations higher than 0,05%, giving rise to a detectable hybridization signal, revealed that PB treatment produces a significant change (P=0,01) on the relative abundance of 15% of the polysomal mRNA sequences in rat liver.

These findings prove that PB produces a prompt phenotype shift in the liver, since the statistical difference between the relative propor-tions of active mRNA species populations before and after PB administra-tion is of the same order of magnitude of the one described when fetal and adult rat liver are compared by a similar experimental approach[22].

The changes in abundance which were found are consistent with the findings from different laboratories showing that PB increases the level of specific mRNA species such as P450 IIB1 and 2, NADPH-cytochrome c reductase, epoxide hydratase[18] as well as glutathione S-transferase[23].

Interestingly, our results showed that a number of repressions are concomittantly produced, demonstrating that PB acts not only as a speci-fic inducer of the mono-oxygenases but also by repressing a wide number of other mRNA species, substantially changing the overall pattern of gene expression products in the hepatocytes[21].

These important number of mRNA species which were revealed to undergo repression may explain the puzzling questions why no increase in the incorporation of nucleotide precursors is found in the nuclear, nucleolar or nucleoplasmic neo-transcribed RNA[24-25] and why no stimulation of the liver RNA polymerases arises during the hyperthrophic and enzyme induc-tive response to PB[26].

Induction of Cytochrome P450 and other responsive gene products by PB puts in motion the mobilization of mRNA into ER membrane-bound polysomes

Early studies on the induction mechanisms of the mono-oxygenases by PB demonstrated that this agent stimulates a marked increase in the concen-tration of mRNA species encoding specific PB-inducible P450 forms[27]. Synthesis in vitro followed by immunoprecipitation of the cell-free translation products by specific antibodies led to the identification of cytochromes P450 b and e (IIB1 and 2, in the recommended nomenclature)[11] as the major PB inducible P450 forms[28]. Other forms, belonging to P450 gene sub-fam ilies IIC and IIIA are both constitutively expressed and PB inducible in mammalian liver[4]. We have previously identified, from the above mentioned cDNA library, constructed from PB induced rat liver polysomal poly(A)-rich RNA, a recombinant plasmid proven to correspond to a 2.0kb mRNA, coding for a IICP450 variant, the P450 IGC1[29-30]. Cloning of the P450 IGC1 full length cDNA in a lambda gt10 vector and sequencing revealed its homology with P450 form IIC7 (results not published).

The characterization of another mRNA from the same cDNA library, revealed that alpha-2u globulin, a well known male specific, hormone regulated gene product is inducible by PB[31]. These two mRNA, gene products clearly induced by PB, were used to study the time course variation of their concentration in the whole liver tissue and in the active polysomal mRNA during the onset of the adaptive response[21] in order to evaluate the relative importance of the mRNA mobilization to the endoplasmic reticulum membrane-bound polyribosomes suggested by previous work[24].

Messenger RNA exists in animal cells as RNP complexes in different pools. Informosomes, the mRNP particles in the cytoplasm of secretory cells, exist not only in polyribosomal free and bound mRNPs, but also as free short-term and long- term repressed mRNA, absent from the polyribosomal mRNA population. A kinetic relationship between latent messenger RNA and polyribosomal mRNA, consistent with a precursor- product relationship, has been found in different biological systems. The existence of these potentially functional mRNAs stored in the cytoplasm in a repressed state as mRNP complexes constitutes an important device for translational control mechanisms, and feed-back regulation of the genetic activity, under different physiological situations. This is the case of mRNA species coding for albumin and for ferritin, which have been proved to be differently represented in the two sub-cellular populations in rat liver according to the physiological state of the tissue[32-33].

The results of the dot blot analysis of P450IIC7 and alpha-2u globulin revealed that the relative increases of the PB induced mRNA's in the total liver RNA are less important and later than in the active polysomes, showing a net mobilization of these specific messengers to their increased translation in the polysomes.

These observations emphasize the importance of epigenetic phenomena produced by PB in the liver for the modulation of gene expression and consequent phenotype shift, which might be involved in the promotion of chemical hepatocarcinogenesis by this xenobiotic[20].

PB INDUCIBLE P450 mRNA RELATIVE ABUNDANCE VARIATIONS DURING HEPATOCARCINOGENESIS PROMOTION

The polymorphic expression of P450 has been shown to constitute a key aspect of adverse drug side effects, namely by altering the susceptibility of the animals to environmental toxins and carcinogens. The levels of the different forms present in the liver are strikingly dependent on the animal's age, sex and exposure to xenobiotics[34].

PB, a prototype inducer of the liver microsomal mono-oxygenases Type I, strongly stimulates the biosynthesis of P450 enzymes in the liver. After initiation of a chemical hepatocarcinogenic process, PB acts as a potent promoter of the development of the chemically induced tumors[16-17], most of these rapidly growing PB promoted hepatic lesions revealing to be deficient in microsomal P450.

Also a variety of hepatoma cell lines[35], as well as the putative pre-neoplastic foci[36] promoted by PB, are known to have impaired mono-oxygenase activities.

As postulated by Oesh[37] the observed decreases in P450 isoenzymes in the liver tumors, may not result from alterations in the P450 gene structure but may rather be the consequence of abnormalities in the function of regulatory systems playing a central role in the maintenance of cell homeostasis.

The P450 deficiency in most liver tumors however, does not seems to be an irreversible characteristic, since several authors have recently found evidence for a significant responsiveness of chemically induced pre-neoplastic liver to induction of P450 IIB1 during promotion by PB[38,39].

Other forms of P450, products of distinct gene families which are constitutively expressed in the liver and developmentally regulated, are positively regulated by PB. Among them, P450 IGC1,(IIC7) mRNA accumulates after sexual maturation, attaining higher concentrations in the female liver both in basal and PB induction situations[30], while P450 IGC2 mRNA (IIIA, steroid inducible variant), present in both sex pre-pubertal rat liver, is extinguished in the female liver after sexual maturation. The expression of these forms of P450, probably play important physiological roles in the sex specific differential metabolism of steroids and susceptibility to genotoxic chemicals. P450 mRNAs corresponding to forms IIB1,2, IIC7, and IIIA have been evaluated at succesive stages of the experimental carcinogenesis[41] process using the Solt[42] and Farber initiation/selection protocol as modified by Lans et al, using two distinct groups of male rats at different initial ages (pubertal and adult, 6/7 and 9/10 week old, respectively)

The concentration of the P450 mRNAs was studied in parallel with mammalian liver developmental markers, the albumin and the alpha-fetopro-tein mRNAS, as well as the alpha-2u globulin mRNA, a marker of the adult male liver phenotype differentiation, previously shown to be sensitive to PB stimulation[31].

Dot and northern blot analysis of each mRNA has been performed at different stages of promotion which were controlled by morphological and biochemical marker analysis, the gamma-glutamyl transpeptidase (GGT) and the glutathione-S-transferase (GST) activities[43,44].

The time course development of the typical nodular structures in the liver revealed to be dependent on the animals age at the initiation step. Animals receiving DEN at an age of 6/7 weeks presented highly disturbed morphological pattern of the liver tissue already at 5 weeks promotion and typical nodular structures at the same stage when fed a PB diet, the levels of the biochemical markers being increased to 1900% and 2680% (GST) and to 120 and 170% (GGT), of the normal values (100%) respectively. At 12 weeks promotion, the liver histological changes observed either in the presence or in the absence of PB feeding were comparable to the situation found at later stages of tumor development (17 weeks) showing distinct nodules[43].

Inducibility of P450 IIB 1 is progressively lost during promotion by PB, and inversely related to the progression of the morphological and bioche-mical preneoplastic lesions

As expected, P450 IIB1 mRNA was virtually absent in the liver of the adult and pubertal rats without PB feeding at any stage of the hepatocar-cinogenesis process regardless the increases in the GGT or GST activi-ties.

Promotion by PB resulted in a marked increase in the P450II B1 mRNA, at the earlier promotion stages, attaining the highest level in the liver of the younger animals at 5 weeks, a value which was twice the induced level attained in the elder rats at 8 weeks promotion.

After prolonged PB feeding the inducibility of this P450 mRNA was severely impaired in both groups of rats, undergoing tumor development barely reaching a value of 30% the concentrations attained at the earlier stages of 5 and 8 weeks PB promotion.

PB inducible P450 IGC1 (IIC7) and male development marker alpha-2u globulin mRNAs are repressed during promotion by PB

This constitutive P450 form of the liver microsomes is a member of the IIC subfamily, responding to PB stimulation[11] in function of development and sexual maturation, the P450 IGC1 mRNA starts to accumulate in rat liver after puberty, the basal and PB induced levels in the young adult animals being respectively sixfold and threefold higher in the females than in the males[30]. Controlled by the hormonal status of the animals this mRNA may play an important role in sex differential steroid metabolism and susceptibility to genotoxic chemicals.

The alpha-2u globulin, a secreted protein which is synthesized in male liver under the control of numerous hormones, has been previously shown to be markedly induced by PB[31].

During tumor promotion, both P450 IGC1 and alpha-2u-globulin mRNA were shown to be spontaneously depressed. When under PB feeding, an over-depression of both mRNAs was observed which was progressively accentuated along promotion. In the younger animals the mRNA concentration attained at 5 and 12 weeks (alpha-2u globulin) or at 12 weeks (P450 IGC1) were approximately tenfold lower than in the healthy controls, at the same developmental age[44].

Developmentally regulated induction and PB stimulation of P450 IGC2, is markedly impaired in pre-neoplastic liver

Cytochrome P450 IGC2 mRNA a member of the P450 IIIA gene family is a steroid inducible enzyme, sensitive to both PCN and PB stimulation[4,45]. The study of the time course variation of the mRNA concentration in the liver of the male rats undergoing a carcinogenic process revealed that a strong reduction in the constitutive mRNA concentration was observed namely in the younger animals, the more sensitive to the hepatocarcinogenesis. In these animals, the chemically induced carcinogenic process prevented the developmentally regulated induction to take place, the basal levels remaining approximately 5-6 fold lower than in the young adults of the same age, which were submitted to DEN initiation after puberty. However a positive response was observed, to PB prolonged administration, which was progressively impaired as tumor promotion progressed in the adults, the mRNA levels in the pubertal rats remaining substantially lower (4-10 fold) under prolonged PB feeding.

Concomitantly, mRNA for albumin, the major protein synthesized in mammalian liver, revealed to be spontaneously depressed along promotion showing a drastic decrease under PB feeding. The concentration of albumin mRNA decreases to approximately 30% of its physiological level, in both groups of animals, between 5 and 17 weeks PB promotion[44].

Alpha-fetoprotein mRNA was virtually absent along the chemically induced preneoplastic transformation but in one case when pubertal rats initiated at 6/7 weeks of age were promoted by PB feeding for 17 weeks. These animals showed the more dramatic changes concerning the liver histological alterations, the decrease in albumin, and alpha-2u globulin as well as P450 IIB1 and IIIA mRNAs[44]. In this case the alpha-fetoprotein mRNA was present at a relative concentration of the same order of magnitude of P450 IGC1 mRNA.

DISCUSSION

Although the molecular mechanisms triggered by PB in the initiated livers, leading to tumor promotion, remain to be elucidated it has been suggested that the alterations in foci during experimental chemical hepatocarcinogenesis might bear a phenotypic similarity with the gene program established under PB in a normal liver[46].

The studies on the tumor promoting effect of PB in rat liver, consisting in the evaluation of the preneoplastic stage dependent variations of several tissue specific gene products above described however, do not support this view.

Actually, the study of the time course variations in the concentration of mRNAs coding for PB inducible forms of the mono-oxygenase terminal enzymes, belonging to three distinct sub-families P450IIB1,2, IIC7 and IIIA during the promotion stage of a chemically induced hepatocarcinogenic process, performed in parallel with the study of liver specific development marker mRNAs corresponding to albumin, alpha-fetoprotein and alpha-2u globulin, contradict this hypothesis. On the contrary our data provide experimental evidence for the foci cells being hepatocytes in a new state of differentiation, as evaluated at a molecular level by the direct analysis of critical gene products. In this situation, PB acts by improving the expression of the tumor phenotype which in many aspects reflects an impairment of normal liver functions and PB inducible mRNAs and proteins.

It has been previously shown that liver hypertrophy and specific enzyme induction by PB is due, in a large extent, to epigenetic events which modulate protein synthesis at the cytoplasmic level.

Translational regulation mechanisms in the higher eukaryotic organisms have been demonstrated to play a fundamental role during early embryogenesis. In the adult hepatic tissue, several examples of strong translational regulation phenomena, arising in response to different forms of stress have been clearly demonstrated.

That is the case of ferritin synthesis following iron administration[33], as well as albumin mRNA translational regulation during starvation and feeding[32].

Several P450 have now been proven to be under translational regulation in different experimental situations[4]. Our results demonstrated that during PB action mobilization of P450 IGC1 mRNA into active polysomes arises as an early event, similarly to other mRNA corresponding to gene products positively regulated by the inducer, like the alpha-2u globulin[21-31].

These facts emphasize the importance of epigenetic events for the liver adaptive response to PB and are in agreement with the entirely reversible nature of the biochemical and morphological modifications observed in the healthy animals. Also during experimental chemical carcinogenesis, after discontinuation of PB administration, it has been described that the majority of foci and nodules stop growing and many of them disappear[47]. Thus, even during carcinogenesis, the effects of PB, as a promoter, increasing the expression of the altered phenotype foci, seem to be reversible.

Differentiated cells in mammalian organisms are characterized by a high phenotype stability, precluding the existence of accurately programmed mechanisms to regulate the relative amounts of the different proteins which are synthesized and their steady-state.

Induction of P450 mono-oxygenases, particulary P450IIB1, is a property which is shared by PB and a large number of other tumor promoters. This particular form of P450 has been proven by Stadmam and co-workers to be very active in the inactivation of several key enzyme, namely the enzymes of the fosforilation - defosforilation cascade systems[49], which represent the major mechanisms of cellular metabolic regulation, acting through the modulation of protein function. These cyclic fosforilation - defosforilation cascades are demonstrated to correspond to biological integration systems, controlled by hormones and other endogenous regulators, and designed for the fine regulation of numerous key enzymes[50].

It has been shown that P450 mono-oxygenases catalyze histidine residues modification in many protein molecules, leading to the formation of oxidized carbonyl containing derivatives. For many enzymes this mechanism constitutes the inactivation reaction that marks the enzyme for proteolytic attack, underlying the normal catabolic reactions governing protein turnover in the cell. Many enzymes exhibiting age dependent changes are particularly sensitive to this inactivation by P450[51].

All the enzymes inactivated by P450 are either kinases or dehydrogenases bearing substrate binding sites for NAD, NADPH or ATP. They are protected from oxidation by the presence of these substrates or co-enzymes[51].

Interestingly it has been previously observed in our Laboratory that the administration of Nicotinic Acid, Nicotinamide or the synthetic derivative 5' methylated, can prevent in a certain extent the adaptive response of the liver to PB, in the healthy animals[52], the same a pronounced decrease in the liver microsomal RNAse activity is brought about by PB administration[53], which is not explained by a complexation with its physiological inhibitor, like it is the case for the reduction of RNAse activity during the liver regeneration period post hepatectomy, nor to a competitive inhibition by PB or its metabolites. Since RNAse is demonstrated to be susceptible of inactivation by the P450 mono-oxygenase systems[53], the loss of activity observed under PB treatment, which is inversely related to the increase in the microsomal P450, may be a consequence of its oxidation by the excess P450 IIB.

In this perspective, we admit that induction of CP450IIB1 at the early stages of tumor promotion by PB may lead to an over oxidation of regulatory enzymes. This may contribute to the cell to escape the physiological controls which assure the maintenance of the liver normal phenotype, as a dynamic steady-state as well as the quiescence of the chemical induced lesions, enhancing the cellular responsiveness to endogenous growth stimuli and favouring tumor development.

This interpretation is supported by the facts recently reported by several groups concerning the disappearance of hepatic foci after prolonged treatment with certain antioxidant drugs, the anti-promoters[54-56].

These anti-promoters could act by preventing the oxidation of critical proteins by the promoter induced P450 mono-oxygenases, therefore protecting the regulatory enzyme systems which control the physiological equilibrium of the cells and assure the quiescence of the chemically induced lesions.

REFERENCES

1. V. Armuth and I. Berenblum, Systemic promotion action of phorbol in lung and liver carcinogenesis in AKR mice, Cancer Res.,32:2259 (1972)
2. V. Armuth and I. Berenblum, Promotion of mammary carcinogenesis and leukemogenic action by phorbol in virgin female Wistar rats, Cancer Res.,34:2704 (1974)
3. C. Peraino, R.J.M. Fry, E. Staffeldt, and J.P. Christopher, Comparative enhancing effects of phenobarbital, aminobarbital, diphenylhydantoin and dichlorodiphenyltrichloro-ethane on 2-acetylaminofluorene-induced hepatic tumorigenesis in the rat, Cancer Res.,35:2884 (1975)
4. D. W. Nebert, F. J.Gonzalez, P450 Genes: Structure, Evolution and regulation, Ann. Rev. Biochem.,56:945 (1987)
5. M.C,Lechner, Controls of gene expression in chemical carcinogenesis: Role of cytochrome P450 mediated mono-oxygenases, in "Cell Transformation", J. Celis and A. Graessmann ed., Plenum Press, New York, (1986)
6. D. W. Nebert, J. R. Robinson, A. Niwa, K.Kumaki, and A.P.Poland, Genetic expression of aryl hidrocarbon hydroxylase activity in the mouse, J.Cell Physiol.,83:393 (1975)
7. A.P. Poland, E. Glover, A.S Kende, Stereospecific high affinity binding of 2,3,7,8, tetrachlorodibenzo-p-dioxin by hepatic cytosol: evidence that the binding species is the receptor for the induction of aryl-hidrocarbon hydroxylase, J. Biol. Chem.,251:4936(1976)
8. L.A. Neuhold, F.J. Gonzalez, A.K. Jaiswal. D.W. Nebert, Dioxin-Inducible Enhancer Region Upstream from the Mouse P450 Gene and Interaction with a Heterologus SV40 Promoter, DNA, 5:403 (1986)
9. A.P. Poland, E.Glover, J.R. Robinson and D.W.Nebert, Genetic expression of aryl hidrocarbon hydroxylase activity. Induction of mono-oxygenase activities and cytochrome P1-450 formation by 2,3,7,8-tetrachlorodibenzo-p-dioxin in mice genetically "non-responsive" to other aromatic hydrocarbons, J.Biol.Chem.,249:5599 (1974)
10. E.C.Miller, Some current perspectives on chemical carcinogenesis in humans and experimental animals, Cancer Res.,38:1479 (1978)
11. D.W.Nebert, M.Adesnik, M.J.Coon, R.W.Estabrook, F.J.Gonzalez, F.P.Guengerich, I.C.Gunsalus, E.F.Johnson, B.Kemper, W.Levin, I.R. Phillips, R.Sato, and M.R.Waterman, The P450 gene superfamily: Recommended nomenclature, DNA,1:11 (1987)
12. D.W.Nebert, Genetic differences in susceptibility to chemical induced myelotoxicity and leukemia, Environm.Health Perspectives,39:11 (1980)
13. D.W. Nebert and F.J.Gonzalez, Cytochrome P450 gene expression and regulation, TIPS, 6:160 (1985)
14. C.Peraino, R.J.M.Fry, E.Staffeld and W.E.Kisieleski, Effects of varying the exposure to phenobarbital on its enhancement of 2-acetylaminofluorene-induced hepatic tumorigenesis in the rat, Cancer Res. 33:2701 (1973)
15. C.Peraino, R.J.M.Fry, E.Staffeldt, and J.P.Christopher, Enhancing effects of phenobarbitone and butylated hydroxytoluene on 2-acetylaminofluorene-induced hepatic tumorigenesis in the rat, Food Cosmet. Toxicol.,15:93 (1977)
16. C.Peraino, R.J.M.Fry and E.Staffeldt, Reduction and enhancement by phenobarbital of hepatocarcinogenesis induced in the rat by 2-acetylaminofluorence,Cancer Res., 31:1506 (1971)

17. H.C.Pitot, L.Barsness, T.Goldsworthy and T.Kitagawa, Biochemical cha-
    racterisation of stages of hepatocarcinogenesis after a single dose
    of diethylnitrosamine, Nature,271:456 (1978)
18. J.P.Hardwick, F.J.Gonzalez, and C.B.Kasper, Transcriptional Regula-
    tion of rat liver epoxide hydratase, NADPH-Cytochrome P450 Oxido-
    reductase, and Cytochrome P450b Genes by Phenobarbital, J.Biol.
    Chem.,258:8081 (1983)
19. A.M.Cohen, and R.W.Ruddon, The Metabolism of Ribonucleic Acid in Rat
    Liver after Phenobarbital Administration, M.Pharmacol.,6:540 (1970)
20. M.C.Lechner, and C.M.Sinogas, Changes in gene expression during liver
    microsomal enzyme induction by phenobarbital, in "Biochem. Biophys.
    and Regulation of Cytochrome P450", Gustafsson et al., ed., Else-
    vier/North-Holland.,405 (1980)
21. M.C.Lechner, C.Sinogas, M.L.O.Almeida, M.T.Freire, P.C.Riffaud,
    M.Frain, and J.M.S.Trepat, Phenobarbital-mediated modulation of
    gene expression in rat liver, Analysis of cDNA clones, Eur.J.Bio-
    chem.,163:231 (1987)
22. M.Frain, Structure and expression of the genes coding to two pro-
    teins, markers of the hepatic differentiation in the humans: the
    albumin and the alpha-fetoprotein, Ph D thesis. University of Paris
    VII (1984)
23. V.Daniel, S.Sarid, S.Bar-Nun, and G.Litwack, Rat Ligandin mRNA Mole-
    cular Cloning and Sequencing, Arch. of Biochem. and Bioph.,227:266
    (1983)
24. M.Lechner, C.M.Sinogas, M.T.Freire, and J.Braz, Expression of liver
    mono-oxigenase functions induced by xenobiotics, in "Somatic Cell
    Genetics", C.T. Caskey, ed., Plenum Publishing Corporation, 69
    (1982)
25. A.Kumar, R.Satyanarayana Rao, and G. Padmanaban, A comparative study
    on the early effects of phenobarbital and 3-methycholanthrene on
    the synthesis and transport of ribonucleic acid in rat liver, Bio-
    chem.J.,186:81 (1980)
26. T.J.Lindrell, R.Ellinger, J.T.Warren, D.Sundheimer and A.F.O'Malley,
    The effect of acute and chronic phenobarbital treatement of the
    activity of rat liver DNA dependent RNA polymerases, Molec.
    Pharm.,13:426 (1977)
27. M.C.Lechner, M.T.Freire and B.Groner, In vitro biosyntesis of liver
    cytochrome P450 mature peptide sub-unit by translation of isolated
    poly(A)$^+$ mRNA from normal and phenobarbital induced rats, Biochem.
    Biophys. Res. Commun., 90:531 (1979)
28. R.N.Dubois and M.R. Waterman, Effect of phenobarbital administration
    to rats on the level of the in vitro synthesis of cytochrome P450
    directed by total rat liver RNA, Biochem.Biophys.Res.Commun.,90:150
    (1979)
29. M.C.Lechner, C.Sinogas, Identification of new form of rat liver Cyto-
    chrome P450. cDNA cloning and characterizaction of the mRNA nucleo-
    tide sequence, Biological Chemistry Hoppe-Seyler,367, Suppl.,123
    (1986)
30. M.Barroso, O.Dargouge and M.C.Lechner, Expression of a constitutive
    form of cytochrome P450 during rat-liver development and sexual
    maturation, Eur.J.Biochem,172:363 (1988)
31. M.L.O.Almeida, C.Sinogas, M.Ludovice and M.C.Lechner, Induction of
    alpha-2u-globulin mRNA by phenobarbital in rat liver: Characteri-
    zation of a cDNA clone, Biochem. and Bioph. Res.,134:1182 (1986)
32. S.H.Yap, R.K.Strair, and D.A.Shafritz, Effect of a short term fast on
    the distribution of cytoplasmic albumin messenger ribonucleic acid
    in rat liver, J.Biol.Chem.,253:4944 (1978)
33. J.Zahring, B.S.Baliga, and H.N. Munro, Novel mechanism for transla-
    tion control in regulation of ferritin synthesis by iron, Proc.
    Natl.Acad. Sci.,73:857 (1976)

34. M. Adesnik, M. Atchison, Genes for cytochrome P450 and their regulation, C.R.C. Biochem.,19:147 (1986)
35. F.J.Wibel, S.S.Park, F.Diefer, and H.V.Gelboin, Expression of cytochromes P450 in rat hepatoma cells: analysis by monoclonal antibodies specific for cytochrome P450 from rat liver induced by 3-menthylcholanthrene or phenobarbital, Eur.J.Biochem., 145:455 (1983)
36. E.Farber, Cellular biochemistry of the stepwise development of cancer with chemicals. Cancer Res.,44:5463 (1984)
37. A.Buchmann, M.Schwarz, R.Schmitt, C.R.Wolf, F.Oesch, and W.Kunz, Development of cytochrome P450 altered preneoplastic and neoplastic lesions during nitrosamine-induced hepatocarcinogenesis in the rat, Cancer Res.,47:2911 (1987)
38. R.Schulte-Herrmann, N.Roome, I.Timmermann-Troisiener, and J.Schuppler, Immunocytochemical demonstration of a phenobarbital inducible cytochrome P450 in putatite preneoplastic foci of rat liver, Carcinogenesis,5:149 (1984)
39. M.Schwarz, G.Peres, A.Buchmann, T.Friedberg, D.J.Waxman, and W.Kunz, Phenobarbital induction of cytochrome P450 in normal and preneoplastic rat liver: comparison of enzyme and mRNA expression as detected by immunohistochemistry and in situ hybridization, Carcinogenesis, 8:1355 (1987)
40. H.W.Kunz, A.Buchmann, M.Schwarz, R.Schmitt, W.D.Kuhlmann, C.R.Wolf, and F.Oesch, Expression and inducibility of drug metabolizing enzymes in preneoplastic and neoplastic lesions of rat liver during nitrosamine-induced hepatocarcinogenesis, Arch. Toxicol.,60:189 (1987)
41. D.B.Solt, and E.Farber, New principle for the analysis of chemical carcinogenesis, Nature,263:702 (1976)
42. M.Lans, J. de Gerlache, H.S.Taper, V.Preat, and M.Roberfroid, Phenobarbital as a promoter in the initiation/selection process of experimental rat hepatocarcinogenesis, Carcinogenesis,4:141 (1983)
43. F.Decloitre, C.Lafarge-Frayssinet, M.Ouldelhkim, C.Frayssinet, M.Barroso and M.C.Lechner, Tumor promoting effect of phenobarbital in pubertal and adult male rat liver: preneoplastic stage dependent variations of enzimatic markers and expression of cytochrome P450 b+e mRNA, submitted to Carcinogenesis, (1988)
44. M.C.Lechner, M.Barroso, F.Decloitre, C.Lafarge-Frayssinet, M.Ouldelhkim, C.Frayssinet, and I.Chouroulinkov, Tumor promoting effect of phenobarbital in pubertal and adult male rat liver: Studies on gene expression of phenotype markers and phenobarbital inducible CP450 isoenzyme mRNAs, submitted to Eur.J.Biochem (1988)
45. V.L.Ribeiro, M.Barroso, and M.C.Lechner, Regulation of the expression of a P450 PCN variant mRNA in rat liver,as a function of the age and sex, 3rd Portuguese-Spanish Congress of Biochemistry, Santiago de Compostela, Spain (1988)
46. R.Schulte-Hermann, Tumor promotion in the liver, Arch Toxicol,57:147 (1985)
47. M.A.Moore, H.J.Hacker, P.Bannasch, Phenotypic instability in focal and nodular lesions induced in a short term system in rat liver, Carcinogenesis 4:595, 1983
48. L.Fucci, C.N.Oliver, M.J.Coon, and E.R.Stadtman, Inactivation of key metabolic enzymes by mixed-function oxidation reactions: Possible implication in protein turnover and ageing, Proc.Natl.Acad.Sci. USA.,80:1521 (1983)
49. E.Shacter-Noiman, P.B.Chock and E.R.Stadtman, Protein phosphorylation as a regulatory device, Phil.Trans.R.Soc.Lond.,B 302:157 (1983)
50. E.R.Stadtman, Oxidation of proteins by mixed-function oxidation systems: implication in protein turnover, ageing and neutrophil function, TIBS (1986)

51. C.N.Oliver, B.Ahn, M.E.Wittenberger, R.L.Levine, and E.R.Stadtman, Age-related alterations of enzymes may involve mixed-function oxidation reactions, in: "Modification of Proteins During Aging", R.C.Adelman, E.E. Dekker, ed., Alan R.Liss, Inc., New York (1985)

52. M.C.Lechner and J.Braz, Nuclear ADP-ribosyl transferase activity correlates wicth induction of P-450 monooygenases by phenobarbital in rat liver microsomes, Eur.J.Biochem.,151:621 (1985)

53. M.C.Lechner and C.R.Pousada, A possible role liver microsomal alkaline ribonuclease in the stimulation of oxidative drug metabolism by phenobarbital, chlordane and chlorophenothane (DDT), Biochem. Pharmacol.,20:3021 (1971)

54. H.Tsuda, R.Hasegawa, K.Imaida, T.Masui, M.A.Moore, N.Jto, Modifying potencial of 31 chemicals on the short-term development of GGT-positive foci in diethylnitrosamine - initiated rat liver, Gann 75:876 (1984)

55. W.Staubli, P.Bentley, F.Bieri, E.Frohlich, F.Waechter, Inhibitory effect of nafenopin upon the development of diethylnitrosamine-induced enzyme-altered foci within the rat liver, Carcinogenesis 5:41 (1984)

56. A.B.Deangelo, C.T.Garrett, Inhibition of development of preneoplastic lesions in the livers of rats fed a weakly carcinogenic environmental contaminant, Cancer Lett. 20:199 (1983)

AN IN VITRO APPROACH FOR INTERSPECIES EXTRAPOLATION

USING ANIMAL AND HUMAN AIRWAY EPITHELIAL CELL CULTURE

M. Emura[a], M. Riebe[a], U. Mohr[a],
J. Jacob[b], G. Grimmer[b], J. Wen[a],
and M. Straub[a]

[a]Institut für Experimentelle Pathologie
Medizinische Hochschule Hannover
D-3000 Hannover 61, FRG and [b]Biochemisches
Institut für Umweltcarcinogene, D-2070
Grosshansdorf, FRG

INTRODUCTION

To assess the risk of cancer development we usually need to extrapolate data from laboratory experiments to the human situation. There is, however, a wide variety of both qualitative and quantitative results from studies with different mammalian species. To cite but a few examples, incubation of benzo(a)pyrene (BaP) with the microsomal preparations from respiratory organs produced predominantly trans-4,5-dihydro-4,5-dihydroxybenzo(a)pyrene (trans-4,5-diol) in rats and rhesus monkeys, while in Syrian hamsters and humans trans-7,8-diol was produced (see review by Cohen and Ashurst, 1983). Polycyclic aromatic hydrocarbons (PAHs) and cigarette smoke induce tumors of the respiratory organs in the pulmonary peripheral region in rats, in the pulmonary hilar region in humans and in the upper respiratory tract in Syrian hamsters (see review by Mohr and Dungworth, 1988). In the respiratory tract cell cultures, 12-0-tetradecanoylphorbol-13-acetate (TPA) enhanced colony formation of rat cells, while it was inhibitory to hamster and human cells (Beeman et al., 1987). We should, therefore, recognize such species-dependent variations and try to understand the mechanisms underlying their occurrence to make the extrapolation more accurate.

One possible approach for achieving this might be to use in vitro cell culture techniques. But these should enable the in vitro circumstances to mimic those in vivo as closely as possible. In this approach, interspecies comparisons would have to be made between each target cell type, because the microanatomical characteristics peculiar to each seem to be so conspicuous and critical from species to species (Plopper et al., 1983). In addition, certain specific physiological

This work is dedicated to Prof. Dr. Rolf Preussmann, German Cancer Research Center, Heidelberg, FRG on the 60th anniversary of his birth.

parameters will be required to monitor whether the selected cell culture conditions are working optimally for the comparison of cells from different species. Our efforts in this regard have concentrated on comparing fetal Syrian hamster and human pulmonary epithelial cells for their specific in vitro functions including the capacity to metabolize several PAHs and be transformed to a state of anchorage independency (AI).

Specific Aspects of Culture Techniques

The basis of the techniques is the use of a collagen (type I) gel as a contact substratum and an assortment of hormones and growth factors in medium. Synergistic or complementary interaction of collagen gels and other biological matrices with various hormones in culture have been reviewed with specific regard to the growth and differentiation of various epithelial cell types (Reid and Jefferson, 1984). For the in vitro growth of human respiratory tract epithelial cells in particular, the presence of insulin, hydrocortisone, epidermal growth factor (EGF), transferrin and cholera toxin seemed essential or at least quite favourable (Minna et al., 1982; Lechner et al., 1984; Wu and Wu, 1986). For Syrian hamster cells of the same tissue type to grow, a similar supplement of hormones and factors was necessary in the medium (Wu et al., 1985; McDowell et al., 1987), whereas rat and mouse respiratory cells did not require EGF (Wu et al., 1982). Furthermore, in combination with a collagen gel substratum, supplementation of the culture medium with these hormones and factors and additional vitamin A (VA) enabled the tracheal epithelial cells of hamsters (Wu et al., 1985; McDowell et al., 1987) and rabbits (Kim, 1985) to undergo differentiation to mucous synthesis. Similar differentiation-promoting effects of collagen gel were also demonstrated for in vitro isolated pancreatic islet cells in a recent publication (Amory et al., 1988). The above-cited studies have been undertaken using primary to quite early passage cells, which presumably still retain at least a proportion of differentiated phenotypes. In contrast to these, our present paper will demonstrate that, when the culture conditions are adequate, cells of a cloned permanent cell line or at relatively later passages can be stimulated to differentiate for mucous secretion from a completely undifferentiated state. Such dedifferentiation is very common in cells under long-term cultivation. A pilot study was started with a clonal permanent epithelial cell line (M3E3/C3) obtained from the fetal Syrian hamster lung at day 15 of gestation (Emura et al., 1982). The main components of the medium used in this study are given in Table 1. Most of them have also been used in the already mentioned media for primary to early passage cells apart from estradiol. Collagen gel was prepared using basically the same technique as described by Elsdale and Bard (1972), but a small amount of gelatin was mixed as shown in Table 1 (see also Emura et al., 1987). The M3E3/C3 cells grew undifferentiated and rapidly (with a population doubling-time of 11 hours) on the conventional plastic surface of culture vessels containing the conventional medium RPMI 1640 supplemented only with serum (FBS) and pyruvate (Emura et al., 1982). This medium is referred to as CM from here onwards in this paper. For these cells to be differentiated toward mucous synthesis they must first be plated on a collagen gel in CM, then 4 days later there is the option to choose between two other types of

Table 1. Supplements for Inducing Cell Differentiation

Medium

CM ⎡ RPMI 1640 + Na-pyruvate (ml)		78.1
⎣ FBS (ml)		20
Insulin (mg)		0.8
Hydrocortisone (mg)		0.18
17ß-Estradiol (mol)		10^{-9}
EGF (mg)		0.002
Transferrin (mg)		2.5
Cholera toxin (mg)		0.1
$CaCl_2$ (mg)		5.16
Trace elements		
All-trans-retinol (mg)		0.8

Substratum

Collagen gel	
Gelatin (%)	0.003

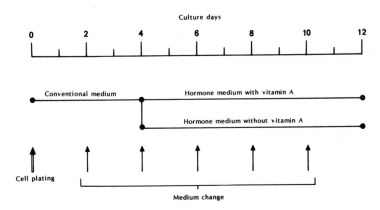

Fig. 1. Outline of Culture Schedule

medium (Fig. 1). One type (referred to as HMA) consists of CM and all
the other medium factors listed in Table 1. The other is practically
the HMA deprived of all-trans-retinol and is referred to as HM. The
most important point with this cell system is that two successive stages
of mucous cell differentiation can be achieved separately by altering
the culture conditions (Emura et al., 1988). In HM (of course on
collagen gel), the cells were differentiated (step-1 differentiation) to
a stage where large volumes of rough endoplasmic reticulum (rER) and

Golgi apparatus developed in the cytoplasm with occasional small mucous
granules. Such ultrastructural features closely resemble those of a
metaplastic, polygonal, secretory type of cell (SMGC), which has been
regarded as an intermediate precursor of columnar secretory cells and
also as a most likely target of carcinogens in the regenerating hamster
and human airway epithelium (McDowell and Trump, 1983; McDowell et al.,
1984). Indeed, it was these cells at step-1 differentiation that showed
capacity to metabolize certain PAHs as will be discussed later.
At this stage the cells grow very slowly with a population doubling-time
of about 158 hrs, and the ^{14}C-thymidine incorporation reduces
continually with a small peak on day 8 (Fig. 2). When cultivated in
HMA, the M3E3/C3 cells undergo mucous synthesis and secretion with the
uptake/cell of radioactive glucosamine reaching its peak on day 8 (step-
2 differentiation); and the cell growth and thymidine uptake are much
more stimulated than at the step-1 differentiation (Emura et al., 1988).

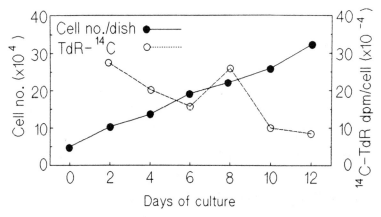

Fig. 2. Kinetics of cell growth and thymidine uptake in M3E3/C3 cells
at step-1 differentiation

The human pulmonary epithelial cells used in this system are
derived from fetal bronchi at 16-22 weeks of gravidity. The fetuses are
obtained from patients for whom continued pregnancy is contraindicated.
The bronchi are removed only when the fetuses are normal on routine
checking. The epithelial cells (FHBE) were prepared and examined for
fibroblast contamination as previously published (Emura et al., 1985).
During the cultivation under our conditions a portion of the cells
become dedifferentiated around 4-6 passages giving a few rapidly
proliferating populations, and only these populations of cells are
frozen-stocked at passages 5-8. Thus, FHBE cells at these passages grow
completely undifferentiated in CM just like the hamster M3E3/C3 cells.
We studied the kinetics of cell growth and thymidine uptake under the
same conditions as for M3E3/C3 cells again at step-1 differentiation

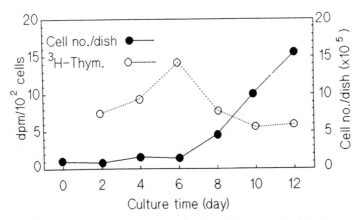

Fig. 3.   Kinetics of cell growth and thymidine uptake in FHBE cells at
step-1 differentiation

(Fig. 3). Being quite different from M3E3/C3 cells the peak of
thymidine uptake was on day 6 in these cells and the population
doubling-time was about 41 hours at the exponential phase, although the
thymidine uptake had reduced slightly with time of culture and the cell
growth was prolonged when compared with the 23 hours population
doubling-time in CM on the conventional plastic surface (Wen et al.,
1988). The difference in speed of cell proliferation between these
hamster and human cells may influence considerably the pattern of PAH
metabolism (Milo et al., 1980). Nevertheless, the ultrastructural
features were comparable with those of M3E3/C3 cells at step-1
differentiation. Furthermore, in HMA (vitamin A-containing), FHBE cells
undergo mucous secretory differentiation (Fig. 4) just as the hamster
M3E3/C3 cells do. Thus, our techniques have now probably reached a
level where we can, at least to a certain extent, establish the same
physiological situations in hamster M3E3/C3 and human FHBE cells, which
are in turn rendered amenable for comparison of carcinogen metabolizing
capacity under the same in vitro conditions.

Response of Hamster Cells to PAH at Step-1 Differentiation

For technical ease we chose NADPH-dependent cytochrome c reductase
(NCcR) and ethoxycoumarin deethylase (ECD) as marker enzymes to monitor
whether the cultures were working correctly after they were set up for a
series of experiments. We are well aware that ECD does not reflect all
aspects of the monooxygenase system. For example, when incubated with
pyrene (PYR), the M3E3/C3 cells growing on plastic in HM produced
completely different types of compounds (a major type was a quinone
derivative of PYR) than the 1-pyrenol (1-hydroxyPYR), which is usually
produced by lung microsomes or by M3E3/C3 cells on collagen gel in HM
(namely, the cells at step-1 differentiation). Nevertheless, the PYR
introduced initially was metabolized to the same extent both by the
cells on plastic and on collagen gel, and ECD also showed practically

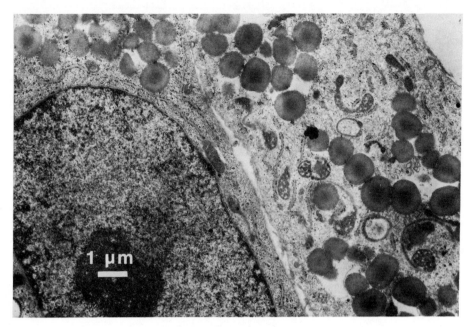

Fig. 4 Electron micrograph demonstrating mucus granules (about 1 μm in average size) in FHBE cells at step-2 differentiation on day 8. For detailed techniques see Emura et al., 1988.

the same activity in these differently cultured cells (unpublished results).

Interestingly, correlating well with the morphological features at step-1 differentiation previously mentioned, the basal (non drug-induced) levels of both NCcR and ECD in M3E3/C3 cells at this stage of differentiation were considerably higher than in the cells at the undifferentiated stage (Table 2). When the cells were pretreated with chrysene (CHR) for 6-8 days (drug-induced), the enhancement at step-1 differentiation was several fold greater. Breakdown of benz(a)anthracene (BaA) by M3E3/C3 was also examined in terms of the intact recovery of initially introduced BaA (Table 3). The results clearly show that the cells at step-1 differentiation metabolized BaA most effectively. They also show that collagen gel alone can stimulate the BaA metabolism to some degree.

In addition, the M3E3/C3 cells at step-1 differentiation showed anchorage-independent (AI) transformation after treatment (from day 6 to day 10 in Fig. 1) with benzo(a)pyrene (BaP) whereas the undifferentiated

Table 2.   Activities of Cytochrome c Reductase (NCcR) and Ethoxycoumarin
           Deethylase (ECD) Measured on Day 9 at Different Cell
           Physiology

	Undifferentiated	Step-1 Differentiated
NCcR (n mol/min/ mg protein)	2.5	3.8
ECD (p mol/min/ mg protein)	11.9	21.7

Data from Emura et al. (1987) with permission of the publisher.

Table 3.   Recovery of Intact BaA at Different Incubation Times under
           Different Culture Conditions

| | Unmetabolized BaA (µg/flask) | | |
	6-h	22-h	48-h
Undifferentiated		49	48
Collagen gel + CM	49.3	42.9	34.6
Step-1 differentiated	48.8	34.5	29.5

50 µg BaA was initially introduced in each flask on day 9.   Data
from Emura et al. (1987) with permission of the publisher.

cells showed practically no AI transformation (Table 4).   We further
compared the frequencies of BaP-induced point mutation at HGPRT locus in
undifferentiated and step-1 differentiated M3E3/C3 cells.   There was
clearly a dose-dependent increase in the frequencies (0.003, 0.013 and
0.615% at 0, 4 and 8 µg/ml, respectively) in step-1 differentiated
cells, while the frequencies in undifferentiated cells were no greater
than 0.005%.

    Quite recently, we also found that BaP (1 µg/ml, treated from day
6-12) yielded 0.005-0.009% of AI transformation in FHBE cells at step-1
differentiation, while in the undifferentiated state the AI frequency
was practically nil (unpublished results).   This FHBE response is
extremely low being almost at the untreated control level of M3E3/C3 at
step-1 differentiation given in Table 4.

Table 4. Percentage of Anchorage Independent Transformation Induced by
BaP in M3E3/C3 at Different Cell Physiology

BaP µg/ml	Undifferentiated	Step 1-Differentiated
0	0.0001 - 5	0.009
2	0.0001 - 5	0.2
4	0.0005 - 9	0.9
8	0.0005 - 9	0.8

BaP treatment was carried out from day 6-10. See also Emura et al.
(1987) for details of experiment.

CHR transformed M3E3/C3 at step-1 differentiation in a dose-
dependent manner; however, neither the cells growing in HM (on plastic
instead of collagen gel) nor those growing undifferentiated were
transformable (Table 5). These findings, together with the previous
observation that M3E3/C3 cells without collagen gel did not metabolize
PYR into 1-pyrenol but into a primarily quinone derivative, suggest that
collagen gel has a steering role enabling the cell to determine which
intermediates, carcinogenic or noncarcinogenic, are to be converted from
PAH.

CHR and PYR Metabolism in Hamster and Human Cells

To see whether the AI transformability of M3E3/C3 and FHBE cells by
PAH at step-1 differentiation is at least partly related to the
production of carcinogenic intermediates, cells from both species were
incubated with CHR (10 µg/flask/5 x 10^5 initial cells) from day 8 of the
step-1 differentiation regimen over various periods up to 8 days (Jacob
et al., 1987).

Fig. 5 compares quantitatively the recovery of unmetabolized CHR
and the total 1,2-oxidized and 3,4-oxidized metabolites of CHR, as
measured by gas-liquid chromatography after aryl sulfatase/glucuronidase
treatment of the culture. The hamster M3E3/C3 cells already metabolized
about 90% of initial CHR after 3 days of incubation, and in 8 days 97%
of CHR was metabolized. Since the total metabolites recovered as
organo-soluble compounds were only about 44% of the initial CHR after 8
days of incubation, the difference between 97% and 44%, namely 53%,
remained partly as water-soluble conjugates of other forms than sulfates
and glucuronides. They are most likely glutathione conjugates and
lesser amounts of other highly polarized conjugates (Autrup, 1979).
Moreover, 1,2-oxidation is moderately stronger than 3,4-oxidation. By
contrast, the human FHBE cells metabolized only about 25% of CHR after 8
days of incubation, the total metabolites being as little as 18%. The
difference of 7% again appears to be conjugated in other forms than

Table 5. Percentage of Anchorage Independent Colonies Induced by
CHR in M3E3/C3 at Different Cell Physiology

CHR µg/ml	Undifferentiated	Step 1-Differentiated
0		0.005
1		0.01
2	0.005 >	0.03
4		0.01

CHR treatment was carried out from day 8-16. AI colony numbers
counted per dish were directly changed into percentages. Other
experimental conditions are the same as in the BaP experiments.

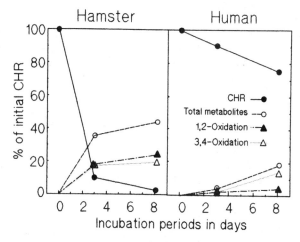

Fig. 5 Kinetic illustration of CHR breakdown and metabolite
        production relative to the initial amount of CHR in the
        hamster M3E3/C3 and human FHBE cells. CHR, intact CHR
        recovered; total metabolites, sum of water-insoluble,
        sulfated and glucuronated metabolites; 1,2-oxidation, sum
        of 1- and 2-hydroxyCHR and 1,2-dihydroxy-1,2-dihydroCHR
        together with their sulfates and glucuronides; 3,4-oxidation,
        analogous to 1,2-oxidation. Data from Jacob et al. (1987)
        with permission of the publisher.

sulfate esters and glucuronides. In addition, 3,4-oxidation is much
stronger than 1,2-oxidation being in direct contrast to the hamster
cells. Especially noteworthy is the very low activity of 1,2-oxidation
in human cells as compared with hamster cells, because the proximate
carcinogen of CHR is produced through this reaction (Jacob et al.,

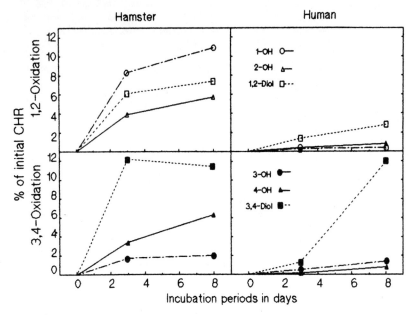

Fig. 6 Individual metabolites in the kinetics illustrated in Fig. 5.
1-OH (3-OH), total of 1 (3)-hydroxyCHR and its sulfates and
glucuronides; 2-OH (4-OH), analogous to 1-OH; 1,2 (3,4)-diol,
total of 1,2 (3,4)-dihyroxy-1,2 (3,4)-dihydroCHR and its
sulfates and glucuronides. Data from Jacob et al. (1987) with
permission of the publisher.

1987). In Fig. 6 individual metabolites are detailed. Under the 1,2-
oxidation the supposedly carcinogenic proximate, trans-1,2-dihyroxy-1,2-
dihydrochrysene (1,2-diol), was the second largest population in the
hamster cells, while it was the largest in the human cells. However,
the rate of 1,2-diol production is far slower in human cells than in
hamster cells. Particularly interesting is that while the ratio of the
supposedly non-carcinogenic intermediate, 3,4-diol, to the supposedly
carcinogenic, 1,2-diol, is not very high (1.5 at 8 days) in hamster
cells, that of human cells is remarkably high (4.3 at 8 days). Whether
this sort of considerably biased oxidation pattern leading to the
production of a less harmful CHR intermediate remains consistent in
every human (fetal) individual is a challenging question. In view of
the general acceptance of the relative resistance of human cells to
carcinogenic effects of diverse chemicals (DiPaolo, 1983), this point
appears to warrant further investigation. On these bases one may assume
these human FHBE cells to be much more resistant to AI transformation by
CHR than the hamster M3E3/C3 cells.

For the non-carcinogenic (supposedly) pyrene (PYR) we have made the
same comparison (unpublished results). The breakdown of PYR is very

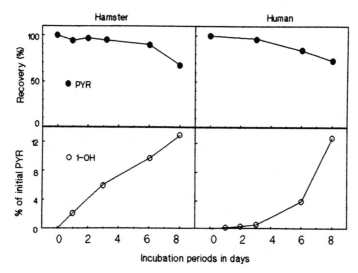

Fig. 7 PYR breakdown and metabolite production relative to the
initial PYR in the hamster M3E3/C3 and human FHBE
cells. PYR, intact PYR recovered; 1-OH, 1-hydroxyPYR. The
experiments were carried out using exactly the same methods
as for CHR.

slow both in hamster and human cells, and 1-hydroxyPYR was the primary
metabolite in both cell types (Fig. 7). In the hamster cells 1-
hydroxyPYR was practically the single product up to 6 days, but at 8
days about 19% of the metabolites were conjugated in forms other than
the sulfates or glucuronides. In the human cells such unidentified
conjugated metabolites are already produced at 3 days and increase with
time, being about 15% at 8 days. Again, hamster and human cells show
different oxidation patterns for PYR, although the speed of breakdown
appears quite similar. In addition to CHR, we have another example
which shows a great difference in the speed of breakdown between hamster
and human cells (Fig. 8). This was obtained in the experiments with
benzo(b)naphtho-(2,1-d)thiophene (2,1-BNT), the results of which have
not been published. Because of lack of availability of appropriate
reference samples the identification of individual metabolites is at
present suspended. At any rate, 2,1-BNT was metabolized much more
rapidly by the hamster cells than by the human cells. The reported
influence of cell proliferation on the rate of PAH metabolism (Milo et
al., 1980) has also to be investigated in this system (refer to Figs. 2
& 3).

Thus our new cell culture system enables us to compare the
metabolic fates of test chemicals in hamster and human respiratory
target (epithelial) cells on the basis of an equivalent state of cell
differentiation. For the chemicals whose metabolites are not known or
available, the rate of breakdown will be the primary parameter. If some
of the metabolites happen to be known or available, the rate of

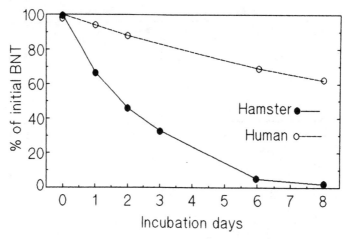

Fig. 8   Breakdown of 2,1-BNT in M3E3/C3
and FHBE cells, as illustrated by
the recovery (% of initial BNT) of
intact BNT. Experimental conditions
are exactly the same as for CHR.

production of individual metabolites and how it balances with each
metabolite will be additional indicators. As far as the available
literature is concerned, our report (Jacob et al., 1987) has for the
first time dealt with the metabolic comparison of CHR in the airway
epithelial cells of Syrian hamsters and humans. For BaP, another PAH,
there are many comparative studies. But most of them have been done
using explant cultures, in which fibroblasts metabolically different
from epithelial cells (Yamasaki et al., 1977; Milo et al., 1980) co-
exist in considerable numbers. Therefore, the results are not
necesssarily comparable with those for pure epithelial cells. Autrup et
al. (1980) reported that after 24 hrs' incubation hamster tracheobronchial tissues metabolized BaP as a total of metabolites in an almost
comparable amount to human main bronchial tissues, somewhat more (1.3
times) than human secondary and tertiary bronchial tissues, and slightly
less than human tracheal tissues. However, when after digestion with ß-
glucuronidase/aryl sulfatase the production of the supposedly
carcinogenic intermediate of BaP, trans-7,8-diol, was compared to that
of the non-carcinogenic trans-4,5-diol (Harris et al., 1982), the
hamster tracheobronchial tissues had a much higher ratio (5.7) than the
human tracheal (1.3) or bronchial tissues (1.1). In this review, CD
rats had a much lower ratio (0.7). As compared with the sum of both 3-
and 9-hydroxyBaP, trans-7,8-diol also shows a higher ratio of production
in hamster (1.0 times) than in human tracheas (0.8 times) or bronchi
(0.7 times). In CD rats the ratio was 0.4.

In similar experiments carried out by Daniel et al. (1983) human
tracheobronchial explants metabolized BaP (after 24 hrs incubation)

by up to about 85% of its initial amount, while the same hamster and (CDF) rat tissues metabolized it up to about 68%. In this study only the organo-soluble fraction of the culture medium was studied for individual metabolites. The human explants produced about 14 times more trans-7,8-diol than trans-4,5-diol, the hamster explants about 0.9 times and the rat explants about 0.5 times. Nearly comparable data have been observed by Mass and Kaufman (1983) in hamster and rat (F344) tracheal explant cultures. Of interest in this series of explant studies is that the constantly observed low rate of BaP activation in rat tracheobronchial tissues parallels well with the remarkable resistance of the same rat tissues to in vivo tumorigenesis by BaP (Schreiber et al., 1975). The comparable hamster tissues developed a high incidence of squamous metaplasia in response to the same doses of BaP as given to the rat. Recently, similar reluctant activation (of BaP) has been observed in cultured mammary epithelial cells of Sprague-Dawley rats (Gould et al., 1986; Moore et al., 1986). By contrast, the comparative data on hamster and human explants appear to agree to only a limited extent between different authors, although the different procedures and techniques adopted for the experiments should be taken into consideration. In this respect, the data from the experiments with microsomal fractions will show us another aspect of BaP activation. For example, the total capacity for metabolizing BaP is approximately half as much in human lung microsomes as in hamster or Sprague-Dawley rat lung microsomes (Prough et al., 1979). The ratio of 7,8-diol to 4.5-diol was the highest in the human microsomes at 1.9, 1.3 in the hamster, and 0.8 in the rat. These results coincide to some extent with those obtained by Daniel et al. (1983) in explant cultures, in which only organo-soluble metabolites released in the medium were determined.

In the light of the observations cited so far, it will be clear that the metabolic capacity of the airway epithelium can be compared more precisely by measuring the products of both oxidative and conjugative reactions. Additionally, human airway epithelial cells appear to metabolize BaP more effectively than CHR and PYR. At present comparative studies on metabolic capacity for BaP between hamster and human airway epithelial cells are underway in our laboratories using our newly developed system.

In this article we have so far exclusively discussed a few aspects of carcinogen metabolism as one of the factors which would probably determine the susceptibility of a species to PAH. Today, however, there is mounting evidence that there are additional factors which should necessarily be responsible for the interspecies differences in susceptibility to carcinogens. These would include the ease of carcinogen-DNA adduct formation, the effectiveness or fidelity of repairing adduct-bound DNA, and the chromosomal stability.

Recently, we have carried out a series of experiments to compare the chromosomal stability and the effectiveness of DNA repair in hamster M3E3/C3 cells and in human FHBE/21 cells (derived from another individual). The results (Wen et al., 1988) showed that the human cells possess a remarkably higher resistance to the induction of chromosomal aberrations and sister-chromatid exchanges by ethylnitrosourea (ENU) than the hamster cells. This mutagen was particularly chosen because it works directly (or through spontaneous activation) without itself being activated by the monooxygenase system discussed previously; we can therefore possibly neglect the interspecies differences in ENU metabolism due to any enzyme systems. Additional results have shown that the human cells showed much lower frequencies of mutation at HGPRT locus than the hamster cells (manuscript in preparation).

Thus, based on the data presented by our research group one might conclude that human cells are more resistant to certain carcinogens than hamster cells. However, these studies have been done using only a few human subjects. In view of the reported very wide variation in the metabolic capacity of human cells (Harris et al., 1982) these studies should be performed for much greater numbers of different individuals. Our present aim is, therefore, to conduct a set of comparative hamster-human cell investigations comprising metabolism analysis and tests for chromosome stability, mutation inducibility and AI-transformability using our new system on as many fetal human subjects as possible.

CONCLUSION

We have developed a new target cell culture system by which the response to a carcinogen of the airway epithelium in different species, including humans, can be compared. Such responses include the time-dependently changing capacity to metabolize carcinogens, feasibility for AI-transformation, chromosome stability and mutation inducibility. A distinguishing characteristic of this system is that through manipulation of culture conditions fetal epithelial cells growing undifferentiated are brought to a pre-stage (step-1 differentiation) of mucous cell differentiation, where the cells closely resemble a cell type postulated to be a carcinogen target in the in vivo epithelium. At this particular in vitro stage the cells demonstrate sufficiently recognizable capacity for PAH metabolization including both phase-I and phase-II activities. This cell system has a few additional advantages over other systems with similar aims. Unlike the hepatocyte or S9 mix-mediated system, the carcinogen-metabolizing cells themselves are simultaneously the target of the carcinogen for transformation, mutation or chromosome aberration. In contrast to the tissue explant method, the cells under observation are purely epithelial; this avoids the possibility that the coexisting stromal cells produce different types of metabolites than the epithelial cells. As compared with adult tissues, fetal tissues (especially of humans) are less exposed to environmental burden and consequently less artificially activated or depressed for drug-metabolism with the amplitude of interindividual variation most likely reduced. Good reproducibility for the induction of two successive (step-1 and step-2) stages of epithelial mucous cell differentiation would enable mechanistic studies of the interrelationship between differentiation and neoplastic transformation. Notwithstanding such pronounced properties, this system has limitations, too. The major one is the lack of whole body environments, such as immunodefence mechanisms and hormonal or nervous homeostasis.

This limitation is commonly seen in almost every in vitro system and is not specific to our system. By contrast, animal bodies as such are a very well organized integral experimental system. One can see in it practically all the events which occur in human bodies. The problem is, however, that such events occur in animals and humans on quantitatively different bases. Since most of these differences have still not been analysed, we are forced to make a large number of assumptions when extrapolating from animal studies to human situations. These assumptions can present a serious pitfall for threshold or minimal safety dose assessment.

It is indeed to this process that our new approach should be applied in order to avoid any false decisions. The collection of more quantitive data on in vitro comparisons between human and animal cells will reduce the number of uncertain assumptions concerning extrapolation.

ACKNOWLEDGEMENTS

The data presented are partly derived from studies supported by the Bundesministerium für Forschung und Technologie. We thank Ann Borchert for editing the manuscript.

REFERENCES

Amory, B., Mourmeaux, J.-L., and Ramacle, C., 1988, In vitro cytodifferentiation of perinatal rat islet cells within a tridimensional matrix of collagen, In Vitro Cell. Dev. Biol, 24:91.

Autrup, H., 1979, Separation of water-soluble metabolites of benzo(a)pyrene formed by cultured human colon, Biochem. Pharmacol., 28:1727.

Autrup, H., Wefald, F.C., Jeffrey, A.M., Tate, H., Schwartz, R.D., Trump, B.F., and Harris, C.C., 1980, Metabolism of benzo(a)pyrene by cultured tracheobronchial tissues from mice, rats, hamsters, bovines and humans, Int. J. Cancer, 25:293.

Beeman, D.K., Siegfried, J.M., and Mass, M.J., 1987, Effect of phorbol esters on clonal cultures of human, hamster, and rat respiratory epithelial cells, Cancer Res., 47:541.

Cohen, G.M., and Ashurst, S.W., 1983, The metabolism of chemical carcinogens by human and rodent respiratory tissues in vitro, in: Comparative Respiratory Tract Carcinogenesis, Vol. 2, H.M. Reznik-Schüller, ed., pp. 135, CRC Press, Boca Raton.

Daniel, F.B., Schut, H.A.J., Sandwisch, D.W., Schenck, K.M., Hoffmann, C.O., Patrick, J.R., and Stoner, G.D., 1983, Interspecies comparisons of benzo(a)pyrene metabolism and DNA-adduct formation in cultured human and animal bladder and tracheobronchial tissues, Cancer Res., 43:4723.

DiPaolo, J.A., 1983, Relative difficulties in transforming human and animal cells in vitro, J. Nat. Cancer Inst., 70:3.

Elsdale, T., and Bard, J., 1972, Collagen substrata for studies on cell behavior, J. Cell Biol., 54:626.

Emura, M., Mohr, U., Kakunaga, T., and Hilfrich, J., 1985, Growth inhibition and transformation of a human fetal tracheal epithelial cell line by long-term exposure to diethylnitrosamine, Carcinogenesis, 6:1079.

Emura, M., Mohr, U., Riebe, M., Aufderheide, M. and Dungworth, D.L., 1987, Predisposition of cloned fetal hamster lung epithelial cells to transformation by a precarcinogen, benzo(a)pyrene, using growth hormone supplementation and collagen gel substratum, Cancer Res., 47:1155.

Emura, M., Mohr, U., Riebe, M., Aufderheide, M., and Dungworth, D.L., 1988, Regulation of growth and differentiation by vitamin A in a cloned fetal lung epitehlial cell line cultured on collagen gel in hormone-supplemented medium, In Vitro Cell. Dev. Biol, in press.

Emura, M., Richter-Reichhelm, H.-B., Böning, W., Eichinger, R., Schoch, C., Althoff, J., and Mohr, U., 1982, A fetal respiratory epithelial cell line for studying some problems of transplacental carcinogenesis in Syrian golden hamsters, J. Cancer Res. Clin. Oncol., 104:133.

Gould, M.N., Grau, D.R., Seidman, L.A., and Moore, C.J., 1986, Interspecies comparison of human and rat mammary epithelial cell-mediated mutagenesis by polycyclic aromatic hydrocarbons, Cancer Res., 46:4942.

Harris, C.C., Autrup, H., Haugen, H., Lechner, J., Trump, B.F., and Hsu, I.C., 1982, Studies of host factors in carcinogenesis using cultured human tissues and cells, IARC Sci. Pub., 39:497.

Jacob, J., Grimmer, G., Raab, G., Emura, M., Riebe, M., and Mohr, U., 1987, Comparison of chrysene metabolism in epithelial human bronchial and Syrian hamster lung cells, Cancer Lett., 38:171.

Kim, K.C., 1985, Possible requirement of collagen gel substratum for production of mucin-like glycoproteins by primary rabbit tracheal epithelial cells in culture, In Vitro Cell. Dev. Biol., 21:617.

Lechner, J.F., Haugen, A., McClendon, I.A. and Shamsuddin, A.M., 1984, Induction of squamous differentiation of normal human bronchial epithelial cells by small amounts of serum, Differentiation, 25:229.

Mass, M.J., and Kaufman, D.G., A comparison between the activation of benzo(a)pyrene in organ cultures and microsomes from the tracheal epithelium of rats and hamsters, Carcinogenesis, 4:297.

McDowell, E.M., Ben, T., Coleman, B., Chang, S., Newkirk, C., and De Luca, L.M., 1987, Effects of retinoic acid on the growth and morphology of hamster tracheal epithelial cells in primary culture, Virchows Arch. B, 54:38.

McDowell, E.M., Keenan, K.P., and Huang, M., 1984, Effects of vitamin A-deprivation on hamster tracheal epithelium, Virchows Arch., Cell Path., 45:197.

McDowell, E.M., and Trump, B.F., 1983, Histogenesis of preneoplastic and neoplastic lesions in tracheobronchial epithelium, Surv. Synth. Path. Res., 2:235.

Milo, G.E., Trewyn, R.W., Tejwani, R., Oldham, J.W., and Douglas, W.H.J., 1980, Intertissue variation in benzo(a)pyrene metabolism by human skin, lung and liver in vitro, in: NATO Advisory Group for Aerospace Research and Development, Conf. Proc. No. 309, Toxic Hazards in Aviation, Vol. B7, pp. B7-1, London.

Minna, J.D., Carney, D.N., Olie, H., Bunn, P.A., Jr., and Gazdar, A.F., 1982, Growth of human and small-cell lung cancer in defined medium, in: Growth of Cells in Hormonally Defined Media, G.H. Sato, A.B. Pardee, and D.A. Sirbasku, ed., pp. 627, Cold Spring Harbor Laboratory, Cold Spring Harbor.

Mohr, U., and Dungworth, D.L., 1988, Relevance to man of experimentally induced pulmonary tumours in rats and hamsters, in: U. Mohr, D. Dungworth, G. Kimmerle, J. Lewkowski, R. McClellan, and W. Stöber, ed., Springer-Verlag, Berlin-Heidelberg, in press.

Moore, C.J., Tricomi, W.A., and Gould, M.N., 1986, Interspecies comparison of polycyclic aromatic hydrocarbon metabolism in human and rat mammary epithelial cells, Cancer Res., 46:4946.

Plopper, C.G., Mariassy, A.T., Wilson, D.W., Alley, J.L., Nishio, S.I., and Nettesheim, P., 1983, Comparison of nonciliated tracheal epithelial cells in six mammalian species: Ultrastructure and population densities. Exp. Lung Res., 5:281.

Prough, R.A., Patrizi, V.W., Okita, R.T., Masters, B.S.S., and Jakobsson, S.W., 1979, Characteristics of benzo(a)pyrene metabolism by kidney, liver, and lung microsomal fractions from rodents and humans, Cancer Res., 39:1199.

Reid, L.M., and Jefferson, D.M., 1984, Cell culture studies using extracts of extracellular matrix to study growth and differentiation in mammalian cells, in: Mammalian Cell Culture, J.P. Mather, ed., pp. 239, Plenum Press, New York.

Schreiber, H., Martin, D.H. and Pazmiño, N., Species differences in the effect of benzo(a)pyrene-ferric oxide on the respiratory tract of rats and hamsters, Cancer Res., 35:1654.

Wen, J., Emura, M., Riebe, M., and Mohr, U., 1988, Toxicity and chromosomal damage in fetal Syrian hamster and human pulmonary epithelial cells, Cancer Lett., 41:37.

Wu, R., Groelke, J.W., Chang, L.Y., Porter, M.E., Smith, D., and Nettesheim, P., 1982, Effects of hormones on the multiplication and differentiation of tracheal epithelial cells in culture, in: Growth of Cells in Hormonally Defined Media, G.H. Sato, A.B. Pardee, and D.A. Sirbasku, ed., p. 627, Cold Spring Harbor Laboratory, Cold Spring Harbor.

Wu, R., Nolan, E., and Turner, C., 1985, Expression of tracheal differentiated functions in serum-free hormone-supplemented medium, J. Cell. Physiol., 125:167.

Wu., R., and Wu, M.M.J., 1986, Effects of retinoids on human bronchial epithelial cells: Differential regulation of hyaluronate synthesis and keratin protein synthesis, J. Cell Physiol., 127:73.

Yamasaki, H., Huberman, E., and Sachs, L., 1977, Metabolism of the carcinogenic hydrocarbon benzo(a)pyrene in human fibroblast and epithelial cells. II. Differences in metabolism to water-soluble products and aryl hydrocarbon hydroxylase activity, Int. J. Cancer, 19:378.

ASSESSMENT OF LOW-EXPOSURE RISK FROM CARCINOGENS:

IMPLICATIONS OF THE KNUDSON-MOOLGAVKAR

TWO-CRITICAL MUTATION THEORY

James D. Wilson

Monsanto Company
St. Louis, MO U.S.A.

ABSTRACT

The two-critical-mutation carcinogenesis theory of Knudson and Moolgavkar seems to provide solutions to some of the most contentious problems in cancer risk assessment. It describes a class of agents which increase tumor incidence without being reactive toward DNA: these nongenotoxic agents act through increases in cell birth rate. Because mutations occur when DNA lesions are not repaired before mitosis, increasing the mitotic rate increases the probability that a critical mutation will occur. Agents which affect mitotic rate can act either on normal cells or on those which have undergone one of the two critical mutations ("initiated"). Those acting on initiated cells are identified with the class called "promoters" by experimentalists. No unequivocal examples of agents acting solely on normal cells have yet been reported, although some are postulated.

Exposure limits for nongenotoxic agents should be set based on the dose-response for mitotic rate increase, since this is the determining step in the process.

Genotoxic agents act directly on DNA; their hazard is proportional to cumulative exposure when acting in this mode. However, all such agents will also increase mitotic rate under some conditions and, in addition, many are believed also to act as promoters. The two kinds of activity are synergistic; where both occur, the dose-response curve is much steeper than would otherwise be expected. Incidence data from this regime (i.e., high dose or dose-rate experiments) cannot be used to estimate low-exposure hazard through the conventional "linearized multistage" technique, because effect cannot be taken to be simply proportional to dose. A mathematically correct version of this method would be appropriate for estimation of low-dose hazard, if applied to data from experiments where mitotic rate is not elevated. Unfortunately, conventional lifetime bioassays do not provide the information needed to ascertain if their output can be so used; additional experiments must be done.

Also discussed are recommendations for improving toxicity testing so that better low-exposure hazard estimates can be made.

INTRODUCTION

Few recent problems have challenged scientists from industry and government more than regulating exposure to low doses of carcinogens. Nearly all scientists who work in relevant disciplines recognize the limitations of current methodologies and most support efforts to improve them. It is now clear that the theory which underlies current methodology is not consistent with much of the growing body of experimental evidence developed by cancer researchers over the last twenty years (Moolgavkar, 1986; Trosko, 1987); long ago it became obsolete in the world of cancer research. What is just as clear is that successful science-based risk assessment must derive from a successful theory.

A new theory of carcinogenesis began to emerge from that evidence in the late 1970s, and was first given its present form by Alfred Knudson and Suresh Moolgavkar (Moolgavkar and Knudson, 1981; Moolgavkar, 1983; Knudson, 1987). (Essentially the same theory was articulated by Greenfield, et al. [1984] and in somewhat different form by Potter [1981].) This theory seems to provide a sound basis for moving forward. It derives from the "multistage" theory of Armitage and Doll (1954) and the long line of research into somatic mutations and the chemical structures of carcinogens (Miller and Miller, 1977) which culminated in identification of the genotoxic pathway to carcinogenesis. However, by incorporating several other concepts also accepted by cancer researchers by the mid-1970s, (Trosko and Chang, 1978) the new theory profoundly alters the concept of a "stage" and gives definition to other processes susceptible to outside influence. Gone is the sequential nature of the several stages, central to the Armitage-Doll model. Introduced is the idea -- still somewhat controversial -- that exactly two irreversible genetic changes lie on the critical path for conversion of normal cells to cancer.

This Knudson-Moolgavkar paradigm, based first on epidemiological and clinical evidence but now strongly supported by experiment, successfully rationalizes most of the observations regarding carcinogenesis which have been reported.[1] In contrast, the multistage paradigm in which conventional risk assessment methodologies are based cannot account satisfactorily for several important phenomena. In particular, it provides no guidance for treating the diverse phenomena loosely grouped together under the term "promotion" (Moolgavkar, 1986).

The Knudson-Moolgavkar paradigm is being explored by the U.S. EPA and others as the basis for "biologically based models" of dose-response (Mauskopf, 1986; Bayard and Thorslund, 1987; Thorslund, et al., 1987; Conolly, et al., 1987; Travis, 1988). Extension of this work, now underway, will test the utility of the paradigm for routine use in risk assessment. However, the theory itself has several implications for risk assessment and public policy generally, which this paper explores.

BACKGROUND: THE THEORY

Conventional techniques for estimating low-exposure carcinogenic hazard are all based on the Armitage-Doll theory, as that was understood about 1970. It assumes the existence of a number of independent "stages" through which normal cells pass on the way to cancer; some or all of these stages may be speeded up by chemical or physical agents. In the mathematical model used

---

[1] Excellent summaries of the theory, listing the phenomena it rationalizes, are given by Moolgavkar (1986) and by Thorslund, et al. (1987).

for regulatory purposes, the interaction is assumed to be first order in the agent (per stage) and the hazard proportional to cumulative exposure. This theory and set of assumptions lead to a mathematical expression in which the hazard is estimated as an exponential function of $(\text{dose})^n$, in which n is the number of stages believed to be effected by the agent.

The Knudson-Moolgavkar theory adds three concepts to the Armitage-Doll framework and subtracts one. Added are these:

- Increases in the rate at which cells divide (more precisely, their net birth rate) in any tissue will increase the probability of a tumor's arising in that tissue.

- "Background" mutations (i.e., those occurring as a result of cosmic rays, oxidation, irreducible errors of transcription, etc.) play an important role in cancer.

- Only two "irreversible genetic events" (which can only loosely be called "mutations") are on the critical path for transformation of a normal cell to a cancerous one.[2]

The concept subtracted, that the stages must be sequential and proceed in a definite order, had only the status of a postulate in the Armitage-Doll model. It makes the mathematics work, and was not inconsistent with what was known about cancer in the mid-1950s. However, it is not necessary for the Knudson-Moolgavkar theory, and it is not consistent with some observations. (One example: single-exposure carcinogenesis studies with rapidly-cleared agents, such as those reported by Isaacs [1984] and Driver, et al. [1987].)

Once stated, the first of the added concepts is almost self-evident. For one thing, it is well known that the majority of adult human tumors arise in epithelial tissues; (Moolgavkar, 1986) these continue to undergo mitosis throughout life. Tumors associated with scars (wound healing) are also common: cells adjacent to a wound proliferate during healing (Alexander, 1988). Further, childhood cancers arise in tissues undergoing growth and terminal differentiation, while breast cancer exhibits an unusual pattern of age dependence which this theory rationalizes (Moolgavkar, 1986). In addition, it is recognized that cell division is necessary for DNA lesions to be "fixed" as mutations (Trosko and Chang, 1978). The more rapid is cell division, the more cells will be at risk for this process. More cells at risk implies, all else being equal, that more mutations will occur.

The influence of mitotic rate on tumor yield in the rat bladder has been studied in some detail by Cohen, Ellwein, and their co-workers (Greenfield, et al., 1984; Hasegawa, et al., 1988; Cohen and Ellwein, 1988; Ellwein and Cohen, 1988). They have shown that sodium saccharin, the complex heterocycle "FANFT", and other bladder carcinogens all increase the mitotic rate in the bladder epithelium (as does freeze-wounding), and that the tumor yield can be modelled using mitotic rate as a critical variable. (FANFT also acts through a genotoxic mechanism in this system.) It is also worth noting that many compounds considered to be "promoters" have been found to increase mitotic rate.[3]

---

[2] In some mathematical explorations of the theory and its implications, it has also been assumed that the time from "birth" of a cancerous cell to detectability of a tumor is constant, and that each cancerous cell born becomes a tumor. Obviously, neither of these is correct. (For discussions of the two points, see Thorslund, et al. [1987], Whittemore and Keller [1978], and Den Otter [1985]). However, making these assumptions simplified the mathematics and did not materially affect the conclusions.

Recently, the importance of the second concept to human cancer has become apparent. We now know of a very large number of natural substances with substantial human exposure that are mutagens (Ames, 1983), some of them very potent. The process by which ionizing radiation induces mutations is understood (Simic, and Karel, 1980; Ames and Saul, 1988), and recognized to be virtually identical to that followed by components (superoxide, hydrogen peroxide) of normal oxidative metabolism. Ames and Saul (1988) have estimated the rate of DNA lesions from oxidative pathways alone (by chemical analysis of excretion of DNA oxidation products) to be ca. 10^3 per cell per day in humans. Lesions arising from other chemical mutagens and from irreducible errors of transcription add an unknown number to this quantity.

Essentially all of these DNA lesions are repaired; the efficiency in vivo is not known, but in certain cell lives in vitro it exceeds 0.9999.[4] Nevertheless, any lesion unrepaired at mitosis will lead to genetic change becoming established in the daughter cell. While the probability is very low that such a change will be on a critical path to cancer (the probability is estimated[5] to be 10^{-5} to 10^{-6} per mitotic event), it is clear that that is high enough to account for essentially all human cancer.[6]

The third element, that only two mutations lie on the critical path between normal and cancerous cells, remains a postulate at this time. It has been shown rigorously to hold for retinoblastoma and certain other cancers of childhood (Moolgavkar, 1986). Good genetic evidence supports its correctness in some forms of colon cancer. Age-specific incidences of common adult cancers are consistent with the postulate (Moolgavkar, 1986). Similarly, tumor incidences in several experimental systems are consistent with a two-"hit" theory, including FANFT and sodium saccharin in the rat bladder (Greenfield, et al., 1984), N-methyl-N'-nitrosourea and 7,12-dimethylbenz[a]anthracene in the rat mammary gland (Isaacs, 1985), N,N-dimethylnitrosamine in the immature rat kidney (Driver, et al., 1987), benzo[a]pyrene in the rat forestomach (Zeise and Crouch, 1985), vinyl chloride in the rat liver (Bois, 1985), and N,N-diethylnitrosamine in the rat liver (Travis, 1988). Furthermore, the plethora of results from the initiation-promotion literature are consistent with this postulate, as Potter pointed out (1981).

Knudson (1987) has outlined an attractive hypothesis to explain the postulate. It assumes the existence of regulatory substances ("chalones" in the pre-1980 literature [Potter, 1981; Potter, 1988]) which inhibit cell division and/or stimulate differentiation, whose action at the cellular level is under genetic control. When the copy of this gene on each chromosome is deleted or otherwise disabled by mutation or other genetic change, the daughter cell bearing these changes will be able to escape from control, and unlimited growth will result. It is now believed that for retinoblastoma the critical

---

[3] This is true, for example, for the classic promoters phorbol myristate acetate (also called "TPA") (Parkinson, et al., 1983) and 2,3,7,8-tetra-chlorodibenzodioxin (Hudson, et al., 1986).

[4] In culture, the efficiency is strongly dependent on both species and organ type.

[5] This estimate is model-dependent, that is, it was derived by Greenfield, et al. (1984) from their studies of saccharin in the rat bladder, through application of a mathematical model based on the K-M theory.

[6] This conclusion is implied by Moolgavkar's (1986) discussion.

control substance is the protein "transforming growth factor β_1", and that the critical genetic events result in retinoblasts becoming unable to bind this factor (Kimchi, et al., 1988).

Argument against the two-event model could be derived from observations that most solid tumors differ by many more than two mutations from the normal tissue from which they evolved. However, such mutations need not be on the critical path. Their occurrence in a group of cells undergoing continuous division is easily understood, expecially if their consequence is increased survivability of the daughter cell. These changes are assigned to the progression phase of cancer (Klein and Klein, 1985; Iannacone, et al., 1987). We note here that such change could, in fact, precede either (or both) of the two critical events. In the theory described here, carcinogenesis -- the birth of the cancer -- ends with the second critical event.

To summarize, when merged with retained elements of the conventional theory the new carcinogenesis paradigm can be described as follows:

• Tumors start from one (or a few) cells which have undergone two critical irreversible genetic changes (Iannacone, et al., 1987). It is hypothesized that these changes may involve alteration in both copies of a single critical gene, possibly that coding for (or regulating the expression of) a "growth factor" receptor protein. (How this hypothesis relates to what is known about oncogenes remains to be worked out.)

• Carcinogenesis occurs only in tissues whose cells are undergoing division; in the process critical genetic events are "fixed" during mitosis. A variety of such changes have been observed to be associated with the process, including point mutations, deletions, chromosomal rearrangements, etc. (Klein, 1987).

• There exists a background process of genetic change due to irreducible errors of transcription, cosmic irradiation, natural mutagens, etc. (Den Otter, 1985). The probability is very low that any one DNA lesion will survive to mitosis and be fixed as a critical mutation.[7] However, that probability is large enough that no other mutations need to be invoked to explain most of the incidence of cancer in the human population.

---

[7] By one estimate, it could be as small as 10^{-20}: If the DNA lesion rate is 10^3/cell/d, given ca. 10^{13} cells/person and 2.7×10^4 d/lifetime, then an individual suffers ca. 3×10^{20} DNA lesions per lifetime. The number of lesions transformed (i.e., not repaired at mitosis) and critical for cancer, p, will be approximated by a Poisson distribution with $\lambda = Np$, where $N \cong 3 \times 10^{20}$. If two critical transformations are required for cancer, and the probability of any individual's suffering a cancer (including nonfatal tumors) in a lifetime is 0.3, then

$$Pr(cancer) = Pr(\geqq 2 \text{ critical transformations}) = 0.3 = 1 - Pr(0) - Pr(1)$$

From $Pr(k \text{ transformations}) = \dfrac{\lambda^k}{k!} e^{-\lambda}$

$$Pr(cancer) = 1 - e^{-\lambda} - \lambda e^{-\lambda} = 0.3$$
$$\lambda = 1.1$$

and

$$p = \frac{\lambda}{N} \cong 10^{-20}$$

On the other hand, in Isaacs' (1985) single-exposure studies, 10^{16} to 10^{17} molecules were dosed per tumor observed. This difference may be due in part to the differences in repair efficiency among different kinds of DNA lesions.

• Once a cancerous cell is born, its daughters accumulate genotypic and phenotypic changes which confer survival advantages on the population.

Chemical (and other) agents can influence cancer incidence through at least two different and independent processes. First, the agent may react directly with DNA, increasing the number of lesions and thus increasing the probability that a critical genetic event will occur. Second, the agent may react with some other component of the cell, increasing the rate at which mitosis occurs and thus increasing the probability of a critical genetic event. (Note that extensive cell killing will induce compensatory hyperplasia and thus increase mitotic rate, at least temporarily). Both of these will increase cancer incidence. In addition, the agent may react with some component of a cell which results in an increased tendency for that cell to undergo terminal differentiation (and death). If this occurs only in normal cells, it will tend to increase tumor incidence; if, however, it occurs in cells which have undergone one or more critical mutations, it will decrease incidence.

Note that some chemical agents require metabolic transformation before becoming active; most of the active transformation products which have been identified can be classified as chemical electrophiles (Miller and Miller, 1979).

Note also that the form of the theory described by Potter (1981), and widely accepted as a rationalization of initiation-promotion experiments (Thorslund, et al., 1987; Nettesheim, et al., 1987; Swenberg, et al., 1987; Barret and Wiseman, 1987) is actually a special case of this paradigm. In this form, the two genetic events are assumed to be sequential, and that in between their occurence, the singly-mutated cell undergoes "clonal expansion" to an intermediate lesion, out of which cancers may (or may not) grow (Trosko and Chang, 1980). Agents which increase growth of singly-mutated, or "initiated", cells have been identified with what are called "promoters" by experimental-ists. It is known, for instance, that the classic promoters in mouse skin, such as phorbol ester (or "TPA"), increase mitotic rate in skin cells in culture; the mechanism by which TPA does this is now reasonably well understood. Phenobarbital, the classic rat liver promoter, is also known to induce hyperplasia. However, some phenomena are not adequately described by this special case. Single-exposure carcinogenesis is one example. Another is carcinogenesis following chronic hyperplasia of normal cells, such as is believed to be the process by which goitrogens cause thyroid follicular tumors in rodents, and by which intubation of BHA, ethyl acrylate, etc., leads to rat forestomach tumors.[8]

---

[8] Considerable confusion is engendered by nomenclature in this field, that we would do well to end. For instance, the term "stage": Moolgavkar (1986) explicitly and Cohen and Ellwein implicitly identify it with the critical genetic events which transform cells. Others, influenced by the obsolete paradigm, include clonal expansion and even progression as separate stages. Under the K-M theory, clonal expansion/promotion are important only because the probability of the second stage's occurring is thereby increased; thus they are part of the second stage, or not a "stage" at all. Similarly, "progression" follows carcinogenesis. It might be better to drop "stage" altogether and return to Moolgavkar's original term, "event". Similarly, both Moolgavkar and Cohen and Ellwein use the term "initiated" to describe singly-transformed cells; Moolgavkar uses "completion" to describe the second event, while Cohen and Ellwein use "transformation". Although it is desirable to have a term describing singly-transformed cells, attaching different names to the two steps obscures their essential similarity.

Under the K-M theory (Moolgavkar, 1986) at low incidence the direct action of genotoxic agents is mathematically described as an increase in a proportionality constant in the age-specific incidence equation. When age and exposure regimen are held constant, the dose-response curve will thus be approximately a linear-quadratic expression in dose. Under experimental conditions which minimize differences in the accumulated number of cell divisions among treated and control animals, we can expect to see a dose-response curve of this form. The incidence of liver tumors in the "ED01" experiment fits a linear model (Littlefield and Gaylor, 1985) and may be an example of this phenomenon. However, when age and exposure are not held constant, or at high (>ca. 25%) incidence, this no longer holds and more complex equations must be used. In general, at low incidence the age-specific incidence depends upon the product of the probability of transformation times a function of the net birth rate of cells in both the normal and initiated states. [At high incidence, only the probability of the first transition is independent of net birth rates, and the incidence function becomes very complex (Moolgavkar, 1988)]. Thus there is a synergistic interaction between formation of DNA lesions and mitotic rate in target cells. Under exposure conditions which increase both, the dose-response will be a very rapidly-rising curve; Ellwein and Cohen (1988) have shown this behavior for the bladder carcinogen "FANFT".

IMPLICATIONS

• Conventional methods for estimating dose-respones, based as they are on the Armitage-Doll model, can no longer be considered generally valid. They probably are appropriate under one set of circumstances, to which their use should be restricted. Agencies which have made the policy decision to prefer one of these models because of its supposed "biological plausibility" should reconsider that decision.

As noted above, the Armitage-Doll model assumes a definite sequence of steps between normal and cancerous cells (without necessarily specifying the identity of those "stages"). It is now known that while the two irreversible genetic events usually proceed one at a time, they can and do occur simultaneously. Cells which have been born possessing the two mutations are fully capable of proceeding through the progression phase into a tumor. Further, the "promotion" stage -- clonal expansion of initiated cells -- need not necessarily occur. Thus, that assumption is contradicted by data and must be abandoned.

Furthermore, the "linearized multistage" (LMS) procedure of Crump, et al., (1977) tacitly assumes that the interaction between agent and cell is kinetically first order, i.e., that effect is directly proportional to dose. This assumption probably is valid for DNA lesions caused by the electrophilic chemicals thought typical of "carcinogens" in the early 1970s. However, it clearly is not valid for promoters. As we have seen, the effect of a promoter

---

8   (cont.) The term "promoter" is much abused and misunderstood. Because of the restricted sense in which "promoter" is used by most experimentalists, I propose restricting its use to compounds which effect the clonal expansion of initiated cells. Both phorbol ester and phenobarbital are well described by this notation. Doing this would require a new name for agents which act only on the mitotic rate of normal cells (if these turn out to be common enough to warrant a special name).

Finally, the term "complete carcinogen" is redundant: genotoxic carcinogens can also promote or cause cell killing at high dose rates. "Genotoxic carcinogen" conveys the essence of the class more readily and is to be preferred.

is to increase the probability that a critical genetic change will occur. Since the increase in that probability is time-dependent, the apparent order of reaction will be time-dependent, as well. In addition, it need not be integral. Put another way, the Crump model assumes that the dose-dependence of tumor incidence can be described by an equation exponential in a polynomial of $(dose)^n$, where $n = 1,2,3, \ldots$ up to the number of "stages" assumed. Instead, the synergy of genotoxic and nongenotoxic effects allows n to take any value, one that depends on the duration of exposure. Thus, the LMS procedure is not generally valid.

The procedure is valid when applied to a data set obtained from experiments in which the mitotic rate of cells in the target organ is essentially the same in all treated and control groups. There may be no data set extant for which this condition is known to be met. However, there may be a few for which this is probably true: the 2-AAF-associated liver tumors from the "ED01" study, and the rat forestomach tumors caused by benzo[a]pyrene treatment at low dose rate, identified by Zeise and Crouch (1985), may be two such.

- In the absence of enough data to estimate the dose-response with an appropriate model, exposure standards should be set using accepted toxico logical practice. In addition, the K-M theory suggests approaches to minimum-data approximations to low-exposure hazard, which deserve exploration.

Clearly it is preferable to obtain separate estimates of the dose-response for genotoxic and nongenotoxic activities -- i.e., for the increases in incidence implied by direct reaction of agents with DNA and by increases in mitotic rate -- and use an appropriate model to estimate the hazard function. (Several different models, all based on the Knudson-Moolgavkar theory, are now being explored by Ellwein and Cohen [Greenfield, et al., 1984], Thorslund, et al., [1987], Conolly, et al. [1987], and Travis, et al. [1988].) From the work done so far by Ellwein and Cohen, it appears that the genotoxic component will be the more important in low-exposure regimes.

When such data are not available (nor likely soon to be), we believe that risk assessors should make no pretense about estimating "risk". Standards should be set using traditional toxicological approaches. Many critics have observed that applying LMS methodology to data sets from typical "maximum tolerated dose" (MTD) bioassays is functionally equivalent to a traditional approach, differing only in the magnitude of the (here, implicit) "uncertainty factor" used. This opinion is supported by the rather surprising discovery of Zeise, et al. (1984) that there exists a very good correlation between the apparent "carcinogenic potency" of an agent (as calculated using Edmund Crouch's version of the LMS methodology) and its median lethal dose in the same strain of animal.[9] This being the case, we recommend explicit recognition of the uncertainty; it has the advantages of clarity and honesty, and does not alter the degree of protection afforded the public.

As noted, studies by Cohen and Ellwein and their co-workers suggest that the low-exposure hazard is dominated by genotoxic effects. Other work (Littlefield and Gaylor, 1985; Zeise and Crouch, 1985) is consistent with that conclusion. In principle, it should be possible to estimate the genotoxic hazard from short-term in vitro and/or in vivo dose-response.

---

[9] The validity and meaning of this correlation have been strenuously debated in the pages of Risk Analysis, and elsewhere. The K-M theory suggests the following interpretation: since all of the incidence data treated were obtained from MTD experiments and since the criterion for identifying the maximum tolerated dose requires some evidence for chronic toxicity (reduced weight gain) in the highest dose tested, it is almost

Now that their original purpose is recognized as not useful (Trosko, 1987), attention of the environmental mutagenesis community should turn toward extracting from this kind of experiment the valuable information which resides there. When appropriate tests have been developed and validated, their results should be used for risk assessment and standard-setting purposes.

- Assessment based on increase of mitotic rate for dose-response assessment of nongenotoxic activity over normal or some surrogate for that quantity should be preferred. When such data are unavailable, nongenotoxic carcinogens should be considered chronic toxicants, and exposure standards set using traditional toxicologic methods.

Because nongenotoxic agents increase tumor incidence through their action on the net birth rate of normal or initiated cells, it is that rate which should form the basis of a hazard assessment. This will be true no matter which of the many possible mechanisms by which mitotic rate can be affected operates in any particular case. The implications of this for the design of toxicology experiments is discussed below. Here, we note only that such data are to be preferred whenever available.

An argument can be made (see Appendix) that the nature of the biochemical system which regulates cell division and differentiation requires that a true threshold of action exists for nongenotoxic agents. (That is, for them there exists some exposure for which the incremental risk is zero.) Whether that turns out to be accepted or not, it remains true that the "threshold" exposure can never be determined experimentally; all that can be measured is the exposure at which elevation of mitotic rate is less than or equal to the uncertainty of measurement. There is need for agreement on how to extract an "acceptable risk" (or "no significant risk") value from this condition. A proposal for this will be made elsewhere.

Unfortunately, at present mitotic rate data seldom are available. In a few instances, it is known that there exists a dose-response relationship between mitotic rate and some physiologic parameter or chemical species concentration for which data are available. (For example, Anderson [1987] has shown that rat urinary tract epithelial hyperplasia depends on blood zinc levels, and has linked that to kidney tumors associated with heavy exposure to the sequestrant NTA.) In these instances, the data should be examined to see if they give a useful surrogate for mitotic rate elevation, and used wherever possible.

For true promoters (i.e., agents which affect only the initiated cell population), mitotic rate elevation data will be directly measurable only in favorable circumstances -- only when clones of initiated cells can be identified under appropriate experimental conditions. Such clones have tentatively been identified in two cases: "enzyme-altered foci" of the rat liver and colon polyps in humans. The rat-liver system may turn out to be a particularly favorable one for obtaining data on the dose-response for action in initiated cell populations, as the discussions in this symposium have suggested. (See also Pitot, et al., 1987.)

---

[9] (cont.) certain that in these experiments mitotic rate increases occur. In addition, promotional effects may also be present. Thus, the potency rarely (if ever) reflected only the genotoxic component of the dose-response. Mitotic rate increase is a cellular phenomenon and thus resembles ordinary chronic toxicity, which is known to correlate with acute lethality. If this interpretation is correct, including data sets from experiments done under conditions where no chronic toxicity is evident should make the correlation poorer; Metzger, et al. (1987) have found this to be the case.

In the absence of data on dose-response for mitotic rate elevation, nongeno-toxic carcinogens should be evaluated like ordinary chronic toxins for standard-setting purposes.

Implications for Toxicology Testing

Although the conventional bioassay does not, by itself, yield enough infor-mation to permit estimation of low-exposure hazard, this kind of experiment will remain important. However, its value can be greatly increased by incorporating the following changes into the experimental design.

First, small numbers of animals from each dose group should be tested to allow evaluation of mitotic rates in key organs at intervals in the experiment. Since subchronic experiments do not reliably predict target organs for cancer, choosing the tissues to examine will necessarily be arbitrary. (Clearly, the prevalence of liver tumors in experimental animals suggests that this organ ought to be routinely included.)

Second, a dose group with exposure at least an order of magnitude less, preferably two, than the MTD should be included. Compounds which are dangerous at exposures orders of magnitude less will still be "positive" under these conditions. At worst, inclusion of such exposures will reduce the error introduced by low-dose extrapolation if it is used as the base for the calculation.

Third, inclusion of groups receiving single or pulsed exposures should be considered.

Data obtained from short-term mutagenicity tests needs to be taken into account when the bioassays are designed. For instance, a potency estimated from short-term results should figure into the identification of exposures in the low-dose or periodic-exposure experiments.

Conclusions

Two decades of advances in our knowledge of cancer and carcinogenesis require changes in the paradigm on which we base our procedures for cancer risk assessment. The paradigm used since the early 1970s arose from the knowledge base of the 1960s. Since then scientists have learned three things which necessitate modifying that paradigm. First is the importance of cell division to mutation, and the recognition that a speeding up of cell division increases cancer risk. Second, DNA lesions are very common (even though mutations are rare); thus, chemical agents (or radiation) can increase cancer risk indirectly by influencing mitotic rate. In effect, this action serves to accelerate the natural process. Third, only two mutations -- "irreversible genetic changes" -- appear to be <u>required</u>, <u>i.e.</u>, to be on the critical path for conversion of normal cells to cancerous ones, at least for most cancers which have been studied.

This new paradigm implies several changes in the way cancer risk is assessed. First, we understand clearly now that the response of an animal to high exposures of carcinogens does not reliably predict the response to very low exposures. Most genotoxic carcinogens behave differently at high dose rates -- "MTD" conditions -- because toxicity which occurs under these conditions exaggerates mutation rates. Thus, low-exposure risks estimated only from high-dose carcinogenic "potencies" will be too large. Further, we know that "LMS" dose-response estimating methodology is valid only when applied to data generated in experiments exhibiting negligible mitotic rate increases.

For nongenotoxic carcinogens, on the other hand, the linearized low-dose procedure is almost certainly never appropriate. The dose-response for mitotic rate increase, integrated over the duration of treatment, needs to be taken into account during standard setting. Some kinds of nongenotoxins, those which affect hormone-mediated responses, are widely believed to exhibit true thresholds of action, and should be regulated on that basis. There is, in fact, some evidence that all agents which act via mitotic rate increases behave similarly. There is need for research to determine how best to identify "acceptable risk" exposures for this class of agents.

The design of lifetime animal bioassays needs to be changed to yield information on mitotic rate increases.

APPENDIX: Outline of an Argument for a Threshold of Action for Nongenotoxic Carcinogens

Nongenotoxic carcinogens increase tumor incidence by increasing the net birth rate of normal or initiated cells. Because DNA lesions unrepaired at mitosis transform to mutations, any elevation in mitotic rate amplifies the activity of any genotoxic agents present. Most biologists believe that organisms possess some capacity to absorb external insult without injury, i.e., that a "threshold" of action exists for physiologically active substances. Physical scientists and mathematicians usually are reluctant to accept this belief, in part because no mechanism has been described which includes buffering capacity against small change. The mechanism by which mitotic rate is regulated may well provide exactly such a buffering capacity, and thus support the existence of thresholds for nongenotoxic carcinogens.

Mitotic rate is one of the physiologic functions closely regulated by any organism. The processes through which this regulation occurs are just beginning to be understood. We know that control is partly genetic, in that certain genes must be caused to express before division can proceed. Some oncogene products may modulate this expression. Further, we know of an extensive family of polypeptide hormones, some called "growth factors", which seem to be involved in regulation of cell growth. (A good introduction to the recent literature on these topics can be found in the recent collection edited by Bradshaw and Prentis [1987].)

Growth factors and related proteins (e.g., interferons, interleukins) bind to cell-surface receptors; their varied effects follow from this. They can be roughly divided into two groups, those which always stimulate division, and those which sometimes inhibit it. The protein "epidermal growth factor", EGF, represents the first group; it stimulates division of cells of epithelial, endodermal and neural origin in culture, and appears to be widely distributed in the body. A widely-distributed representative of the mitostatic group is "transforming growth factor-beta", TGF-β; less well studied than EGF, it inhibits cell division in certain epithelial and endothelial cells in culture (Takehara, et al., 1987).

We know from control and chemical theory that two substances are required for the organism to regulate cell division: one to signal "divide", one to signal "stay". We also know that both will ordinarily be present in the extracellular fluid, and thus that the signal being received by a cell will depend on the relative concentrations (and thus ratios of receptors occupied) of the two substances. The apparent ubiquity and spectrum of activities of EGF and TGF-β make it tempting to identify them as the two universal signalling substances. This hypothesis is supported by two observations: Inman and Colwick reported (1985) that both EGF and TGF-β must be occupied for glucose uptake to occur; this provides mechanistic support for the observation by Takehara, et al. (1987) that cultures containing both TGF-β and EGF

sustained cells for long periods, while in those lacking EGF, cells slowly
die off.

Clearly the foregoing hypothesis is far too simple. The enormous number of
these "growth factor" proteins now known, by itself, tells us that. In
particular, it seems likely that tissue-specific factors will exist. It also
neglects control exerted through intercellular communication (Trosko, et al.,
1983). Nevertheless, it is consistent with what is known and suggests
experiments which can test it.

We postulate the existence of a chemically-based system by which the organism
regulates mitosis. It relies on the relative concentrations of two (or more)
circulating hormones, with the receptor binding and subsequent events being
responsible for signal transduction. (The regulation is dynamic, in that a
continuous flux of transduction is required to maintain control of gene
expression.) Cells will begin mitosis when the ratio of the two substances
exceeds some value; we identify the growth condition as

$$[EGF]/[TGF-\beta] > Q.$$

In mature or quiescent tissues, this ratio will be maintained within a range
at some difference from Q:

$$[EGF]/[TGF-\beta] = N \pm \partial N < Q, \ |\partial N| < |Q-N|$$

The difference, Q-N, will be a balance between the contradictory needs for
system stability and responsiveness. It is also this difference which
provides the buffering capacity required for a threshold.

REFERENCES

Alexander, P., 1988. In: "Theories of Carcinogenesis", O. H. Iversen, ed.,
    Hemisphere Publishing Co., Washington, DC, 293-294.
Ames, B., 1983, Science, 221:1256-1264.
Ames, B. and R. L. Saul, 1988. In: "Theories of Carcinogenesis", O. H.
    Iversen, ed.; Hemisphere Pub. Corp.; Washington; 203-220.
Anderson, R. L., 1987. In Banbury Report 25: Nongenotoxic Mechanisms in
    Carcinogenesis, Cold Spring Harbor Laboratory, 277-283. Also
    R. L. Anderson, C. L. Alden, manuscript submitted for publication.
Armitage, P. and R. Doll, 1954. Brit. J. Cancer
Barrett, J. C. and R. W. Wiseman, 1987. Environ. Health Perspect., 76:65-70.
Bayard, S. and T. W. Thorslund, 1987. Paper given at "Dioxin 87", Las
    Vegas, NV; Chemosphere, 17 (in press).
Bois, F., 1985. Private communication (poster presented at symposium, "Human
    Risk Assessment -- The Role of Animal Selection and Extrapolation",
    St. Louis, MO; October 28-31, 1985.
Bradshaw, R. A. and S. Prentis, eds., 1987. "Oncogenes and Growth Factors",
    Elsevier, Amsterdam.
Cohen, S. M., and L. B. Ellwein, 1988. Tox. Letters (in press).
Conolly, R. B., R. H. Reitz, and M. E. Andersen, 1987. In: "Pharmaco-
    kinetics in Risk Assessment", National Academy Press, Washington, DC;
    273-285.
Den Otter, W., 1985. Cancer Immunol. Immunother., 19:159-162.
Driver, H. E., I. N. H. White, W. H. Butler, 1987. Br. J. Exp. Path., 68:
    133-143.
Ellwein, L. B., and S. M. Cohen, 1988. Risk Analysis, 8:215-221.
Greenfield, R. E., L. B. Ellwein, and S. M. Cohen, 1984. Carcinogenesis,
    5:437-445.
Hasegawa, R., S. M. Cohen, M. St. John, M. Cano, and L. B. Ellwein, 1986.
    Carcinogenesis, 7:633-636.
Hudson, L. G., W. A. Toscano, Jr., and W. F. Greenlee, 1986. Tox. Appl.
    Pharm., 82:481-492.

Iannaccone, P. M., W. C. Weinberg, and F. D. Deamant, 1987. Int. J. Cancer 39:778-784.
Inman, W. H. and S. P. Colowick, 1985. Proc. Natl. Acad. Sci. USA, 82:1246-1349.
Isaacs, J. T., 1985. Cancer Res., 45:4827-4832.
Kimchi, A., X. -F. Wang, R. A. Weinberg, S. Cheiftez, and J. Massague, 1988. Science, 240:196-199.
Klein, G. and E. Klein, 1984. Carcinogenesis, 5:429-435.
Klein, G., 1987. Science, 238:1539-1545.
Knudson, A. G., 1985. Cancer Research, 45:1437-1443.
Knudson, A. G., 1987. Adv. Viral Oncology, 7:1-17.
Littlefield, N. A. and D. W. Gaylor, 1985. J. Tox. Env. Health, 15:545-550.
Mauskopf, J., 1986. Paper given at the annual meeting of the Society for Risk Analysis; Boston, MA. Proceedings (in press).
Metzger, B., E. A. C. Crouch, and R. Wilson, 1987. Manuscript submitted for publication.
Miller, J. A. and E. C. Miller, 1977. In: "Origins of Human Cancer", H. H. Hiatt, J. D. Watson, and J. A. Winsten, eds., Cold Spring Harbor Laboratory, 605-627.
Moolgavkar, S. H., 1979. J. Nat. Cancer Inst., 61:49-52.
Moolgavkar, S. H., 1983. Env. Health Perspectives, 50:285-291.
Moolgavkar, S. H., 1986. Ann. Rev. Pub. Health, 7:151-169.
Moolgavkar, S. H. and A. Dewanji, 1988. Risk Analysis, 8:5-7.
Moolgavkar, S. H. and A. G. Knudson, 1981. J. Nat. Cancer Inst., 66:1037-1052.
Moolgavkar, S. H. and D. J. Venzon, 1979. Math. Biosci., 47:55-77.
Parkinson, E. K., P. Grabham, A. Emmerson, 1983. Carcinogenesis, 4:857-861.
Pitot, H. C., T. L. Goldsworthy, S. Moran, W. Kennan, H. P. Glauert, R. R. Maronpot, and H. A. Campbell, 1987. Carcinogenesis, 8:1491-1499.
Potter, V. R., 1981. Carcinogenesis, 2:1375-1379.
Potter, V. R., 1988. Advan. Oncology, 4(1):3-8.
Saul, R. L., Ames, B. N., 1985. Paper given at the International Conference "Mechanisms of DNA Damage and Repair", Gaithersburg, Maryland. Proceedings (in press).
Simic, M., and M. Karel, eds., 1980. "Autoxidation in Food and Biological Systems", Plenum Press, New York.
Takehara, K., E. C. LeRoy, and G. R. Grotendorst, 1987. Cell, 49:415-422.
Thorslund, T. W., C. C. Brown, and G. Charnley, 1987. Risk Analysis, 7:109-119.
Travis, C., 1988. This volume.
Trosko, J. E., 1988. Mutagenesis, 3:363-364.
Trosko, J. E. and C. -C. Chang, 1978. Quart. Rev. Biology, 53:115
Trosko, J. E. and C. -C. Chang, 1980. Med. Hypotheses, 6:455-468.
Trosko, J. E., C. -C. Chang, and A. Medcalf, 1983. Cancer Investigation. 1:511-526.
Whittemore, A., and J. B. Keller, 1978. SIAM Rev., 20:1-30.
Zeise, L., E. A. C. Crouch, and R. Wilson, 1984. Risk Anal., 4:187-199. Also, Risk Anal., 5:265-270 (1985) and J. Tox. Environ. Health, 20:1-10 (1987).
Zeise, L. and E. A. C. Crouch, 1985. Private communication (unpublished manuscript).

A BIOLOGICAL DATA BASE FOR METHYLENE CHLORIDE RISK ASSESSMENT

Trevor Green

ICI Central Toxicology Laboratory
Alderley Park
Macclesfield
Cheshire, U.K.

INTRODUCTION

Methylene chloride is used extensively in industry and in a variety of consumer products. Its solvent properties and volatility have led to its use in paint strippers, in aerosol preparations, and in the decaffeination of coffee in addition to a wide range of industrial applications. Methylene chloride has low acute toxicity, its metabolism to carbon monoxide and the formation of carboxyhaemoglobin being the basis of current occupational exposed limits.

In 1986 the United States National Toxicology Program reported a significantly elevated incidence of lung and liver cancer in mice exposed to 2000 and 4000ppm of methylene chloride for a lifetime (NTP 1986). Increased incidences of lung and liver cancer were not seen in rats in the same study at these dose levels nor in rats or hamsters exposed at similar dose levels in a previous study (Burek et al 1984). Low doses of methylene chloride given to mice in drinking water (Serota et al 1986) or by oral gavage (Maltoni et al 1986) also failed to cause an increase in either tumour type.

The finding of high incidences of lung and liver cancer in mice exposed to high doses of methylene chloride caused considerable concern to both regulators and manufacturers alike, particularly because of the availability of methylene chloride to the general public through its use in paint strippers and aerosols. At the same time the marked qualitative species differences in response seen in the cancer bioassays left considerable doubt about the relevance of the mouse data to man. This paper presents details of a series of studies undertaken to explain the species differences in the carcinogenicity of methylene chloride and the relevance of the mouse data to man. The work consisted of four parts, firstly an investigation of the mechanism of action of methylene chloride in mice, secondly a study of the in vivo pharmacokinetics of methylene chloride in rats and mice, thirdly, comparative in vitro metabolism in rat, mouse, hamster and human tissues and finally the use of this data in risk assessment. The paper concentrates on the biological basis for the risk assessment rather than the risk assessment itself.

Mechanism of Carcinogenicity in Mice

Two aspects were considered; firstly the genotoxicity was evaluated in a series of short term tests, and secondly the cytotoxicity of methylene chloride was determined in rat and mouse liver and lung tissues under the conditions of exposure used in the NTP bioassay.

Methylene chloride has been known to be mutagenic in the Ames bacterial mutation assay for many years (Kirwin and Thomas 1980, Nestmann et al, 1980, Gocke et al 1981, Jongen et al 1978, 1982, Green 1983). It also appears to have activity in some strains of E.Coli (Osterman-Golkar 1983) and yeast (Callen et al 1980) but not in others (Osterman-Golkar 1983, Simmon et al 1977, Callen et al 1980). Tests for chromosomal effects have shown methylene chloride to cause chromosomal aberrations, but not sister chromatid exchanges, in vitro (Thilager et al 1984, Thilager and Kumaroo 1983), but not in vivo (Gocke et al 1981, Kramers et al 1983, Burek et al 1984, Sheldon et al 1987). In contrast a large number and variety of short term tests in mammalian cells, both in vitro and in vivo, have failed to find evidence of genotoxicity (Jongen et al 1981, Perocco and Prodi 1981, Andrae and Wolf 1983, Thilager et al 1984). It could be concluded from these studies that methylene chloride is a mutagen in micro-organisms (bacteria and yeast) but not in mammalian cells. Further studies were undertaken to attempt to clarify this position, namely a DNA binding study (Green et al 1987), unscheduled DNA synthesis assays (Ashby and Trueman 1987) and the mouse micronucleus assay (Sheldon et al 1986). The ability of methylene chloride to stimulate cell division (S-phase) was also determined. All of these studies failed to detect a response, even in the strain of mouse used in the cancer bioassay.

The effects of methylene chloride on lung and liver cells was investigated following 6hr exposures of F344 rats and $B_6C_3F_1$ mice to 2000 or 4000ppm for either 1 or 10 days. The livers and lungs of rats were unaffected by exposure to these dose levels nor were there any morphological changes seen in the livers of mice. The most significant findings from these studies were liver growth in mice and a marked lesion in the Clara cells of the mouse lung. This lesion, seen after a single exposure, involved extensive vacuolation, or balloon degeneration of the Clara cells and had largely recovered after 10 days of exposure.

Although there is clear evidence that both target organs respond differently to methylene chloride in the mouse than they do in the rat, the relevance of these observations to the subsequent development of lung and liver tumours is unclear. The lesion in the Clara cell of the mouse lung has been shown to have a marked effect on the metabolism of methylene chloride in this cell type. The changes in metabolism are believed to lead to those cells being at greater risk than other lung cell types suggesting that the Clara cell may be the cell of origin of the lung tumours seen in exposed mice. Details of these changes and their impact on risk assessment are given later in this paper.

Following these studies the mechanism of action in mice still remains unclear. The positive results in prokaryotic micro-organisms and chromosomal effects in vitro provide evidence that methylene chloride has mutagenic potential. The negative results in mammalian in vitro mutation assays and the lack of in vivo chromosomal effects or damage to DNA lead to the conclusion that methylene chloride is not a somatic cell mutagen and is therefore non-genotoxic in vivo. At the present time no alternative mechanism is apparent, although the liver growth and pulmonary toxicity seen specifically in mice may be contributory factors, particularly in a strain of mouse ($B_6C_3F_1$) which has significant incidences of both lung and liver tumours in control animals.

Metabolism and Pharmacokinetics

The metabolism of methylene chloride (Fig 1) has been known for many years, the metabolic pathway to carbon monoxide having first being discovered in man (Stewart et al 1972). This pathway which leads to carbon monoxide and elevated levels of carboxyhaemoglobin in blood involves the cytochrome P-450 mixed function oxidase system (Kubic and Anders, 1975, 1978) and has been shown to occur in the microsomal fraction of several organs including liver, kidney and lung. More recent studies using metabolic inhibitors have suggested that significant amounts of carbon dioxide are also derived from this pathway (Gargas et al 1986). The other metabolic pathway for methylene chloride, catalysed by a soluble glutathione-S-transferase enzyme, leads to formaldehyde and the subsequent formation of carbon dioxide in vivo (Ahmed and Anders 1976, 1978, Neely 1964). In addition to being metabolised to both carbon monoxide and carbon dioxide large amounts of the dose are exhaled unchanged (Riley et al 1966, McKenna and Zempel 1981). In vitro the two pathways may be studied independently using microsomal and cytosolic fractions from the organs of interest. The pathways have been investigated in a number of experimental animals and the cytochrome P-450 pathway to carbon monoxide has been extensively studied in man. Prior to the studies described in this paper there was no information about the fate of methylene chloride in the mouse.

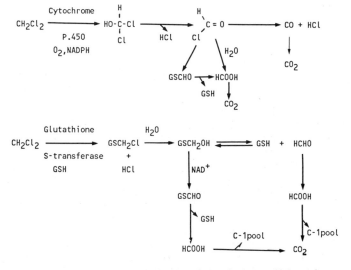

Fig. 1. The Metabolism of Methylene Chloride

In the present studies the metabolism and pharmacokinetics of methylene chloride have been investigated in vivo in F344 rats and $B_6C_3F_1$ mice and in vitro in rat, mouse, hamsters and human tissues. The objective of these studies was to determine if there was a correlation between the rate of metabolism by either of the pathways, or in the circulating levels of the parent chemical, and the species-specific cancer seen in mice. If such a correlation could be established the extent of metabolism in each species by, for example, one of the pathways, could be used as the basis of a risk assessment.

Access to human data with chemicals such as methylene chloride can only be obtained by in vitro studies using human tissues. Consequently the rate of metabolism of methylene chloride was measured in vitro in lung and liver tissue from each of the animal species and in human liver. Because the extrapolation across species to man is based on these in vitro measurements it was considered essential that the process of in vitro extrapolation should be shown to be an accurate representation of the in vivo species differences. A full comparison of the fate of methylene chloride was therefore made in vivo and in vitro in two species, rats and mice.

In Vivo Studies

The in vivo studies involved a full kinetic profile of methylene chloride and its metabolites in $B_6C_3F_1$ mice and F344 rats, both during and after 6hr exposures in the range 100 to 4000ppm. Blood levels of methylene chloride and carboxyhaemoglobin were measured together with the rates of elimination in exhaled air of methylene chloride, carbon monoxide and carbon dioxide. Because carbon dioxide is a metabolite of both metabolic pathways in vivo (Fig 1), stable isotopes were used to quantify the amount of carbon dioxide from each pathway. The rate of metabolism of methylene chloride by the cytochrome P-450 pathway, involving the oxidation of a C-H bond, occurs at a slower rate with the stable isotope form CD_2Cl_2 than with the normal isotopic form CH_2Cl_2. Consequently carbon dioxide and carbon monoxide from this pathway will be formed at a slower rate with deuterated methylene chloride than with the protonated form. However, carbon dioxide from the glutathione-S-transferase pathway, which involves the breaking of a C-Cl bond in the rate determining step, will not be affected by the use of deuterated methylene chloride. Thus the impact of the use of CD_2Cl_2 on the rate of formation of carbon dioxide was used to quantify the source of carbon dioxide in vivo over the range of dose levels used.

The steady state blood levels of methylene chloride during exposure were up to five-fold higher in rats than in mice at the higher dose levels, suggesting a significantly higher rate of metabolism in mice at high dose levels (Table 1). However, comparison of carboxyhaemoglobin levels showed that this was not due to differences in cytochrome P-450 metabolism between rats and mice. The levels of carboxyhaemoglobin were identical (8-16%) and saturation of the pathway was shown to occur at an exposure level of less than 500ppm in both species (Table 1). Saturation of the pathway was also confirmed by the levels of carbon monoxide in exhaled air. Quantitative analysis of carbon dioxide exhaled from mice during exposure to 100, 500 or 4000ppm of either C-14 CH_2Cl_2 or C-14 CD_2Cl_2 revealed that at 100ppm 62% of the carbon dioxide was obtained from the cytochrome P-450 pathway whereas at 4000ppm the glutathione-S-transferase pathway was the major source of carbon dioxide (90%).

Comparison of carbon dioxide levels exhaled from rats and mice at the 4000ppm dose level showed a ten-fold higher level in mice than rats, suggesting a ten-fold higher rate of glutathione-S-transferase metabolism since this is the major source of carbon dioxide at this dose level. The data obtained from these studies enabled the utilisation of the two pathways to be calculated over the range of dose levels from 100 to 4000ppm (Table 2). The metabolic rate constants Km and Vmax were also obtained from this data for each pathway by computer optimisation of the data.

Table 1. Methylene Chloride and Carboxyhaemoglobin Levels in Rats and Mice Exposed to Methylene Chloride

Exposure Level (ppm)	Rats			Mice		
	Blood[a] Levels (μg/ml)	AUC	COHb[a] (%)	Blood[a] Levels (μg/ml)	AUC	COHb[a] (%)
500	6	0.1	15	6	0.2	16
1000	62	1.0	14	31	1.0	13
2000	125	2.1	12	40	1.3	14
4000	230	3.7	10	54	2.1	8

[a]Average levels between 3 and 6 hours after exposure commenced.
AUC - Area under the blood level curve.

In conclusion, these in vivo studies provided evidence that the major species difference between rats and mice was the difference in rates of metabolism by the glutathione-S-transferase pathway. They also provided metabolic rate constants and the ability to extrapolate accurately from high to low dose, this extrapolation being one of the key aspects of risk assessment.

Table 2.   The Rates of Metabolism of Methylene Chloride in Mice
by the Cytochrome P-450 and Glutathione-S-Transferase
Pathways at Different Dose Levels

Exposure (ppm)	Rate of metabolism by	
	Cytochrome P-450 Glutathione-S-transferase (μmol/kg bodyweight/hr)	
100	183.8	63.5
500	228.4	159.0
4000	228.4	456.5

In Vitro Studies

The human liver samples (n = 12) used in these studies were
obtained from renal transplant donors and were used either
immediately or stored at -70°C before use. Each tissue was
homogenised and fractionated by centrifugation into microsomal and
cytosolic fractions prior to determining the metabolic rates for
each pathway independently. A comparison of the rates of metabolism
by each pathway in liver fractions from rats, mice, hamsters and
humans is shown in Fig 2. The ten-fold difference in the rate of
metabolism by the glutathione-S-transferase pathway in vivo between
rats and mice was confirmed in vitro. It is clear from this figure
that there is an excellent correlation between glutathione-S-
transferase metabolism and the outcome of the cancer bioassays in
the three animal species. No such correlation exists for the
cytochrome P-450 pathway where for example, the metabolic rate in
the hamster is very similar to that in the mouse.

Cytochrome P-450 mediated metabolism of methylene chloride could
be detected in lung tissues from all three animal species, the
relative activities being similar to those in the liver.
Glutathione-S-transferase activity was only detectable in mouse lung
cytosol.

The low rates of metabolism of methylene chloride by the
glutathione-S-transferase pathway in human liver samples have been
attributed to a deficiency in the transferase enzyme responsible.
The same liver samples had similar activity to rat liver when
assayed with 1-chloro-2,4-dinitrobenzene, a substrate for other
glutathione-S-transferase iso-enzymes.

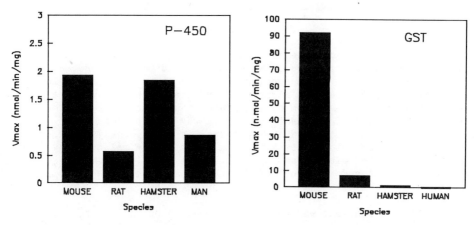

Fig. 2. The rates of metabolism of methylene chloride in the livers
of different species in vitro.

Metabolism in the Mouse Lung

The type of lesion observed in the Clara cell after a single
exposure to methylene chloride has been reported for a number of
other unrelated chemicals and has been associated with a loss of
cytochrome P-450 from affected cells (Boyd et al 1980, Forkert et al
1982, 1985, Krijgsheld et al 1983).

It was not surprising therefore to find that Clara cells damaged
by exposure to methylene chloride no longer contained cytochrome
P-450 iso-enzymes as determined using polyclonal antibodies. Using
microsomes prepared from whole lung homogenates the metabolism of
methylene chloride to carbon monoxide was reduced by 50%, suggesting
that 50% of the cytochrome P-450 responsible for metabolising
methylene chloride is found in the Clara cells, which themselves
comprise only 5% of the total cell types in the mouse lung. Assay
of the glutathione-S-transferases with methylene chloride,
chlorodinitrobenzene or with antibodies revealed that these enzymes
were not affected either in Clara cells or whole lung homogenates.
After 10 days of exposure (6hr/day) to methylene chloride the lesion
recovered, as did the iso-enzymes of cytochrome P-450 with the
exception of the one responsible for methylene chloride metabolism.
On a whole lung basis, metabolism of methylene chloride remained
reduced by 50%.

As a result of these changes a cell type in the mouse lung is
no longer able to metabolise methylene chloride by the cytochrome
P-450 pathway, but remains fully competent for the glutathione-S-
transferase pathway, the one associated with cancer.

These studies suggest that Clara cells damaged in this way are
at increased risk and may well be the population of cells from which
tumours develop.

Risk Assessment

As a result of these studies a comprehensive set of
experimental animal and human data now exists to enable the species
differences in metabolism and pharmacokinetics to be incorporated
into a risk assessment. The species difference that correlates with
the observed cancer has been identified and the risk assessment is
therefore based on metabolism by the glutathione-S-transferase
pathway. The metabolic rates for this pathway are known in each
species of interest and the dose-dependency of this pathway is known
over a range of dose levels from those used in the animal bioassay,
to those associated with human exposure. Full details of this risk
assessment are beyond the scope of this paper and are given only in
outline.

The risk assessment was made using a physiologically based
pharmacokinetic model very similar to that described by Andersen et
al (1986). The internal dose of glutathione-S-transferase
metabolites was calculated for the liver and lungs of each species
using species-specific physiology and the metabolic rate constants
measured experimentally. From this was derived the relationship
between internal dose and tumours for each organ in the mouse using
either Weibull or multistage models to fit the data. From this
relationship the risks associated with the internal dose in human
liver and lung were determined. A summary of the outcome of this
risk assessment is given in Table 3. The predicted risks to man
from exposure to methylene chloride are extremely low and indicate
that man is adequately protected by the current guidelines for safe
exposure and use of this chemical.

In addition to the results given above, the impact of the changes
in the Clara cells of the mouse lung on risk assessment was also
investigated by taking into account the metabolic changes and the
volume of the Clara cells relative to the whole lung. In the model
described by Andersen et al (1986) the internal dose calculations
are based on the volume of the whole lung. This procedure gives an
internal dose for the lung (542mg/l at 4000ppm) which is significantly
below that for the liver (4923mg/l) even though the tumour incidences
were similar in both organs. The internal dose based on the Clara
cells (5501mg/l), taking into account the volume of the cells and
the metabolic changes, is very similar to that in the liver.
Clearly internal dose and risk calculations in extrahepatic organs
have to consider the heterogeneous nature of those organs and the
consequences of cell specific effects on the internal dose.

Table 3. The Risks to Man From Exposure to Methylene Chloride Based on
the Internal Dose of Glutathione-S-Transferase Metabolites

Exposure (ppm)	Risk, Lung + Liver (MLE)	
	Weibull	Multistage
10	3.554×10^{-12}	6.519×10^{-9}
50	5.650×10^{-10}	2.720×10^{-7}
100	4.959×10^{-9}	1.504×10^{-6}

Conclusions

This paper has given an outline of the types of studies necessary to support risk assessment based on the internal dose of key metabolites. Two problems have to be addressed, that of high to low dose extrapolation and that of cross-species extrapolation. The first is complicated in the case of methylene chloride because of competing pathways, different enzyme activities, saturation of one of the pathways and by the formation of common metabolites in vivo. The resolution of these problems involved experiments over a wide range of dose levels and the use of stable isotopes. Cross-species extrapolation in the absence of in vivo human data has to be based on in vitro measurements. The ability of in vitro data to accurately predict the behaviour of a chemical in vivo must be validated, in this case this was done against the in vivo data obtained in rats and mice. The work with Clara cells has illustrated the problems of the use of metabolism and pharmacokinetics in risk assessment where extrahepatic organs are involved. Consequently a considerable amount of information and experimentation has been necessary to provide an adequate data base for the use of metabolism and pharmacokinetics in risk assessment. Many of these studies are unique to methylene chloride and for many chemicals the necessary data can probably be obtained much more expediently.

References

Andrae, U., and Wolff, T., 1983, Dichloromethane is not genotoxic in isolated hepatocytes, Arch. Toxicol., 52:287.

Ahmed, A. E., and Anders, M. W., 1976, Metabolism of dihalomethanes to formaldehyde and inorganic chloride, Drug Met., and Dispos., 4:357.

Ahmed, A. E., and Anders, M. W., 1978, Metabolism of dihalomethanes to formaldehyde and inorganic halide. II. Studies on the mechanism of the reaction, Biochem. Pharmacol., 27:2021.

Andersen, M. E., Clewell, H. J., Gargas, M. L., Smith, F. A., and Reitz R. H., 1987, Physiologically based pharmacokinetics and the risk assessment process for methylene chloride, Toxicol. Appl. Pharmacol., 87:185.

Ashby, J., and Trueman, R. W., 1987, Lack of UDS activity in the livers of mice and rats exposed to dichloromethane, Environ. Mutagen., 10:189.

Boyd, M. R., 1980, Biochemical mechanisms of chemical-induced lung injury: roles of metabolic activation, Critical Reviews in Toxicology, 7:103.

Burek, J. D., Nitschke, K. D., Bell, T. J., Wackerle, D. L., Childs, R. C., Beyer, J. E., Dittenber, D. A., Rampy, L. W., and McKenna, M. J., 1984, Methylene chloride: A two year inhalation toxicity and oncogenicity study in rats and hamsters, Fundam. Appl. Toxicol., 4:30.

Callen, D. F., Wolff, C. R., and Philpot, R. M., 1980, Cytochrome P-450 mediated genetic activity and cytotoxicity of seven halogenated aliphatic hydrocarbons in Saccharomyces cerevisiae, Mut. Res., 77:55.

Forkert, P. G., and Reynolds, E. S., 1982, 1,1-Dichloroethylene induced pulmonary injury, ExpH. Lung Res., 3:57.

Forkert, P. G., Silvestre, P. L., and Polard, J. S., 1985, Lung injury induced by trichloroethylene. Toxicol., 35:143.

Gargas, M. L., Clewell, H. J., and Anderson, M. E., 1986, Metabolism of inhaled dihalomethanes in vivo: differentation of kinetic constants for two independent pathways, Toxicol. Appl. Pharmacol., 82:211.

Gocke, E., King, M. T., Eckhardt, K., and Wild, D., 1981, Mutagenicity of cosmetics ingredients licensed by the European Communities, Mut. Res., 90:91.

Green, T., 1983, The metabolic activation of dichloromethane and chlorofluoromethane in a bacterial mutation assay using Salmonella typhimurium, Mut. Res., 118:227.

Green, T., Provan, W. M., Collinge, D. C., and Guest, A. E., 1988, Macromolecular interactions of inhaled methylene chloride in rats and mice, Toxicol. Appl. Pharmacol., 93:1.

Jongen, W. M. F., Alink, G. M., and Koeman, J. H., 1978, Mutagenic effect of dichloromethane on Salmonella typhimurium, Mut. Res., 56:245.

Jongen, W. M. F., Lohman, P. H. M., Kottenhagen, M. J., Alink, G. M., Berends, F., and Koeman, J. H., 1981, Mutagenicity testing of dichloromethane in short-term mammalian test sytems, Mut. Res., 81:203.

Jongen, W. M. F., Harmsen, E. G. M., Alink, G. M., and Koeman, J. H., 1982, The effect of glutathione conjugation and microsomal oxidation on the mutagenicity of dichloromethane in Salmonella typhimurium, Mut. Res., 95:183.

Kramers, P. G. N., Mout, H. K. A., Mulder, C. R., 1983, Mutagenitiet van dihalogeenalkanen by Drosophila melanogaster, Annual Report National Institute of Public Health and Environmental Hygiene, The Netherlands, 169.

Krijgsheld, K. R., Lowe, M. C., Minnaugh, E. G., Trush, M. A., Ginsburg, E., and Gram, T. E., 1983, Lung-selective impairment of cytochrome P-450 dependent mono-oxygenases and cellular injury by 1,1dichloroethylene in mice, Biochem. Biophys. Res. Comm., 110:675.

Kirwin, C. J., and Thomas, W. C., 1980, In vitro microbiological mutagenicity studies of hydrocarbon propellants, J. Soc. Cosmet. Chem., 31:367.

Kubic, V. L., and Anders, M. W., 1975, Metabolism of dihalomethanes to carbon monoxide. II. In vitro studies on the mechanism of the reaction, Biochem. Pharmacol., 27:2349.

Kubic, V. L., and Anders, M. W., 1978, Metabolism of dihalomethanes to carbon monoxide. III. Studies on the mechanism of the reaction, Biochem. Pharmacol., 27:2349.

Maltoni, C., Cotti, G., and Perino, G., 1986. Experimental research on methylene chloride carcinogenesis. Archives of research on industrial carcinogens, Vol. IV. C. Maltoni and M. A. Mehlman eds. Princeton Scientific Publishing Co. Princeton.

McKenna, M. J., and Zempel, J. A., 1981, The dose-dependent metabolism of [^{14}C] methylene chloride following oral administration to rats, Food Cosmet. Toxicol., 19:73.

Neely, W. B., 1964, Metabolic rate of formaldehyde ^{14}C intraperitoneally administered to the rat, Biochem. Pharmacol., 13:1964.

Nestmann, E., and Kowbel, D. J., 1980, Mutagenicity of paint-removing products detected in a modified Salmonella/mammalian assay [Abstract], Canad. J. Genet. Cytol., 22:673.

NTP (1986-Jan), NTP technical report on the toxicology and carcinogenesis studies of dichloromethane in F344/N rats and $B_6C_3F_1$ mice, NTP TR 306, Final Report.

Osterman-Golkar, S., Hussain, S., Walles, S., Anderstam, B., and Sigvardsson, K., 1983, Chemical reactivity and mutagenicity of some dihalomethanes, Chem-Biol. Interactions, 46:121.

Perocco, P., and Prodi, G., 1981, DNA damage by haloalkanes in human lymphocytes cultured in vitro, Cancer Lett., 13.

Riley, E. C., Fassett, D. W., and Sutton, W. L., 1966, Methylene choride vapour in expired air of human subjects, Am. Ind. Hyg. Assoc. J., 27:341.

Serota, D. G., Thakur, A. K., Ulland, B. M., Kirschman, J. C., Brown, N. M., Coots, R. H., and Morgareidge, K., 1986b. A two year drinking-water study of dichloromethane in rodents, II. Mice, Fd. Chem. Toxicol., 24:959.

Sheldon, T., Richardson, C. R., and Elliott, B. M., 1987, Inactivity of methylene chloride in the mouse bone marrow micronucleus assay, Mutagenesis., 2:57.

Simmon, V. F., Kauhanen, K., and Tardiff, R. G., 1977, Mutagenic activity of chemicals identified in drinking water. In: Scott, D., Bridges, B. A., Sobels, F. H., eds, Progress in genetic toxicology, Elsevier, Amsterdam, 249.

Stewart, R. D., Fisher, T. N., Hasto, M. J., and Peterson, J. E., Baretta, E. D., and Dodd, H. C., 1972. Carboxyhaemoglobin elevation after exposure to dichloromethane, Science, 176:295.

Thilager, A. K., Back, A. M., Kirby, P. E., Kumaroo, V., Pant, K. J., Clarke, J. J., Knight, R., and Haworth, S. R., 1984, Evaluation of dichloromethane in short-term in vitro genetic toxicity assays, Environ. Mutagenesis., 6:418.

Thilager, A. K., and Kumaroo, V., 1983. Induction of chromosomes damage by methylene chloride in CHO cells, Mut. Res., 116:361.

COMPUTER SIMULATION OF CHEMICAL CARCINOGENESIS

Rory B. Conolly[a], Richard H. Reitz[b],
Harvey J. Clewell, III[c], and Melvin E. Andersen[c]

[a]NSI Technology Services, Corp.
101 Woodman Dr., Suite 12
Dayton, OH 45431-1482

[b]Mammalian and Environmental Toxicology
1803 Building
Dow Chemical Company
Midland, MI 48674-1803

[c]Harry G. Armstrong Aerospace Medical Research Laboratory
Toxic Hazards Division
Wright-Patterson AFB, OH 45433-6573

INTRODUCTION

The standard procedure for evaluating carcinogen risk is the rodent bioassay coupled with statistically-based risk extrapolation. Extrapolation serves to bridge the physiological differences between the experimental species and man and between the experimental exposure scenario and that occurring in the 'real world'. Little of what is known, however, about carcinogen pharmacokinetics, biochemical mechanisms of action, and cancer biology in either the experimental species or in man is used in risk assessment because no paradigm has been available to guide the incorporation of this information. Moolgavkar and Venzon (1979), and Moolgavkar and Knudson (1981), have described a biologically structured model of carcinogenesis (M-V-K model) that provides quantitative insights into the relationship between cellular proliferation, mutation, and tumor development. This is not, however, (and was not intended to be) a fully integrated model of chemical carcinogenesis as it lacks a biologically-based description of carcinogen pharmacokinetics, nor does it explicitly define biochemical mechanisms linking target tissue dose with tumorigenesis.

Chemical carcinogenesis is a complex, integrated process involving many highly interdependent events. It encompasses exposure to the chemical, absorption and disposition within the organism, interaction of reactive forms of the chemical with susceptible tissues, alteration of cellular growth induced by this interaction, and the eventual appearance of tumors. Quantification of the relationship between carcinogen exposure and tumor formation depends on an understanding of the interdependencies of these events.

This report describes the numerical implementation of a comprehensive cancer model in which the structure of the M-V-K model was combined with descriptions of carcinogen pharmacokinetics and plausible pharmacodynamic mechanisms of carcinogen action. The design philosophy used was that all model parameters should correspond to physiological or biochemical processes that can be measured in the laboratory. As these data are obtained model behavior will simulate more and more closely that of the actual biological system. The influence of individual events on the overall cancer process can thus be examined quantitatively.

CANCER MODEL STRUCTURE

The overall model (PCM: pharmacodynamic cancer model; Fig. 1) has 3 parts:

(1) A physiologically-based pharmacokinetic portion which defines tissue dose by describing carcinogen absorption, distribution and metabolism (Fig. 1, Part I).

(2) A 2-stage cancer portion in which cells are either normal, intermediate (1 mutation) or malignant (2 mutations). Tumor incidence is a direct function of the number of cells in the normal and intermediate populations, their birth and death rates and of the transition frequencies between stages (Fig. 1, Part III).

(3) Representative biochemical mechanisms of action for DNA-damaging agents, promoters and cytotoxic carcinogens. These mechanisms link the tissue dose of chemical carcinogen to the birth and death rate parameters and transitional probabilities of the 2-stage cancer model (Fig. 1, Part II). (No attempt was made to portray all possible mechanisms by which carcinogens act nor to include every nuance of those mechanisms which are described. Our intent was simply to demonstrate how several, biologically plausible mechanisms can be used to link the pharmacokinetic and cancer sections of the PCM.)

METHODOLOGICAL APPROACH

The PCM consists of a system of differential equations which are solved numerically. Stepwise integration of this initial value problem defines the behavior of the system over time. The model reported on here was written in ACSL (Mitchell and Gauthier, Assoc., Concord MA), a computer program which greatly simplifies the process of writing and exercizing the model. The numerical approach offers certain advantages over the use of analytical forms. For example, there is no need for 'time-slicing' in which time-dependent changes of parameter values must be discretized as constant values within successive time intervals. Rather, model structure stipulates how these values change continuously in response to whatever input is driving behavior. In the case of the PCM, for example, behavior is driven by carcinogen dosing. A further advantage is the relative ease with which complicated biological structures can be explicitly described. In the PCM there is an attempt to maintain a 1 to 1 correspondence between model parameters and specific biological elements. This level of detail incurs a corresponding increase in the requirement for laboratory validation studies but also provides the opportunity, through the model, of learning how these individual elements of the biological structure contribute to its overall behavior. An analytical solution to such a complex mathematical system would require a large number of simplifying assumptions with a concomitant loss of biological realism.

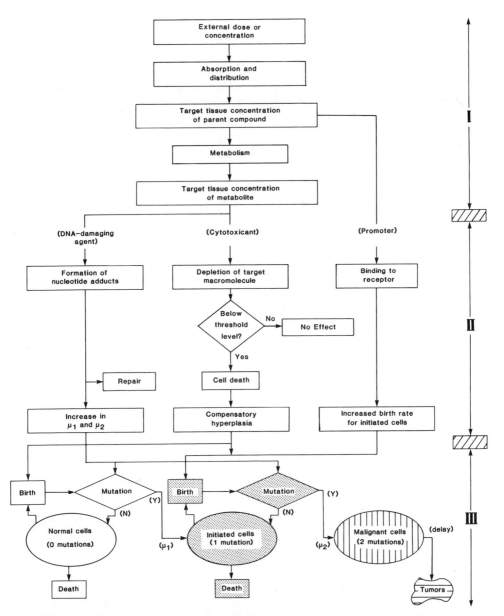

FIGURE 1. Schematic of the Pharmacodynamic Cancer Model (PCM). Part I is a physiologically-based description of the processes controlling carcinogen pharmacokinetics. Its main role is converting external carcinogen dose to a realistic target tissue concentration of either the parent compound or relevant metabolite(s). In Part II, representative biochemical mechanisms are described for 3 distinct classes of carcinogens: DNA-damaging agents, promoters, and cytotoxicants. Part III consists of a 2-stage cancer model where cells are either normal, intermediate or malignant (0, 1 and 2 mutations, respectively). The linkages between Parts II and III specify how the different kinds of carcinogens affect the cell growth and mutation parameters of the cancer model.

PHARMACOKINETICS OF CHEMICAL CARCINOGENS

The full simulation model tracks highly time-dependent changes in tissue concentrations of parent chemical and important metabolites. Pharmacokinetic behavior of drugs and toxic chemicals can be accurately simulated by what are commonly known as physiologically-based pharmacokinetic (PB-PK) models (Bischoff and Brown, 1966; Matthews and Dedrick, 1984; Ramsey and Andersen, 1984; and Andersen et al., 1987). The essence of PB-PK models is an accurate mathematical representation of mammalian architecture and of the actual biochemical processes for metabolism and elimination. A PB-PK model based on that described by Ramsey and Andersen (1984) is part of the PCM (Fig. 1, Part I). This PB-PK component simulates absorption, distribution, metabolism and elimination in order to obtain target tissue concentrations of parent compound and metabolite(s).

NUMERICAL TWO-STAGE CANCER MODEL

The M-V-K model is a two-stage cancer model incorporating basic biological information on the cell growth characteristics of normal, initiated and overtly malignant cells. The M-V-K model is able to describe the complex, age-specific incidence curves for breast cancer (Moolgavkar et al., 1980) and for childhood cancers such as retinoblastoma (Moolgavkar and Knudson, 1981), and has been used to identify different incidence behaviors expected for promoters as opposed to genotoxic chemical carcinogens (Moolgavkar, 1983).

The biological structure of the M-V-K model (Fig. 1, Part III) was encoded as a set of three differential equations describing changes in the numbers of normal (NO), initiated (N1) and malignant (N2) cells over time:

$$dA_{NO}/dt = A_{NO}(a_0 - b_0) \tag{1}$$

$$dA_{N1}/dt = A_{N1}(a_1 - b_1) + u_1 a_0 A_{NO} \tag{2}$$

$$d(N1 \to N2)/dt = u_2 a_1 A_{N1} \tag{3}$$

Turnover rates for normal and initiated cells (equations 1 and 2) are related to birth and death rate parameters (a_0, a_1, b_0, b_1 [events/cell/hr], respectively) and the numbers of cells (A_{NO}, A_{N1}). The term $u_1 a_0 A_{NO}$ in equation (2) describes the rate of production of initiated cells arising through mutation of normal cells; u_1 [mutations/division] is the transitional probability for the normal to initiated cell transition. Integration of these equations gives the numbers of cells at any point in time.

Equation (3) is different from equations (1) and (2). It only tracks the formation of malignant cells from initiated cells. Usually, clinically-evident tumors are assumed to occur with a time delay after appearance of individual malignant cells. For example, the tumor incidence predictions of Moolgavkar et al. (1980) are based on human female breast tumors becoming clinically-evident 5 years after a malignant cell arises. In these simulations we made no distinction between malignant cells and tumors. This is sufficient for illustrating qualitative aspects of model behavior.

In this deterministic implementation of the 2-stage cancer model the number of malignant cells/liver computed by the PCM represents the expected value of the number of malignant cells for a member of the population (or cohort) at risk. The number of tumors in an individual cohort member is, of course, an integer. We assume here that the number of tumors in an individual cohort member is a Poisson random variable. The probability of an individual member of the cohort having 1 or more tumors is then given by:

$$P_{tum} = 1 - e^{-AN2} \qquad (4)$$

where A_{N2} is the expectation for malignant cells, calculated by integrating $d(N1\text{-->}N2)/dt$ over time. Using this approximation, tumor prevalence (# of test animals with 1 or more tumors) is simply P_{tum} times the size of the cohort, and $d(N1\text{-->}N2)/dt$ gives an estimate of the incidence (# previously tumor-free animals getting tumors/time interval/# tumor-free animals at the beginning of the interval). This approximation can be expected to provide useful information in so far as the calculation time interval is sufficiently short and the true distribution of tumors in animals is close to Poisson.

BIOCHEMICAL MECHANISMS OF CARCINOGENS

A major challenge in this work was definition of the linkages between carcinogen pharmacokinetics (Fig. 1, Part I) and the cancer processes (Fig. 1, Part III). This was accomplished by describing discrete biochemical mechanisms for a DNA-damaging agent, a promoter, and a cytotoxic carcinogen (Fig. 1, Part II). In these mechanisms the parent compound or its metabolite(s) interact with specific cellular macromolecules and these biochemical interactions, in turn, directly affect the cell growth parameters of the cancer model.

All the events in this description occur in adult rat liver which contains only normal cells at the start of the simulation. All hepatocytes are stem cells that proliferate without further differentiation. The choice of liver as the target organ is only a matter of convenience, and other tissues could be similarly described.

CARCINOGENS THAT FORM DNA ADDUCTS

In the biochemical mechanism modeled for a chemical that forms DNA adducts (Fig. 1, Part II) the parent compound is a pro-carcinogen metabolized in the liver with Michaelis-Menten kinetics. Metabolite either undergoes first-order elimination or forms adducts with DNA nucleotides. These adducts are repaired by a first-order process. The following differential equation specifies the change in the amount of nucleotide adducts (A_{ANU} in micromoles) as a function of their time-dependent rates of formation and repair:

$$dA_{ANU}/dt = k_{MNU}A_M A_{NU} - k_{RNU}A_{ANU} \qquad (5)$$

The formation of adducts is described by a second-order rate constant (k_{MNU} [L/hr/micromole]), the amounts of reactive metabolite (A_M) and of nucleotides (A_{NU}). The rate of adduct repair is given by the product of a first-order rate constant (k_{RNU} [L/hr]) and the amount of adducts (A_{ANU}). Equation (5) is used to calculate the fraction (F_{AD}) of all nucleotides which have adducts. This fraction is then multiplied by a term (u_{max}) defining the maximum possible increase in transition probabilities due to the particular DNA-damaging agent. In effect, u_{max} reflects the mutational potency of the adducts. The resulting increase ($F_{AD}*u_{max}$) is added to the transitional probabilities u_1 and u_2 (equations 2 and 3). The birth and death rate parameters a_0, b_0, a_1, and b_1 however, are not affected. Both the normal-->initiated cell and initiated-->malignant cell transitions are consequently more likely during and for some time after exposure to the DNA-damaging agent. This mechanism of action is well-supported by the literature (McCann et al., 1975; Weinstein, 1981; Barrett et al., 1978; and Reddy, 1983).

305

PROMOTERS

In the biochemical mechanism for promoters (Fig. 1, Part II) a growth advantage is conferred on intermediate (N1) cells. This is achieved by increasing the birth rate of N1 cells while leaving the death rate unchanged. Equation (6) describes the essential features of this mechanism:

$$P_{KBN1} = F_{PRE}K_{BMAX} \tag{6}$$

The promoter binds reversibly to a receptor which is distributed throughout the cell. The fractional occupancy of the receptor (F_{PRE}) is multiplied by K_{BMAX}, the maximum possible increase in N1 birth rate. P_{KBN1} is added to a_1 (equation 2). In this scheme promoters have no effect on the transitional probabilities u_1 and u_2 (equations 2 and 3) nor on the growth characteristics of normal cells. This mechanism of promotion, only one of several possible that could have been portrayed, is consistent with the experimental observation that cells in preneoplastic foci (intermediate cells in the M-V-K model) grow faster than normal cells (Emmelot and Scherer, 1980) and with postulated biochemical mechanisms for promotion by 2,3,7,8-tetrachlorodi-benzo-p-dioxin (Gasiewicz and Rucci, 1984) and phorbol esters (Weinstein, 1981).

CARCINOGENS WHICH ARE PRIMARILY CYTOTOXIC

For cytotoxicants, binding of a carcinogen metabolite to a target macromolecule (T) is taken to be the primary cytotoxic event. Cell death occurs when T is depleted below some threshold level which is less than its normal level. The threshold level of T is modeled as varying among individual cells in accordance with normal distribution. Alternatively, an experimentally determined relationship between the concentration of T and the probability of cell death could be used. Several equations are used to describe cytotoxicity:

$$dA_T/dt = K_{ST} - K_{LT}A_T - K_{MT}A_M A_T \tag{7}$$

$$A_{CSC} = A_{CO}K_{KILL} - T_X \tag{8}$$

$$dN0/dt = A_{N0}(a_0 - b_0) + F_{N0}(K_{BTX}T_X - A_{CSC}K_{DU}) \tag{9}$$

$$dN1/dt = A_{N1}(a_1 - b_1) + F_{N1}(K_{BTX}T_X - A_{CSC}K_{DU})$$
$$+ u_1(a_0 A_{N0} + F_{N0}K_{BTX}T_X) \tag{10}$$

$$d(N1{-}{-}{>}N2)/dt = u_2(a_1 A_{N1} + F_{N1}K_{BTX}T_X) \tag{11}$$

Change in the amount of target macromolecule (A_T [micromoles]) is described by equation (7). Macromolecule is produced by zero-order synthesis (k_{ST} [micromoles/hr]) and lost either through a basal first-order pathway ($k_{LT}A_T$) or through attack by carcinogen metabolite ($k_{MT}A_M A_T$) where k_{MT} [L/hr/micromole] is a second-order rate constant and A_M is the amount of metabolite.

K_{KILL} represents the fraction of target tissue cells in which the target macromolecule has been depleted below the threshold level. To calculate K_{KILL} a normal distribution is first defined where C_{TM} is the concentration of macromolecule at the mid-point of the normal distribution and $s2_T$ is the variance in units of target macromolecule concentration. K_{KILL} is calculated as the area under the curve from the basal level of macromolecule (C_{T0}) to the concentration at time t (C_T). As configured for most of the simulations presented here the basal concentration of macromolecule was 963 micromolar, the midpoint of the normal distribution was 550 micromolar and the standard deviation was 80 micromolar. These values were set arbitrarily and would be adjusted appropriately for specific compounds as data became available. Validation studies are unlikely to identify a single macro-molecule whose depletion leads to cell death. It is more probable that a correlation will be found between binding to a class of macromolecules, for instance, proteins in a cellular subfraction, and cell death. In any event, validation studies with selected compounds can be reasonably expected to show a correlation between covalent binding and cell death which could be used in place of the normal distribution.

Equation (8) describes the number of cells in the target tissue (A_{CSC}) in which the concentration of T is below threshold and which are therefore 'available' to die. A_{CSC} equals the basal number of cells in the tissue (A_{CO}) times K_{KILL} minus the number of cells (T_X) that are already 'missing' from the tissue due to cytotoxicity. This difference can, of course, have a negative value. When it does A_{CSC} is forced to 0.

Equations (9), (10) and (11) are just equations (1), (2) and (3) modified to account for toxicity-related changes in the birth and death rates of normal, initiated and malignant cells. In equations (9) and (10) the rate of cell killing due to cytotoxicity is given by the product of the first-order term K_{DU} [L/hr] and A_{CSC} [# cells]. These terms are further multiplied by either F_{NO} or F_{N1} which represent the fractions of the whole liver made up of normal and intermediate cells, respectively. The model is structured so that F_{NO} and F_{N1} always sum to 1. Malignant cells are not susceptible to cytotoxicity. Regenerative hyperplasia is described by a first-order term (K_{BTX} [L/hr]) multiplied by T_X [# cells] and F_{NO} or F_{N1}. In equations (10) and (11) the terms containing u generate the number of cells appearing through mutations arising during regenerative hyperplasia.

CANCER MODEL SPECIFICATION FOR SPECIES-SPECIFIC BEHAVIOR

The PCM contains a generic description of mammalian architecture. Simulation of experiments with a particular species requires physiological and biochemical parameter values appropriate for that species. This approach has enabled physiologically-based disposition models like the one incorporated in the PCM to be successful in predicting pharmacokinetic behavior of toxic chemicals across various mammalian species (Ramsey and Andersen, 1984; Andersen et al., 1987). Some PCM parameters, such as cardiac output and the sizes of major organs, are already well known and also scale between species according to well-defined allometric relation-ships. However, while allometry is often useful, it is preferable to set species-specific parameter values using data obtained from the target species. This practice precludes the possibility that unnoticed failure of an allometric relationship might invalidate model behavior. Some parameter values in the PCM, for example, the birth and death rates of initiated cells, are not yet known with accuracy. We have consistently found, however, that data are available in the literature which allow rough estimates of these values.

The simulations described here were for a 250 gm rat. Physiological parameters controlling carcinogen disposition throughout the organism were set to realistic values as described by Ramsey and Andersen (1984). The liver was modeled as the target organ for carcinogens and specific hepatic parameter values were obtained whenever possible. Hepatocyte volume was set at $5.608*X*10^{-12}$ L/cell (de la Iglesia et al., 1975) and the total number of hepatocytes/liver was calculated based on the liver being 4% of body weight. Hepatocyte birth and death rates were set at $1.7*X*10^{-4}$ events/cell/hr based on microautoradiography data collected by Reitz (unpublished). The number of nucleotides per hepatocyte was calculated based on 2.9 X 10^9 base pairs per human cell (Darnell et al., 1986). The basal transition probabilities u_1 and u_2 were $1.0*X*10^6$ per cell generation (Elmore et al., 1983; Tsutsui et al.,1981).

The mathematical descriptions used for the DNA-damaging agent, promoter, and cytotoxicant were partly realistic and partly hypothetical. Actual tissue:blood and blood:air partition coefficients and metabolic rate constants for a representative volatile organic chemical in male Fisher-344 rats were used in each case. The pharmacokinetic portion of the PCM (Fig. 1, Part I) has been well validated for these types of exposures (8,9) and the simulated pharmacokinetic behavior should be reasonable.

For simulated experiments with a DNA-damaging agent and with a promoter, appropriate parameter values were set so that the test chemical had the capacity either to damage DNA or to act as a promoter. Parameter values were always set such that the test chemical only worked by one mechanism of action at a time. Specific chemicals may well exhibit multiple mechanisms of action. While the PCM could be configured for use with such chemicals, these more complex behaviors will not be addressed in this paper.

Structurally-simple volatile toxicants offer certain advantages for model validation studies. Inhalation exposures with these compounds are relatively easy to conduct and detailed pharmacokinetic data can be obtained with closed, recirculating inhalation chambers (Andersen et al., 1987). Moreover, these compounds have simple kinetic behavior and well-understood metabolic pathways. Several, including vinyl chloride, are directly carcinogenic. Some, like chloroform, appear to be cytotoxic and others, such as trichloroethylene, or more correctly its metabolite trichloroacetic acid, seem to induce cancer by promotional mechanisms.

BIOCHEMICAL EFFECTS OF CARCINOGENS

The PCM can be used to examine time-dependent macromolecular interactions comprising the biochemical mechanisms of carcinogens. The ease with which simulation models can be exercised and parameter values changed makes it relatively simple to evaluate behavior of a given mechanism for different chemicals over a range of conditions. The basic description of a mechanism can also be readily changed. This allows the implications of different mechanisms for biochemical parameters and tumor incidence to be examined.

For DNA-damaging agents, the relationship between rate of carcinogen metabolism in target tissue and concentration of DNA adducts is illustrated when all model parameter values are held constant except for the rate of DNA repair (Fig. 2). Rate of carcinogen metabolism is an index of tissue exposure and is a better predicitor of intensity of effect than, for example, the concentration external to the organism (Andersen, 1987). The simulated exposure regimen was 6 hr/day, 5 days/week for 2 weeks. The daily rise and fall in rate of metabolism is clearly seen as is the corresponding fluctuation in concentration of DNA adducts. When the rate of DNA repair was 0.01 hr (upper curve), DNA adducts accumulated during the week and were not completely repaired during the weekend. With the repair rate set at 0.05 hr (lower curve), adduct accumulation during the week was diminished and repair was nearly complete on the weekend.

Simulations were also conducted for the interaction of a promoter with its receptor and the consequence of this interaction for the growth of initiated cells (Fig. 3). The exposure regimen was 2 years at 6 hr/day, 5 days/week. An interval late in the simulation (day 700 through day 712) was chosen since effects on initiated cells are more clearly illustrated once a

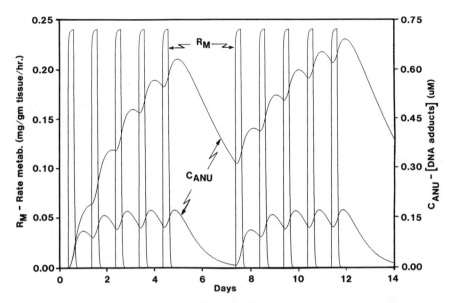

FIGURE 2.   Kinetics and DNA-binding behaviors for a DNA-damaging agent.   The
relationship between the rate of carcinogen metabolism (R_M) and the concentration of DNA adducts (C_{ANU}) is illustrated when all model parameter values
are held constant except the rate of DNA repair (K_{RNU}).   The simulated
exposure regimen was 6 hr/day, 5 days/week for 2 weeks.   The rate of repair
was 0.01 hr^{-1} (upper curve) or 0.05 hr^{-1}.

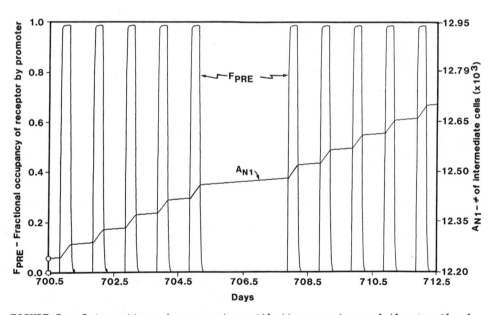

FIGURE 3.   Interaction of a promoter with its receptor and the growth of
initiated cells (A_{N1}).   The exposure regimen was 2 years at 6 hr/day, 5
days/week.   Daily spikes in the fraction of receptor molecules occupied by
promoter (F_{PRE}) mirror the daily 6 hr exposure to promoter.   Each spike of
receptor occupancy is accompanied by a sharp increase in the number of
initiated cells.

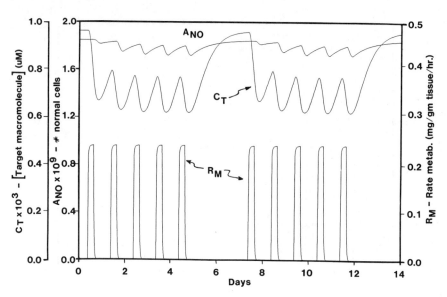

FIGURE 4. Cytotoxicant metabolism (R_M), depletion of target macromolecule (T) and effect on number of normal cells (A_{NO}). Two weeks of exposure at 6 hr/day, 5 days a week were simulated. Cytotoxicant metabolism generates a reactive metabolite which depletes the target macromolecule. Death of normal cells is followed by regenerative hyperplasia.

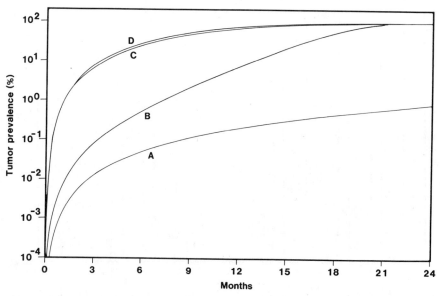

FIGURE 5. Tumor prevalence curves for a DNA-damaging agent, a promoter, and a cytotoxicant. The exposure regimen was 6 hr/day, 5 days/week for 2 years. Prevalence elicited by each agent at 2 years was close to 100%. This allows a comparison of the shapes of the curves. Curve A is background prevalence (about 0.8%). Curves B, C and D are for a promoter, cytotoxicant and DNA-damaging agent, respectively.

significant population of these cells has developed. Daily spikes in the
fraction of receptor molecules occupied by promoter mirror the daily 6 hr
exposure to promoter. Each spike of receptor occupancy is accompanied by an
increased rate of appearance of initiated cells.

Cytotoxicant exposure depletes target macromolecule and thereby leads
to a decrease in the number of normal cells (Fig. 4). Two weeks of exposure
at 6 hr/day, 5 days a week were simulated. The daily spikes in rate of
metabolism of cytotoxicant are followed by a corresponding decline in the
level of target macromolecule. The macromolecule is destroyed by a reactive
metabolite of the cytotoxicant. Resynthesis of macromolecule is not complete within 24 hr but full recovery does occur over the weekend. A similar
pattern of daily fluctuation is seen for the number of normal cells, illustrating how viability of normal cells depends on the concentration of target
macromolecule.

TUMOR PREVALENCE AND DOSE-RESPONSE CURVES

Tumor prevalence curves for a DNA-damaging agent, a promoter, and a
cytotoxicant have significantly different shapes (Fig. 5). The exposure
regimen was 6 hr/day, 5 days/week for 2 years. Parameter values were set to
provide a tumor prevalence close to 100% for each agent at 2 years. Curve A
shows the background prevalence, which totaled about 0.8% at 2 years.
Background prevalence was due solely to the regular turnover of normal and
initiated cells. Curve B shows tumor prevalence for a promoter while curves
C and D are for cytotoxicants and DNA-damaging agents, respectively. The
shapes of the curves for cytotoxicants and DNA-damaging agents are similar,
as would be expected given the interactions of these agents with parameters
controlling cell dynamics (Fig. 1, Part III). The transition frequencies
(N0-->N1 and N1-->N2 [cells/hr]) are determined by the product of the transitional probability (u_1 or u_2 [mutations/division]), the birth rate (a_0 or
a_1 [divisions/cell/hr]), and the number of cells (A_{N0} or A_{N1}). DNA-damaging
agents affect the transitional probabilities while cytotoxicants affect the
birth rate but these effects are not distinguishable at the level of the
transition frequency. With the promoter, tumor prevalence rises more slowly
in the early months of the simulated experiment. The shape of the prevalence curve for the promoter reflects the fact that a promoter has a minimal
effect on tumor development until a relatively large population of initiated
cells has developed.

Carcinogen dose-response curves can also be generated (Fig. 6). These
curves represent tumor prevalence at the end of a 2-year bioassay for a
range of exposure concentrations. For these simulations continuous exposure
was modeled in order to save computer time (Simulations run much faster when
abrupt changes in parameter values, as occurs with intermittent exposure,
are avoided). Switching between intermittent and continuous exposure
affects the magnitude but not the shape of these dose-response curves. To
obtain low-dose tumor prevalence due to carcinogen exposure the background
prevalence was subtracted from each data point.

Dose-response curves for a DNA-damaging agent are affected by enhanced
mutational frequency and repair rates (Fig. 6a). The basal transition
probabilities (u_1 and u_2) were 1.0×10^{-6} [mutations/division] in all cases.
Maximum possible increases in transition probabilities due to the carcinogen
were 0.1, 0.1 and 1.0 [mutations/division], for curves A, B and C, respectively. (This maximum possible increase can be thought of as a measure of
mutational potency.) The actual increase in transition probability due to
carcinogen was obtained by taking the product of maximum possible increase
with the fraction of all nucleotides having adducts. The first order rates
of DNA repair were 1.0, 0.1 and 0.1 [L/hr] for curves A, B and C, respec-

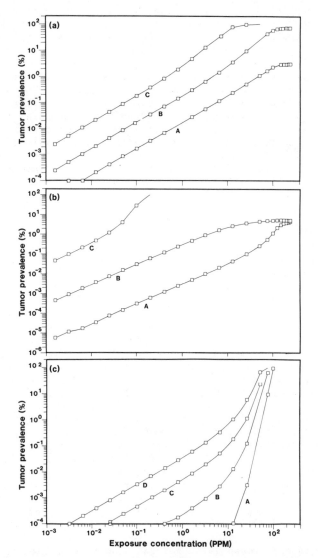

FIGURE 6. Dose-response curves for a DNA-damaging agent (6a), a promoter
(6b) and a cytotoxicant (6c). These curves represent tumor prevalence at
the end of a simulated 2-year bioassay over a range of exposure concentrations. In order to see low-dose tumor prevalence due to the carcinogen,
background prevalence (~0.8%) was subtracted from the calculated curves.

DNA DAMAGE (6a): The maximum possible increases in transition probabilities due to carcinogen exposure were 0.1, 0.1 and 1.0 [mutations/
division], for curves A, B and C, respectively. The corresponding, first-
order rates of DNA repair were 1.0, 0.1 and 0.1 [L/hr].

PROMOTION (6b): Maximum possible increases in intermediate cell birth ra*
due to the promoter were $1.7*X*10^{-4}$, $1.7*X*10^{-4}$ and $1.7*X*10^{-2}$ [divisions
/cell/hr] for curves A, B and C, respectively. The corresponding dissociation constants for the promoter-receptor complex were 10.0, 0.1 and 0.1
micromolar.

CYTOTOXICITY (6c): These dose-response curves were generated by
changing the standard deviation of the normal distribution (s_T). For curves
A-D the standard deviation was set at 80, 100, 120 and 140 micromolar of
target macromolecule, respectively. The midpoint of the normal distribution
was 550 micromolar.

tively. Increasing the rate of DNA repair decreased tumor prevalence (B vs. A) while increasing mutational potency increased tumor prevalence (B vs. C) had the opposite effect. The linearity of these dose-response curves on log-log plots reflects the lack of a threshold in the mechanism modeled for DNA-damaging agents.

Dose-response curves for a promoter (Fig. 6b) were generated with a constant basal birth rate for intermediate cells. The maximum possible increases in this birth rate due to the promoter were $1.7*X*10^{-2}$, $1.7*X*10^{-4}$ and $1.7*X*10^{-2}$ [divisions/cell/hr] for curves A, B and C, respectively. (This maximum possible is as a measure of the potency of the promoter.) The dissociation constants for promoter-receptor complex were 10.0, 0.1 and 0.1 for curves A, B and C, respectively. The actual increases in birth rate were obtained by taking the product of the maximum possible increase in birth rate and the fractional occupancy of the receptor. Decreasing the affinity of the promoter for the receptor decreases tumor prevalence while increasing promoter potency increases prevalence. There is no suggestion of a threshold for these curves. This result is, of course, a consequence of the mechanism modeled in the PCM where all concentrations of promoter have proportional effects. Promotional mechanisms where some minimum occupancy of the receptor is required before any effect occurs would show a threshold and such biological information could be readily incorporated into the model.

The family of dose-response curves for a cytotoxicant (Fig. 6c) were generated by changing the standard deviation of the normal distribution (s_m). For curves A-D, the standard deviation was set at 80, 100, 120 and 140 micromolar of target macromolecule, respectively and the midpoint of the normal curve at 550 micromolar. These parameters together determine the number of cells that will die from cytotoxicity at a particular concentration of macromolecule. For example, for the simulations shown in Fig 6c the basal number of cells in the liver was $1.85*X*10^{9}$ and the basal concentration of target macromolecule was 963 micromolar. At 16 ppm inhalation exposure concentration, the concentration of target macromolecule was 888 micromolar and the number of cells/liver below threshold was 1102, 93177, $1.104*X*10^{6}$ and $5.091*X*10^{6}$ for curves A-D, respectively. The PCM demonstrates that the slope of the dose-response curve can become quite steep in some instances (Fig. 6c, curve A), suggesting that chemicals which influence the carcinogenic process through induction of recurrent cytotoxicity may have different dose-response curves than chemicals which interact directly with DNA.

There has been a long debate over the shape of carcinogen dose-response curves in the low dose region where experimental investigation is not practical. A fully validated version of the PCM could be used to explore this issue (Fig. 6). Dose-tumor prevalence curves for different biochemical mechanisms are simulated over a range of exposure concentrations extending from those commonly used for rodent carcinogen bioassays down to the parts-per-billion concentrations often found at sites of environmental pollution.

LABORATORY VALIDATION OF THE CANCER MODEL

Much of the structure of the PCM, which has been incorporated from pre-existing models, has already been validated. The major segment of the PCM that is basically without validation at this time is that describing the biochemical mechanisms of action for DNA-damaging agents, promoters and cytotoxicants. Our laboratories are currently attempting to validate the PCM for chloroform using the working hypothesis that chloroform carcinogenesis is secondary to repeated cytotoxic insults. Experimental programs could also be designed for validation of the model with respect to promoters and genotoxicants.

There are many challenges inherent in the laboratory studies needed to validate any portion of this PCM. Necessary experiments include quantitation of rates of DNA adduct formation and repair, identification of initiated cells, quantitation of initiated cell birth and death rates, and definition of the relationship between first appearance of a malignant cell and of a clinically-observable tumor. These experiments are, however, feasible with currently-available technology (Freidberg, 1985;Peraino et al., 1986; Rushmore et al., 1987; and Digernes, 1983).

An important aspect of simulation models with a biologically-based structure is that they assist in their own validation. For example, simulated experiments can be run using a range of initial conditions to determine which experimental design is most likely to provide useful output. This facet of simulation modeling helps to emphasize the iterative nature of model validation. The model actually becomes a form of working hypothesis guiding the laboratory work and being refined in response to it.

DISCUSSION

The obvious complexity of the carcinogenic process underscores the need for models which balance necessary detail with purposeful simplification. Moolgavkar et al. (1980) have shown that a biologically-based 2-stage model is sufficient to model human cancer incidence and to provide insight to the consequences of different carcinogenic mechanisms (Moolgavkar, 1983). The physiologically-based description of pharmacokinetics works well for a variety of compounds. The mechanisms described for DNA-damaging agents, promoters and cytotoxicants are well-supported by the literature though they are not, by any means, the only such mechanisms which could be modeled. While the PCM incorporates a substantial level of biological detail it is still tractable. Tumor prevalence curves for 2-years of intermittent exposure (Fig. 5) can be generated in about 15 minutes of VAX 8530 (Digital Equipment Co.) cpu time. Dose-response curves for 2 years of continuous exposure (Fig. 6) take about 3 minutes each. Many aspects of model behavior can also be readily studied with microcomputers.

In the calculations performed for this paper, we used a simple approximation to estimate the tumor prevalence from the rate of appearance of tumor cells. Rigorously, the quantity we would like to compute is the true incidence, the expected rate of appearance of tumor cells in previously tumor-free animals. The quantity $d(N1-->N2)/dt$ used in the approximate method here is the average rate of appearance of tumor cells in all animals. Moolgavkar (et al., 1988) has demonstrated that the approximate solution can overestimate tumor incidence when the birth-rate of initiated cells is high. We have recently developed a correction term for equation (2) which properly adjusts for this discrepancy in the case where the cellular dynamic parameters (birth rates, death rates, and transition rates) are constant or cyclic (e.g. for an intermittent exposure). We are now comparing the predictions of this 'corrected approximation' with the exact solution for cases where the cellular dynamic parameters vary over the course of the animal's lifetime. The basis for comparison is a newly-derived solution for the two-stage model with time-dependent parameters based on the method of characteristics (Quinn, 1988).

Alternatively, these deterministic formulations could be replaced with a stochastic approach in which the generation of initiated and malignant cells in an individual is predicted by a simulated weighted coin toss and the model is iterated a large number of times. However, this approach would require considerable computer time, and is not practical for running large numbers of cases.

Much, but not all, of what is known about the biology of chemical carcinogenesis is encoded in the PCM. The immune system, for example, is not explicitly described and may kill initiated and malignant cells. At present, any effect of the immune system on tumor prevalence must be implicitly accounted for by the values used for a_1, b_1, u_1 and u_2. Genetic recombination appears to be an important mechanism for some cancers (Friedberg, 1985) but is not described. The current version of the model could not be properly validated for such agents. Age-related changes in % body fat affect pharmacokinetic behavior (Lutz et al., 1977; Yang et al., 1984). Consequently, the target tissue concentration will change over time for a constant external concentration of carcinogen. For quantitatively accurate simulations the PCM will need, therefore, to describe the aging of its encoded biological structures. Each of these factors which is either missing from the current PCM or described implicitly could be explicitly described and would fit easily into the pre-existing structure. Immune system-mediated cell killing could be described as a first-order process acting on initiated and malignant cells in the current deterministic version of the PCM. Genetic recombination could be described as a process increasing u_2 as has been discussed by Moolgavkar (1986). Similarly, the model could be revised to exhibit age related changes in body composition, and biochemical processes simply by including formulae for age-specific values for the affected parameters.

The ease with which foreseeable changes in the PCM fit into its pre-existing structure are characteristic of biologically-based simulation modeling. Computer programs are by their nature easy to change. Because the model explicitly describes biological structure, future insights into chemical carcinogenesis will doubtless lead to additions and refinements but almost certainly not to fundamental changes in model structure.

Each element of the PCM (Fig. 1) has been thoroughly described by other investigators. The innovation in this work is in the consolidation of previously separate elements. This, combined with the use of computer simulation, provides a flexible tool which can be utilized for step-by-step examination of the process of chemical carcinogenesis and, with validation, for rationally estimating the risks of human exposure to chemical carcinogens. Before this or any simulation model can accurately describe the carcinogenicity of real chemicals, appropriate validation studies are necessary. Validated, biologically-structured simulation models will eventually form the cornerstone of risk assessment for chemical carcinogens but more importantly, they will support hypothesis testing for a wide range of studies of chemical toxicity and carcinogenesis.

REFERENCES

Andersen, M.E., Clewell, H.J., III, Gargas, M.J., Smith, F.A. and Reitz, R.H. (1987). Physiologically based pharmacokinetics and the risk assessment process for methylene chloride. Toxicol. Appl. Pharmacol. 87:185-205.

Andersen, M.E. (1987). Tissue dosimetry in risk assessment, or What's the Problem Here Anyway? In: Drinking Water and Health, Volume 8: Pharmacokinetics in Risk Assessment, National Academy Press, Washington, D.C., pp. 8-23.

Barrett, J.C., Tsutsui, T. and Ts'o, P.O.P. (1978). Neoplastic transformation induced by a direct perturbation of DNA. Nature 274:229-232.

Bischoff, K.B. and Brown, R.G. (1966). Drug Distribution in Mammals. Chemical Engineering Progress Symposium Series 62:33-45.

Darnell, J., Lodish, H. and Baltimore, D. (1986). <u>Molecular Cell Biology</u>, Scientific American Books, p. 138.

de la Iglesia, F.A., McGuire, E.J. and Feuer, G. (1975). Coumarin and 4-methylcoumarin induced changes in the hepatic endoplasmic reticulum studied by quantitative stereology. <u>Toxicology</u> 4:305-314.

Digernes, V. (1983). Chemical liver carcinogenesis: Monitoring of the process by flow cytometric DNA measurements. <u>Environ. Hlth. Perspect.</u> 50:195-200.

Elmore, E., Kakunaga, T. and Barrett, J.C. (1983). Comparison of spontaneous mutation rates of normal and chemically transformed human skin fibroblasts. <u>Cancer Research</u> 43:1650-1655.

Emmelot, P. and Scherer, E. (1980). The first relevant cell stage in rat liver carcinogenesis. A quantitative approach. <u>Biochimica Biophysica Acta</u> 605:247-304.

Freidberg, E.C. (1985). <u>DNA Repair</u>, W.H. Freeman and Co., New York, pp. 23-40.

Gasiewicz, T.A. and Rucci, G. (1984). Cytosolic receptor for 2,3,7,8-tetra-chlorodibenzo-p-dioxin. Evidence for a homologous nature among various mammalian species. <u>Molec. Pharmacol.</u> 26:90-98.

Lutz, R.J., Dedrick, R.L., Matthews, H.B., Eling, T.E. and Anderson, M.W. (1977). A preliminary pharmacokinetic model for several chlorinated biphenyls in the rat. <u>Drug Metab. Disp.</u> 5:386-396.

Matthews, H.B. and Dedrick, R.L. (1984). Pharmacokinetics of PCBs. <u>Ann. Rev. Pharmacol. Toxicol.</u> 24:85-103.

McCann, J., Choi, E., Yamasaki, E. and Ames, B.N. (1975). Detection of carcinogens as mutagens in the salmonella/microsome test: Assay of 300 chemicals. <u>Proc. Natl. Acad. Sci.</u> 72:5135-5139.

Moolgavkar, S.H. (1983). Model for human carcinogenesis: action of environmental agents. <u>Environ. Hlth. Perspect.</u>, 50:285-291.

Moolgavkar, S.H. (1986). Carcinogenesis modeling: From molecular biology to epidemiology. <u>Ann. Rev. Public Health</u> 7:151-169.

Moolgavkar, S.H., Day, N.E. and Stevens, R.G. (1980). Two-stage model for carcinogenesis: Epidemiology of breast cancer in females. <u>J.N.C.I.</u> 65:559-569.

Moolgavkar, S.H., Dewanji, A., and Venzon, D.J. (1988). A stochastic two-stage model for cancer risk assessment I: The hazard function and the probability of tumor. To be published in <u>Risk Analysis.</u>

Moolgavkar, S.H. and Knudson, A.G., Jr. (1981). Mutation and cancer: A model for human carcinogenesis. <u>J.N.C.I.</u> 66:1037-1052.

Moolgavkar, S.H. and Venzon, D.J. (1979). Two-event models for carcinogenesis: Incidence curves for childhood and adult tumors. <u>Mathematical Biosciences</u> 47:55-77.

Peraino, C., Carnes, B.A. and Stevens, F.J. (1986). Evidence for growth among foci with different phenotypes in the population of altered hepatocyte foci induced by a single neonatal treatment with carcinogen. Carcinogenesis 7:191-192.

Quinn, D.W. Calculating the hazard function and probability of tumor for cancer risk assessment when the parameters are time dependent. Submitted to Risk Analysis.

Ramsey, J.R. and Andersen, M.E. (1984). A physiological model for the inhalation pharmacokinetics of inhaled styrene in rats and humans. Toxicol. Appl. Pharmacol. 73:159-175.

Reddy, E.P. (1983). Nucleotide sequence analysis of the T24 human bladder carcinoma oncogene. Science 220:1061-1063.

Rushmore, T.H., Sharma, R.N.S., Roomi, M.W., Harris, L., Satoh, K., Sato, K., Murray R.K. and Farber, E. (1987). Identification of a characteristic cytosolic polypeptide of rat neoplastic hepatocyte nodules as placental glutathione S-transferase. Biochem. Biophys. Res. Commun. 143:98-103.

Tsutsui, T., Crawford, B.D. and Ts'o, P.O.P. (1981). Comparison between mutagenesis in normal and transformed Syrian hamster fibroblasts. Difference in the temporal order of HPRT gene replication. Mutation Research 80:357-371.

Weinstein, I.B. (1981). Current concepts and controversies in chemical carcinogenesis. J. Supramolecular Structure and Cellular Biochemistry 17:99-120.

Yang, R.S., Tallant, M.J. and McKelvy, J.A. (1984). Age-dependent pharmacokinetic changes of ethylenediamine in Fisher-344 rats parallel to a two-year chronic toxicity study. Fund. Appl. Toxicol. 4:663-670.

DETERMINATION OF CARCINOGEN EXPOSURE BY IMMUNOLOGICAL TECHNIQUES

Lars O. Dragsted

National Food Agency of Denmark, Institute of Toxicology
Department of Biochemical and Molecular Toxicology, 19
Mørkhøj Bygade, Dk-2860 Søborg, Denmark

INTRODUCTION

Humans are exposed to carcinogens from a variety of sources including food, drinking water, air, and the working environment. A few of these carcinogens have been identified epidemiologically, but the majority have been identified by animal bioassays and their impact on human cancer is not well established. The mathematical quantitation of human cancer risk from exposures to animal carcinogens relies on the validity of animal to man extrapolations. Several pieces of information could increase the validity of such extrapolations. Among these, comparative pharmacokinetic data from the relevant test animals and from man are particularly important because these data will tell to what extent the compound is handled similarly and whether it elicits toxicity by the same mechanism in the two species. The quantitation of human risk is also highly dependent on data providing the actual human exposure levels. Futhermore, large interindividual variations in exposures and in pharmacokinetics are most probably found for most carcinogens in human populations. Therefore this variability should also be validated in order not to underestimate the risk to certain groups or individuals.

Human exposure data can only be obtained in those cases, where populations are actually being exposed to the carcinogen. In the case of carcinogenic environmental pollutants, food contaminants and industrial compounds this will be true in many instances. Even so, exposure data are most often not available even for those carcinogens to which humans are currently being exposed. The reason for this is that exposures are very low and that sufficiently sensitive and quick methods are not presently available for the quantitation of carcinogens in biological samples.

Several sensitive analytical methods have been developed during the last decade to allow quantitation of extremely low concentrations of carcinogens and carcinogen-DNA adducts, see Vainio (1985), Perera (1987), or Ashby (1988) for recent reviews. Among these, the immunoassay techniques are particularly promising because they allow the quantitation of very small amounts of non-radioactive substances, and because large amounts of samples can be processed with relatively little effort. The production of polyclonal sera and monoclonal antibodies (MAb's) to carcinogens and to carcinogen-DNA adducts (see Strickland and Boyle, 1984, and Poirier, 1984 and 1986 for reviews) has allowed quantitation of these compounds in femtomolar or even attomolar concentrations in body fluids, isolated DNA and in tissue preparations. These techniques have been used to enlighten such different questions as the persistence of DNA-adducts in humans (Eggset et al., 1983), the relationship between dose and adduct formation in individuals receiving chemotherapy (Reed et al., 1986) and the frequency of O^6-methyldeoxyguanosine adducts in the target organ of humans living in a high-risk area for oesophageal cancer (Umbenhauer et al., 1985).

ANTIBODIES AND IMMUNOASSAYS

Polyclonal antisera may be raised in rabbits, or monoclonal mouse- or rat-antibodies may be produced by hybridoma technologies. Theoretically, MAb's should have higher specificities to the epitope against which they are raised, i.e. they should have less cross-reactivity with similar structures as compared to the polyclonal sera. This seems, however, to depend on the immunogen used. In a study of polyclonal and monoclonal sera against O^6-ethyldeoxyguanosine (O^6-EtdGuo), Wani et al. (1984) found no major difference in their specificity.

Similar findings have been reported for antisera against O^6-methyldeoxyguanosine (O^6-MeGuo) (Wild et al., 1983) and against aflatoxin M_1 (AFM_1) (Woychic et al., 1984). Also, the polyclonal sera reported in these studies have at least as good affinities as the monoclonals. In a large and systematic study where several MAb's have been raised against alkyldeoxyguanosines and thymidines, extremely good specificities and high affinities (10^8-10^{10} L/mole) have been obtained with MAb's (Rajewsky et al., 1980, Adamkiewicz et al., 1984).

Several immunoassay procedures are available for determination of small compounds, most notably the radioimmunoassay, RIA, and the solid phase enzyme immunoassay, EIA. In the RIA, a radioactively labelled competitor for the antibody is used to determine the amount of unlabelled compound in the sample. In the EIA a solid phase is used to adsorb a fixed quantity of antigen before antibody and sample is introduced. The amount of competitor in the sample will be related to the amount of antibody bound to the solid phase in a reciprocal manner. The bound antibody is determined by the aid of an enzyme-labelled second antibody that binds to the first antibody and allows subsequent colorimetric quantitation. Competitive as well as non-competitive EIA assays have been developed. The RIA as well as the EIA exist in several modifications giving increased sensitivity or other advantages. The RIA appears to be the most sensitive for assays with antibodies to alkylated DNA-bases where radiotracers with specific activities of around 30 Ci/mmol are available (Müller and Rajewsky, 1980, Wani et al., 1984). In several studies comparing different immunoassay procedures with antibodies to more bulky carcinogens or their base-adducts, the EIA procedures were found to give more sensitive assays. Even more sensitive assays are the ultra-sensitive enzyme radioimmunoassay (USERIA), where a radioactively labelled substrate is used in an EIA, and the HS-EIA, where a fluorescent substrate is used. Hsu et al. (1980) compared competitive RIA, EIA and USERIA assays for N-(deoxyguanosin-8-yl)-N-acetyl-2-aminofluorene (AAF-dGuo) and found that the EIA was five times and the USERIA was fifty times more sensitive than the RIA. In a similar study with a polyclonal serum against Benzo[a]pyrenediol-epoxide-DNA adducts, Hsu et al. (1981) found that the RIA was 100 times less sensitive than the EIA and 500 times less sen-

sitive than USERIA. With the most sensitive assays developed
so far, less than one femtomole of a compound can be accurately determined in a 100µl volume. For most carcinogens, this
will allow exposure determination even when exposures are
fractions of a microgram a day.

AVAILABILITY OF ANTIBODIES FOR EXPOSURE STUDIES

Immunoassays are sensitive and efficient methods, but
they are dependent on the availability of specific antibodies.
The formation of antibodies to carcinogens have been described
as early as the nineteen thirties (Strickland & Boyle, 1984),
but most polyclonal sera and MAb's with high specificity to
carcinogens and carcinogen-DNA adducts have been raised much
more recently. Generally, carcinogens are too small molecules
to elicit directly an antigen response in animals, and they
need to be coupled as haptens to carrier molecules, e.g. proteins or DNA, in order to be antigenic. Chemically activated
carcinogens may react with proteins to give adducts containing
10-50 carcinogen molecules for each protein molecule (Santella
et al., 1986; Sizaret & Maleiville, 1983). Very efficient
procedures have also been described for the coupling of carcinogen-nucleoside adducts to proteins (Erlanger and Beiser,
1964) and for electrostatic coupling of highly modified DNA to
proteins (Leng et al., 1978, Haugen et al., 1981). Depending
on the carcinogen or the DNA-modification, polyclonal sera or
MAb's may be more easy to obtain with sufficient specificity
and affinity to give sensitive immunoassays. Generally, affinities in the range, 10^7-10^{10} L/mole are necessary for monitoring studies.

DETERMINATION OF CARCINOGENS IN BLOOD AND URINE SAMPLES

Blood samples and, in particular urine samples, are among
the least objectionable to obtain from healthy individuals for
research purposes. Free carcinogen may be determined in the
serum of individuals following recent exposures. In this way,
carcinogen exposures from complex sources like food may be
quantitated without exact knowledge of all components in the

Table 1. Selected anti-carcinogen antibodies.

ANTIBODY TO	ASSAY	50% INHIBITION pmoles/assay	REFERENCE
4-acetamidobiphenyl	RIA	4.8	Johnson et al. (1980)
actinomycin D	RIA[p]	40	Brothman et al. (1982)
2-amino-3-methyl-imidazo[4,5-f]-quinoline	EIA	20	Vanderlaan et al. (1988)
2-aminoimidazo-quinoxalines	EIA	0.47-4.4	-"-
aflatoxin B$_1$	RIA[p]	0.65	Yang et al. (1980)
-"-	EIA[p]	6.5	Martin et al. (1984)
-"-	RIA	1.0	Groopman et al. (1984)
-"-	EIA[p]	0.1	Wild et al. (1986)
-"-	EIA	0.1	Dragsted et al. (1988)
aflatoxindihydrodiol	EIA	3.2	Pestka and Chu (1988)
aflatoxin M$_1$	EIA	2	Woychik et al. (1984)
-"-	EIA[p]	0.04	-"-
aflatoxin Q$_{2a}$	EIA[p]	0.35	Fan et al. (1984)
mitomycin C	EIA	6	Fujiwara et al. (1982)

[p] polyclonal sera were used.

source. Tsuboi et al (1984) determined the level of free aflatoxin B$_1$ (AFB$_1$) in blood samples from individuals in Japan who had recently ingested an ordinary lunch with no known source of aflatoxin contamination. The AFB$_1$ was isolated by affinity chromatography from the serum samples and identified unequivocally by mass spectrometry. As seen from table 1, antibodies have been developed to several carcinogens. The list is not exhaustive as more examples can be found in the literature. For some carcinogens, notably certain microbial toxins, there is a need to quantify the amount of carcinogen as such in environmental samples, e.g. AFM_1 in milk. In most cases, however, it is more interesting to obtain antibodies to the carcinogen metabolites that may be found in body fluids, e.g. blood or urine.

All of the antibodies listed in table 1 have been tested for their affinity to several chemical analogs of the compound they have been raised against. MAb's may bind to a very small molecular target, and the polyclonal sera of course bind to several such targets, even on small molecules like carcinogens. It is therefore not surprising that monoclonal as well as polyclonal antibodies often bind to several analogs of the primary antigen. Vanderlaan et al. (1988) designed an epitope that would allow the production of a MAb that recognises several of the 2-aminoimidazoarenes formed in the crust of fried meat. Groopman et al. (1984) found that their monoclonal AFB_1 antibody binds to several AFB_1 metabolites, including aflatoxin P_1, an important human metabolite (Groopman et al., 1985). Fan et al. (1984) developed a polyclonal serum directed against aflatoxin Q_1, another important human AFB_1 metabolite (Moss and Neal, 1985). Consequently, these antibodies could prove very useful for monitoring human exposures to AFB_1. Conversely, the AFB_1 MAb raised by Sun et al. (1983) only binds analogs modified in the 8,9-position (Dragsted et al., 1988). As the putative 8,9-oxide of AFB_1 is generally thought to be the ultimate carcinogenic metabolite of AFB_1, the latter MAb may be useful to determine the fraction of an AFB_1 dose that has been activated in this position and further metabolised. The use of two or more MAb's with different specificities may allow delicate toxicokinetic analyses to be performed in human populations exposed to environmental carcinogens.

DETERMINATION OF CARCINOGEN-DNA ADDUCTS IN BLOOD OR TISSUES

It is generally believed that carcinogens initiate the carcinogenic process by binding to DNA, thus interfering with the normal regulation of cellular growth. It is therefore of interest to determine the amount of carcinogen that reacts with DNA in a target organ and relate it to the dose of carcinogen and to cancer risk (Perera et al., 1985, Farmer et al., 1987). Samples of potential target organs are available for studies on humans only from autopsy samples. Though useful for the purpose of quantitating median levels of DNA adducts in different organs, autopsy samples are obviously not useful for biomonitoring purposes. One way to get around this problem is to determine the adduct levels in DNA from peripheral blood, assuming proportionality between levels in blood-DNA and target organ DNA. One good reason to expect proportionality in many cases is that the blood continuosly perfuses the target organ, thus exposing blood cells to the activated carcinogens present there. Good proportionality between adduct levels in hemoglobin and in target organ DNA has been observed for several small alkylating agents (Ostermann-Golkar et al., 1977; Segerbäck, 1983).

High affinity antibodies to a range of carcinogen-DNA adducts have been prepared and selected for high specificities towards their target epitopes, see table 2. Poirier et al. (1985) and Reed et al. (1986) used highly specific antibodies directed against cis-diamminodichloroplatinum(II) (cis-DDP) adducts in DNA to determine the adduct level in cancer patients receiving chemotherapy. They found that patients with detectable adduct levels in blood lymphocytes were more responsive to cis-DDP therapy. Their detection limit was on the order of 25 attomoles cis-DDP per µg of DNA, and the relation between cumulative cis-DDP dose and lymphocyte DNA adduct levels could be established for individual patients. A few studies have also been performed to determine DNA adduct levels in occupational exposure groups. Harris et al. (1985) studied Benzo[a]pyrenediolepoxide-DNA (BPDE-I-DNA) adducts in lymphocytes from coke oven workers, and Shamsuddin et al. (1985) performed a similar study with roofers and foundry workers. They found 2/3 and 1/3 of the workers in the two studies, respectively, were positive for BPDE-I-DNA adducts by EIA or USERIA assays with a lower detection limit in the order of 40 attomoles BPDE-I per µg DNA. Sample requirements were 50µg of DNA per well. Haugen et al. (1986) compared the BPDE-I-DNA adduct levels found in peripheral blood of coke oven workers as determined by USERIA or by synchronous fluorescence

Table 2. Antibodies to carcinogen-DNA or carcinogen-protein adducts.

ANTIBODY TO	ASSAY	50% INHIBITION fmoles/assay	REFERENCE
AAF-dGuo[a] in DNA	USERIA	5[b]	Hsu et al. (1980)
-"- in DS-DNA	RIA[p]	8300	Poirier et al. (1981)
AFB$_1$-dGuo in DNA	EIA	10000	Haugen et al. (1981)
-"-	USERIA	1000	-"-
-"-	EIA	1700[p]	Pestka et al. (1982)
AFB$_1$-FAPYR in DNA	EIA	2000[p]	-"-
-"-	EIA	10000	Hertzog et al. (1982)
BPDE-I-DNA	RIA	5000	Hsu et al. (1981)
-"-	EIA	40	-"-
-"-	USERIA	10	-"-
BPDE-I-dGuo in DNA	EIA	17	Santella et al. (1984)
-"-	EIA	350	Santella et al. (1986)
BPDE-II-RSA	EIA	3000	-"-
BPDE-I-dGuo	EIA	70	Shamsuddin et al. (1985)
-"-	USERIA	9	-"-
cis-DDP-DNA	EIA	50[p]	Poirier et al. (1981)
-"-	EIA	10[p]	Reed et al. (1986)
O^6-EtdGuo in DNA	ISB	0.3[c]	Nehls et al. (1984)
O^4-EtdThd in DNA	ISB	0.1[c]	-"-

[a] Abbreviations: AAF-dGuo, N-(deoxyguanosin-8-yl)-N-acetyl-2-aminofluorene; DS-DNA, double-stranded DNA; AFB$_1$-dGuo, 8,9-dihydro-8-(N^7-deoxyguanosyl)-9-hydroxyaflatoxin B$_1$; AFB-FAPYR, 8,9-dihydro-8-(N^5-formyl-2',5',6'-triamino-4-oxo-N^5-pyrimidyl)-9-hydroxyaflatoxin B$_1$; BPDE-I, 7-beta,8-alpha-dihy-

droxy-9-alpha,10-alpha-epoxy-7,8,9,10-tetrahydrobenzo[a]py-
rene; cis-DDP, cis-diamminedichloroplatinum(II); O^6-EtdGuo, O^6-
ethyldeoxyguanosine; O^4-EtdThd, O^4-ethylthymidine; O^6-
iProdGuo, O^6-isopropyldeoxyguanosine; O^6-MedGuo, O^6-
methyldeoxyguanosine; O^4-MedThd, O^4-methylthymidine.
[b] Detection limit in a non-competitive USERIA assay.
[c] Detection limit by immuno-slot-blot (ISB) in 3µg of DNA.
[p] Polyclonal sera were used.

---

spectroscopy. However, only the most positive samples were
equally identified by both methods, possibly because BP is
only one of many polycyclic aromatic hydrocarbons that these
workers were exposed to, and some of these may interfere with
either assay.

The antibodies to carcinogen-DNA adducts have been used
in several studies to determine adducts at the cellular level
by immunocytochemical methods. By using antibodies labelled
with a fluorescent dye, Adamkiewicz et al. (1985) reported a
detection limit of approximately 700 O^6-EtdGuo residues per
diploid genome as measured in single cells by immunocytolo-
gical analysis. Menkveld et al. (1985) used immunohistochemical double peroxidase anti-peroxidase staining with antibodies to O^6-EtdGuo and to AAF-dGuo to visualize the distribution of DNA adducts in liver slices from rats dosed with diethylnitrosamine or N-acetylaminofluorene. The detection limit
was around 10^4 adducts per nucleus, and they were able to show
differences in distribution as well as in persistence of the
adducts in the liver.

DNA samples may also be hydrolysed to nucleotides or
nucleosides, and the adducts quantitated in the hydrolysate.
Several antibodies to the adducts found in hydrolysed DNA are
presently available, see table 3. This allows preconcentration
of adducts by chromatography, thus increasing the sensitivity
of the procedure, and at the same time decreasing the requirements for specificity. Using this approach, Müller and Rajew
sky (1980) were able to increase the sensitivity of their RIA
assay to O^6-EtdGuo in hydrolysed DNA about 100-fold. With an
initial excess of unmodified guanosine of 5×10^8 fold, they
were able to quantify O^6-EtdGuo by Sephadex G-10 chromato-

Table 3. Antibodies to carcinogen-nucleoside adducts.

ANTIBODY TO	ASSAY	50% INHIBITION pmoles/assay	REFERENCE
AAF-dGuo	RIA[p]	0.46	Poirier et al. (1977)
-"-	RIA	250	Hsu et al. (1980)
-"-	EIA	50	-"-
-"-	USERIA	5	-"-
-"-	RIA	0.15	Van der Laken et al. (1982)
AFB-dGuo	EIA	6	Dragsted et al. (1988)
BPDE-I-dGuo	RIA	5	Poirier et al. (1980)
-"-	EIA	0.15	Santella et al. (1986)
O^6-n-BudGuo	RIA	0.044	Safhill et al. (1982)
O^2-n-BudThd	RIA	0.069	-"-
O^4-n-BudThd	RIA	0.45	-"-
cis-DDP-(dGuo)$_2$	EIA	0.0049-0.009	Plooy et al. (1985)
O^6-EtdGuo	RIA	0.05	Müller & Rajewsky (1980)
-"-	RIA	0.05	Adamkiewicz et al. (1982)
-"-	RIA[p]	0.15	Wani et al. (1984)
-"-	EIA[p]	20	-"-
-"-	RIA	0.63	-"-
-"-	RIA	0.04	Adamkiewicz et al. (1985)
O^4-EtdThd	RIA	0.24	-"-
O^6-iProdGuo	RIA	0.05	-"-
O^6-MedGuo	RIA	0.3	Wild et al. (1983)
-"-	RIA[p]	0.16	-"-

Table 3. Antibodies to carcinogen-nucleoside adducts, continued.

ANTIBODY TO	ASSAY	50% INHIBITION pmoles/assay	REFERENCE
O^6-MedGuo	EIA[p]	1.0	Foiles et al. (1985)
O^6-MedGuo	RIA	0.1	Umbenhauer et al. (1985)
-"-	RIA	0.25	Adamkiewicz et al. (1985)
O^4-MedThd	RIA	7.0	-"-

[a] Abbreviations are as in fig. 2.
[b] Two different platinum-dGuo crosslinks exist, an inter-strand (50% inhibition, 4.9 fmoles/assay) and an intra-strand (50% inhibition, 9 fmoles/assay) crosslink.
[p] Polyclonal antibodies were used.

graphy and RIA. Safhill et al. (1982) have developed antibodies to O^6-n-butyldeoxyguanosine, O^4-n-butylthymidine and O^2-n-butylthymidine. The main cross-reactivities of these antibodies were with the other butyl adducts, and a major increase in sensitivity of the RIA assays by chromatography prior to RIA was suggested.

ANTIBODIES TO CARCINOGENS IN EXPOSED POPULATIONS

The early notion that antibodies protect against infections led to the hypothesis, that anti-carcinogen antibodies might protect against cancer. This hypothesis was discouraged, however, as it was found that tumors could be induced by carcinogens in animals that produced antibodies to those same carcinogens (Creech, 1952). However, it has subsequently been found, that antibodies to a fluorinated analog of 7,12-dime-thylbenz[a]anthracene (DMBA) protected against DMBA-tumorige-nesis on CD-1 mouse skin, decreasing the incidence of tumors by 50% (Moolten et al., 1981). Caviezel et al. (1984) found a more than three fold reduction in the covalent binding of AFB_1 to the liver DNA in rabbits that had previously been immunised against AFB_1. These findings are particularly interesting in the light of the findings by Harris et al. (1985) and Haugen et al. (1986) that coke oven workers, exposed to carcinogenic benzo[a]pyrene may develop antibodies to this carcinogen. Similar findings have been obtained with AFB_1 exposed indivi-duals from Kenya (H. Autrup, personal communication). The finding of anti-carcinogen antibodies in human populations may be used to indicate that carcinogen exposure has taken place, but may also be a parameter indicating a decreased risk of cancer. Thus, the determination of anti-carcinogen antibodies in humans may add important information to be used in risk analysis.

CONCLUSIONS

Immunoassay techniques are versatile and sensitive means of establishing the concentrations of many compounds, inclu-ding carcinogens in biological samples. They do not seem to need any increase in sensitivity to quantify carcinogens and major metabolites in body fluids, as they presently allow pico- or femtomolar concentrations to be determined in body fluids. This level of sensitivity will allow total doses of less than a nanogram a day for most carcinogens to be deter-mined by analysing the urine, provided a high sensitivity and high specificity antibody is available. These assays could be used to add important exposure- and toxicokinetic data to the process of risk analysis. Unfortunately, very few efforts have been done so far to develop antibodies to the major carcinogen metabolites, so only a limited number of carcinogens can pre-sently be evaluated in this way.

A longer range of antibodies have been developed to the carcinogen-DNA adducts and to the isolated carcinogen-nucleo-side adducts. Although very sensitive immunoassays exist to quantify these adducts, the quantitation of adducts from expo-

sures to the public of ambient levels of environmental carcinogens may not presently bee feasible. However, carcinogen-DNA
adducts resulting from occupational exposures, exposures to
cigarette smoke or from medical therapy may be quantified in
some cases. A few pilot studies of this kind have allready
been published, but one major problem is the relatively large
amounts of blood (40-50ml) that has to be collected to perform
these analyses with the present technology.

During the last decade immunoassay procedures with ever
increasing sensitivity have been developed, and it is likely
that the present technical difficulties in determining the
dose of environmental carcinogens to blood DNA will be over-
come in the near future. The dose to target organ DNA will
only be possible to determine when autopsy or biopsy material
is available. In some cases, the urinary excretion of products
resulting from repair or spontaneous depurination of carcino-
gen-guanine adducts has been described. The concentration of
these products from urine samples, followed by immunoassay
quantitation may be another way to quantify the fraction of
carcinogen that has reacted with nucleic acids in the body.
Notice however,that RNA as well as DNA adducts are determined
in this way.

In conclusion, the immunoassay techniques are highly
developed, and could presently add important information to
the process of quantitating risk from carcinogen exposures.
Even data on DNA adduct levels in human risk groups may presently be obtained in some cases, but more sensitive assays
are still needed for most applications. The development of
antibodies that would allow accurate determination of the
exposure levels in humans could be an integrated part of the
carcinogen risk evaluations, and could be used to monitor the
levels of carcinogen exposures actually resulting from
acceptable levels of carcinogens in the environment.

LITERATURE

Adamkiewicz, J., Drosdziok, W., and Eberhardt, W., Langenberg,
    U., and Rajewsky, M. F., 1983, High-affinity monoclonal
    antibodies specific for DNA components structurally modi-
    fied by alkylating agents, Banbury Report 13:265.

Adamkiewicz, J., Nehls, P., and Rajewsky, M. F., 1984, Immuno-
    logical methods for detection of carcinogen-DNA adducts,
    In: "Monitoring human exposure to carcinogenic and muta-
    genic agents," A. Berlin, M. Draper, K. Hemminki, H.
    Vainio, eds., International Agency for Research on Can-
    cer, Lyon.

Ashby, J., 1988, Comparison of techniques for monitoring human
    exposure to genotoxic chemicals, Mutat. Res. 204:543.

Brothman, A. R., Davis, T. P., Duffy, J. J., and Lindell, T.
    J., 1982, Development of an antibody to actinomycin D and
    its application for the detection of serum levels by
    radioimmunoassay, Cancer Res., 42:1184.

Caviezel, M., Aeschbach, A. P., Lutz, W. K., and Schlatter,
    C., 1984, Reduction of covalent binding of aflatoxin B_1
    to rabbit liver DNA after immunization against this car-
    cinogen, Arch. Toxicol., Suppl.7:249.

Creech, H. J., 1952, Chemical and immunological properties of
    carcinogen-protein conjugates. Cancer Res. 12:557.

Dragsted, L. O., Bull, I., and Autrup, H., 1988, Substan-
    ces with affinity to a monoclonal aflatoxin B_1 antibody
    in Danish urine samples, Fd. Chem. Toxic. 26:233.

Eggset, G., Volden, G., and Krokan, H., 1983, U.v.-induced DNA
    damage and its repair in human skin in vivo studied by
    sensitive immunohistochemical methods, Carcinog. 4:745.

Erlanger, B., and Beiser, S., 1964, Antibodies specific for
    ribonucleosides, ribonucleotides and their reaction with
    DNA, Proc. Natl. Acad. Sci. USA, 52:68

Fan, T. S. L., Zhang, G. S., and Chu, F. S., 1984, Produc-
    tion and characterisation of antibody against aflatoxin
    Q_1 , Appl. Environ. Microbiol. 47:526.

Farmer, P. B., Neumann, H.-G., and Henschler, D., 1987,
    Estimation of exposure of man to substances reacting
    covalently with macromolecules, Arch Toxicol 60:251.

Foiles, P. G., Truschin, N., and Castonguay, A., 1985,
    Measurement of O^6-methyldeoxyguanosine in DNA methylated
    by the tobacco-specific carcinogen 4-(methylnitrosamino)-
    1-(3-pyridyl)-1-butanone using a biotin-avidin enzyme-
    linked immunosorbent assay, carcinogenesis 6:989.

Fujiwara, K., Saikusa, H., Yasuno, M., and Kitagawa, T., 1982,
    Enzyme immunoassay for the quantification of mitomycin C
    using ß-galactosidase as a label, Cancer Res., 42:1487.

Groopman, J.D., Trudel, L.J., Donahue, P.R., Marshak-Rothstein, A., and Wogan, G.N., 1984, High-affinity monoclonal antibodies for aflatoxins and their application to solid-phase immunoassays, Proc. Natl. Acad., 81:7728.

Groopman, J. D., Donahue, P.R., Zhu, J., Chen, J., and Wogan, G. N., 1985, Aflatoxin metabolism in humans: Detection of metabolites and nucleic acid adducts in urine by affinity chromatography, Proc. Natl. Acad. Sci. 82: 6492.

Harris, C. C., Vähäkangas, K., Newman, M. J., Trivers, G. E., Shamsuddin, A., Sinopoli, N., Mann, D. L., and Wright, W. E., 1985, Detection of benzo[a]pyrene diol epoxide-DNA adducts in peripheral blood lymphocytes and antibodies to the adducts in serum from coke oven workers, Proc. Natl. Acad. Sci. 82: 6672.

Haugen, Aa., Becher, G., Benestad, C., Vähäkangas, K., Trivers, G. E., Newman, M. J., and Harris, C. C., 1986, Determination of polycyclic aromatic hydrocarbons in the urine, benzo[a]pyrene diol epoxide-DNA adducts in lymphocyte DNA, and antibodies to the adducts in sera from coke oven workers exposed to measured amounts of polycyclic aromatic hydrocarbons in the work atmosphere, Cancer Res. 46:4178.

Haugen, AA., Groopman, J.D., Hsu, I-C., Goodrich, G.R., Wogan, and Harris, C.C., 1981, Monoclonal antibody to aflatoxin B_1-modified DNA detected by enzyme immunoassay, Proc. Natl. Acad. Sci., 78:4124.

Hertzog, P. J., Lindsay Smith, J. R., and Garner, R. C., 1982, Production of monoclonal antibodies to guanine opened aflatoxin B_1 DNA, the persistent DNA adduct in vivo, Carcinog., 3:825.

Hsu, I.C., Poirier, M.C., Yuspa, S.H., Yolken, R.H., and C.C. Harris, 1980, Ultrasensitive enzymatic radioimmunoassay (USERIA) detects femtomoles of acetylaminofluorene-DNA adducts, Carcinog. 1:455.

Hsu, I-C., Poirier, M. C., Yuspa, S. H., Grunberger, D., Weinstein, I. B., Yolken, R. H., and Harris, C. C., 1981, Measurement of benzo[a]pyrene-DNA adducts by enzyme immunoassays and radioimmunoassay, Cancer Res., 41:1091.

Johnson, H. J., Jr., Cemosek, S. F.,Jr., Gutierrez-Cemosek, R. M., and Brown, L. L., 1980, Development of a radioimmunoassay procedure for 4-acetamidobiphenyl, a metabolite of the chemical carcinogen 4-aminobiphenyl, in urine, J. of Anal. Tox. 4:86. Kriek, E., Engelse, L. D., Scherer, E., and Westra, G., 1984, Formation of DNA modifications by chemical carcinogens identification, localisation and quantification, Biochim. Biophys. Acta 738:181.

Leng, M., Sage, E., Fuchs, R. P., and Daune, M. P., 1978, Antibodies to DNA modified by the carcinogen, N-acetoxy-N-2-acetylaminofluorene, FEBS Lett., 92:207.

Malfoy, B., Hartmann, B., Macquet, J-P., and Leng, M., 1981, Immunochemical studies of DNA modified by cis-dichlorodiammineplatinum(II) in vivo and in vitro, Cancer Res. 41:4127.

Martin, C. N., Garner, R. C., Tursi, F., Garner, J. V., Whittle, H. C., Sizaret, R. P., and Montesano, R., 1984, An elisa Procedure for assaying aflatoxin B_1 , in Berlin, A., Draper, M., Hemminki, K. & Vainio, H. cds. Monitoring Human Exposure to Carcinogenic and Mutagenic Agents (IARC Scientific Publications No. 59), International Agency for Research on Cancer, Lyon.

Menkveld, G. J., Van Der Laken, C. J., Hermsen, T., Kriek, E., Scherer, E., and Den Engelse, L., 1985, Immunohistochemical localisation of O^6-ethyldeoxyguanosine and deoxyguanosin-8-yl-(acetyl)aminofluorene in liver sections of rats treated with diethylnitrosamine, ethylnitrosourea or N-acetylaminofluorene, Carcinog. 6:263.

Moolten, F. L., Schreiber, B., Rizzone, A., Weiss, A. J., and Boger, E., 1981, Protection of mice against 7,12-dimethylbenz[a]anthracene-induced skin tumors by immunization with afluorinated analog of the carcinogen, cancer Res, 41:425.

Moss, E. J., and Neal, G. E., 1985, The metabolism of aflatoxin B_1 by human liver, Biochem. Pharmacol. 34:3193.

Müller, R., and Rajewsky, M.R., 1980, Immunological quantification by high-affinity antibodies of O^6-ethyldeoxyguanosine in DNA exposed to N-ethyl-N-nitrosourea, Cancer Res. 40:887.

Nehls, P.,Adamkiewicz, J., and Rajewsky, M. F., 1984, Immuno-Slot-Blot: A highly sensitive immunoassay for the quantitation of carcinogen-modified nucleosides in DNA, J. Cancer Res. Clin. Oncol. 108:23.

Osterman-Golkar, S., Hultmark, D., Segerbäck, D., Calleman, C. J., Gothe, R., Ehrenberg, L., and Wachtmeister, C. A., 1977, Alkylation of DNA and proteins in mice exposed to vinyl chloride, Biochem. Biophys. Res. Commun. 76:259.

Perera, F. P., Santella, R. M., and Poirier, M. C., 1985, Potential methods to monitor human populations exposed to carcinogens: Carcinogen-Dna binding as an example, in: "Risk quantitation and regulatory policy," D. G. Hoel, R. A. Merrill, F. P. Perera, eds., Cold Spring Harbor Laboratory, Cold Spring Harbor.

Perera, F. P., 1987, Molecular Cancer Epidemiology: A new tool in cancer prevention, JNCI 78:887.

Pestka, J. J., Li, Y. K., and Chu, F. S., 1982, Reactivity of aflatoxin B_{2a} antibody with aflatoxin B_1-modified DNA and related metabolites, Appl. Environ. Microbiol. 44:1159.

Pestka, J. J., and Chu, F. S., 1984, Aflatoxin B_1 dihydrodiol antibody: Production and specificity, Appl. Environ. Microbiol. 47:472.

Plooy, A.C.M., van Dijk, M., and Lohman, P.H.M., 1984, Induction and repair of DNA cross-links in Chinese hamster ovary cells treated with various platinum coordination compounds in relation to platinum binding to DNA, cytotoxicity, Cancer Res. 44:2043.

Plooy, A. C. M., Fichtinger-Schepman, A. M. J. ., Schutte, H. H., van Dijk, M., and Lohman, P. H. M., 1985, The quantitative detection of various Pt-DNA-adducts in Chinese hamster ovary cells treated with cisplatin: application of immunochemical techniques, Carcinog. 6:561.

Poirier, M. C., Yuspa, S. H., Weinstein, I. B., and Blobstein, S., 1977, Detection of carcinogen-DNA adducts by radioimmunoassay Nature, 270:186.

Poirier, M.C., Santella, R., Weinstein, I.B., Grunberger, D., and Yuspa, S. H., 1980, Quantitation of Benzo(a)pyrene-deoxyguanosine adducts by radioimmunoassay, Cancer Res. 40:412.

Poirier, M.C., 1981, Antibodies to carcinogen-DNA adducts, JNCI, 67:515.

Poirier, M.C., M.C., Lippard, S.J., Zwelling, L.A., Ushay, H.M., Kerrigan, D., Thill, C.C., Santella, R.M., Grunberger, D., and Yuspa, S.H., 1982, Antibodies elicited against cis-diamminedichloroplatinum(II)-modified DNA are specific for cis-diamminedichloro-platinum(II)-DNA adducts formed in vivo and in vitro, Proc. Natl. Acad. Sci. 79:6443.

Poirier, M. C., 1984, The use of carcinogen-DNA adduct anti-sera for quantitation and localisation of genomic damage in animal and the human population, Environ. Mutagen. 6:879.

Poirier, M. C., Reed, E., Zwelling, L. A., Ozols, R. F., Litterst, C. L., and Yuspa, S. H., 1985, Polyclonal antibodies to quantitate cis-diamminedichloroplatinum(II)-DNA adducts in cancer patients and animal models, Environ. Hlth. Perspect. 62:89

Rajewsky, M. F., Müller, R., Adamkiewicz, J., and Drosdziok, W., 1980, Immunological detection and quantification of DNA components structurally modified by alkylating carcinogens (ethylnitrosourea), In: B. Pullman, P. O. P. Ts'o, H. Gelboin, eds., Carcinogenesis: Fundamental mechanisms and environmental effects, Reidel, Dordrecht.

Reed, E., Yuspa, S. H., Zwelling, L. A., Ozols, R. F., and Poirier, M. C., 1986, Quantitation of cis-Diamminedichloroplatinum II (Cisplatin)-DNA-Intrastrand adducts in testicular and ovarian cancer patients receiving cisplatin chemotherapy, J. Clin. Invest. 77:545.

Safhill, R., Strickland, P. T., and Boyle, J. M., 1982, Sensitive radioimmunoassays for O^6-n-butyldeoxyguanosine, O^2-n-butylthymidine and O^4-n-butylthymidine, carcinogenesis 5:547.

Santella, R.M., Lin, C.D., Cleveland, W.L., and Weinstein, I.B., 1984, Monoclonal antibodies to DNA modified by a benzo[a]pyrene diol epoxide, Carcinogenesis 5:373.

Santella, R. M., Lin, C. D., and Dharmaraja, N., 1986, Monoclonal antibodies to a benzo[a]pyrene diolepoxide modified protein, Carcinogenesis 7:441.

Segerbäck, D., 1983, Alkylation of DNA and hemoglobin in the mouse following exposure to ethene and ethene oxide, Chem. Biol Interact 45:139.

Sizaret, P., Malaveille, C., Montesano R., and Frayssinet, 1982, Detection of aflatoxins and related metabolites by radioimmunoassay, JNCI 69:1375.

Strickland, P. T., and Boyle, J.M., 1984, Immunoassay of carcinogen modified DNA, Prog. Nucleic Acid Res. Mol. Biol. 31:1.

Sun, T., Wu Y., and Wu, S., 1983, Monoclonal antibody against aflatoxin B_1, and its potential applications, Chinese J. Oncol., 5:401.

Tsuboi, S., Nakagawa, T., Tomita, M., Seo, T., Ono, H., Kawamura, K., and Iwamura, N., 1984, Detection of Aflatoxin B_1 in Serum Samples of Male Japanese Subjects by Radioimmunoassay and High-Performance Liquid Chromatography, Cancer Res. 44: 1231.

Umbenhauer, D., Wild, C.P., Montesano, R., Saffhill, R., Boyle, J.M., Huh, N., Kirstein, U., Thomale, J., Rajewsky, M.F. and Lu, S.H., 1985, O^6-Methyldeoxyguanosine in Oesophageal DNA among individuals at high risk of Oesophageal cancer, Int. J. Cancer 36:661.

Vanderlaan, M., Watkins, B.E., Hwang, M., Knize, M. G., and Felton, J.S., 1988, Monoclonal antibodies for the immunoassay of mutagenic compounds produced by cooking beef, Carcinog. 9: 153.

Van der Laken, C. J., Hagenaars, A. M., Hermsen, G., Kriek, E., Kuipers, A. J., Nagel, J., Scherer, E., and Welling, M., 1982, Measurement of O^6-ethyldeoxyguanosine and N-(deoxyguanosin-8-yl)-N-acetyl-aminofluorene in DNA by high-sensitivity enzyme immunoassays, carcinogenesis 5:569.

Vainio, H., 1985, Current trends in the biological monitoring of exposure to carcinogens, Scand J Work Environ Health 11:1

Wani, A. A., Gibson-D'Ambrosio, R. E., and D'Ambrosio, S. M., 1984, Quantitation of O^6-ethyldeoxyguanosine in ENU alkylated DNA by polyclonal and monoclonal antibodies, Carcinog. 5: 1145.

Wild, C. P., Smart, G., Saffhill, R., and Boyle, J. M., 1983, Radioimmunoassay of O^6-methyldeoxyguanosine in DNA of cells alkylated in vitro and in vivo, Carcinog. 4:1605.

Wild, C. P., Umbernhauer, D., Chapot, B., and Montesano, R., 1986, Monitoring of individual human exposure to aflatoxins (AF) and N-Nitrosamines (NNO) by immunoassays, J. Cell. Biochem.., 30:171.

Woychik, N. A., Hinsdill, R. D., and Chu, F. S., 1984, Production and characterisation of monoclonal antibodies Against aflatoxin M_1 , Appl. Environ. Microbiol., 48:1096.

Yang, G., Nesheim, S., Benavides, J., Ueno, I., Campbell, A. D., and Poland, A., 1980, Radioimmunoassay detection of Aflatoxin B_1 in monkey and human urine, Medical Mycology, Zbl. Bakt.. suppl. 8:329.

RISK ESTIMATION FOR LEUKEMOGENIC DRUGS

J.M. Kaldor and D.E.G. Shuker

International Agency for Research on Cancer
Lyon, France

ABSTRACT

A number of drugs used in cancer chemotherapy are known to be highly leukemogenic. Because the cancer risks per unit dose can be estimated more precisely for these drugs than for many other human carcinogens, they provide a unique opportunity to test the predictions of cancer risk models, and bioassay outcomes. The available data on leukemia incidence following cytostatic drug treatment are reviewed, with regard to differences in potency. Quantitative data from animal bioassays are also used as the basis for potency estimates, and the correlation with the human data is examined. Chemical and biochemical properties of several of the drugs are then discussed, with view to explaining some of the observed differences in leukemogenic potency.

QUANTIFICATION OF HUMAN CANCER RISK

The best quantification of cancer risk factors come from epidemiological studies on humans. However, there are very few carcinogens for which accurate quantitative risk information is available from epidemiology. Table 1 summarizes human carcinogens according to the context of exposure, indicating the major sites of action (IARC, 1988).

Table 1. Categories of human carcinogens

Carcinogens	Sites of action
Personal habits (smoking etc.)	lung, larynx, esophagus, oral cavity, bladder
Radiation	probably all sites
Occupational exposures	Nasal sinus, bladder, liver, lung, leukemia
Medical drugs	Leukemia, bladder cancer

The quantification of carcinogenic risk from epidemiological data poses unique problems for each one of these groups. In the case of tobacco smoking, many large studies have been carried out. However, tobacco smoke contains many carcinogens, at levels which vary according to the type of cigarette, and individuals smoke in different ways, all of which could affect exposure levels (IARC, 1986). It is possible to infer important information about temporal patterns of risk (Doll, 1971), but dose-response studies are generally limited to estimation of the risk per number of cigarettes smoked. Similar problems apply for tobacco chewing and alcohol consumption. In the latter case grams of ethanol per day is used to quantify exposure, but it may only be a surrogate for other components of the alcoholic beverage (Tuyns et al., 1977)

The level of occupational exposure can be quantified by environmental sampling. However, the samples obtained may not well reflect the exposures which took place in the past, and in particular during the period which is relevant to the cancer cases under study. Furthermore, in many studies, the major risk is confined to a subgroup of employees within a small number of plants or job categories. Thus while many agents to which workplace exposure has occurred are very potent carcinogens, such as vinyl chloride, BCME, and benzidine, quantification of their effect is still limited by these factors. One exception is asbestos, for which cancer risk in a large number of workers has been studied. Nevertheless, attempts to quantitatively model the effect of exposure are still complicated by poor exposure data, and the possibility that asbestos fibres remain in the lungs for long periods during which they can exert a carcinogenic effect (Peto, 1979).

Exposure to high doses of radiation has occurred in a variety of settings, of which the most important have been occupational, therapeutic, and military. In the latter two cases, where exposure is for a relatively short time period, accurate estimates of dose can be constructed. Studies of the effects of radiation provide perhaps the most comprehensive effort in quantitative risk estimation of carcinogenicity (BEIR, 1980). However, it is not clear how far the quantitative features of radiation carcinogenesis apply to chemical exposures, for which the route of exposure, metabolism, and other physiological factors can all play a role in modifying exposure levels and hence effect.

Among chemical exposures, this leaves the group of carcinogenic medical drugs as potentially the most suitable for quantitative risk evaluation. They are given to individuals at carefully measured doses, and in many cases metabolic and pharmacokinetic pathways have been well studied. Patients often undergo long follow-up and clinical evaluation, and long-term effects of therapy, such as cancer, are naturally an important observation.

The drugs which cause cancer can do so in a variety of ways. Some, such as estrogens used in post-menopausal replacement therapy (Jick et al., 1979), are purely hormonal with an unclear pathway to cancer while others, including azathioprine (Kinlen et al., 1979), used in organ transplants, act as immunosupressors, possibly allowing viral agents to transform the cells. For a number of anticancer agents which react directly with cellular DNA by alkylation (Connors, 1987), it is likely that the carcinogenic mechanism is via mutations induced in cells which survive the cytotoxic action of the drugs. Alkylating drugs appear to be primarily leukemogens (Penn, 1987), although some studies suggest that they can induce tumours at other sites (Tucker et al., 1987).

Quantitative analysis of epidemiological data is important both to improve understanding of the effects of exposures such as those in Table 1, but it must also play a fundamental role in the validation of other means of assessing cancer risk. If our goal is the prediction of risk before exposure occurs, or at least before harm can be observed, we must utilize sources of data other than epidemiological studies, such as animal experiments and short-term tests, combined with whatever human data is available as metabolic and other parameters. However, these sources are ultimately meaningless unless they can be validated against human observation.

In this paper we review published studies on leukemia following alkylating agent therapy for cancers, and summarize the quantitative findings. We then examine the extent to which apparent differences in leukemogenic potency can be attributed to known chemical and biochemical differences among the agents.

LEUKEMIA FOLLOWING CANCER THERAPY

It is now well recognized that a number of the alkylating agents used in the therapy of Hodgkin's disease, ovarian cancer, breast cancer and other malignancies are capable of inducing leukemia several years after treatment. There has been a large number of publications on this subject, but for the moment, only a limited number provide information which could be useful in quantifying the leukemogenic potential of the drugs. In order to do this, it is necessary to formulate an index of potency. For animal carcinogenicity experiments, the TD50, or the dose required to reduce by half the probability of remaining tumour free under a lifetime daily exposure to the test chemicals, has been proposed for this purpose (Peto et al., 1984). In a review of data from the studies in which leukemia incidence was reported for groups of patients who had all received the same single alkylating agent (Kaldor et al., 1988), we proposed an index analogous to the TD50. In fact, the TD50 is simply proportional to the inverse of the slope of the dose-response curve, under the assumption that this curve is linear. In the case of the human leukemia data, there is very little information on the shape of the dose-response curve. If linearity is a valid assumption, and the incidence is constant following exposure, an approximate estimate of the slope would be obtained by subtracting the background incidence of leukemia from the incidence following treatment and dividing by the average dose received in the group of patients under study. In other words, if we believe that Incidence = Background + Slope . dose, a crude estimate of slope is (Incidence - background)/average dose. In practice, the background incidence is so low compared to that in the patient group that it can be ignored. Table 2 gives the result of this calculation for a number of drugs used in cancer therapy. The data come from published studies in which leukemia incidence following treatment with a single alkylating agent was reported (Kaldor et al., 1988). The comparison represented by this table does not take into account several potentially important factors, such as differing age- and sex-composition of the groups reported on, or the possible effect of the first cancer or other therapy such as radiation and non-alkylating agents, on the risk of leukemia. Furthermore,

it requires the assumption that excess leukemia incidence occurs uniformly
following chemotherapy. However, it is clear from the table that there is
an appreciable range in the leukemogenic potency of these drugs, per unit
dose. Melphalan appears to be two orders of magnitude more powerful than
cyclophosphamide, based on administered dose levels. For several of the
drugs in table 2, TD50's have been estimated from carcinogenesis experiments in rats and mice (Gold et al., 1984), and Figure 1 shows the correlation between the TD50's for rats and the human leukemia potency estimate.
The solid bars are potency estimates based on all tumours in the animal
experiment, and the dashes are based on tumours of the hematopoietic system
only. Error bars have not been estimated for the human potency indices,
because of the unquantifiable uncertainties involved. Although the numbers
of drugs with data in common are few, one can see a correlation for the
three related nitrogen mustard compounds, chlorambucil, melphalan and
cyclophosphamide. Neither actinomycin D nor methotrexate is an alkylating
agent, but actinomycin is nevertheless a strong rat carcinogen, based on
experiments in which the route of administration was via intraperitoneal
injection.

CHEMICAL AND BIOCHEMICAL DIFFERENCES AMONG LEUKEMOGENIC DRUGS

Although a great deal of information has been accumulated on various
biological parameters associated with anticancer drugs, in an attempt to
understand and improve their therapeutic activity, many chemotherapeutic
drugs and treatments have been successfully developed with relatively
limited knowledge of therapeutic structure activity relationships. The
amount of information on mechanisms of leukemogenicity, an unwanted side-
effect, is even more limited. Nevertheless, there are studies of chemical
and biochemical characteristics of individual compounds which may provide
some insight into the differences in leukemogenic potency suggested by
Table 2.

The crudest way to compare the alkylating activity of different
chemicals is via the use of a common parameter such as the Epstein test
(e.g. Hemminki et al., 1983), in which 4-(4-nitrobenzyl) pyridine is mixed
with the test compound to give a coloured product indicating the degree of
total alkylation, which is quantifiable by spectroscopy. This test however
does not discriminate between different alkylating species and cannot
detect such subtleties as cross-linking activity. Most alkylating agents
used as anticancer drugs are directly active, being able to react with DNA
without further metabolic activation. There are, however, exceptions, such
as cyclophosphamide, which requires metabolic activation via 4-hydroxyla-
tion to generate the presumed active intermediate, phosphoramide mustard.

Nitrogen mustard (chloromethine hydrochloride), chlorambucil, melphalan and cyclophosphamide are structurally related drugs, each containing
a so-called nitrogen mustard group. However, even closely related drugs
which give rise to qualitatively and quantitatively similar amounts of DNA
modifications may show profound differences with respect to reaction kinetics. For example, although an important route of DNA alkylation by nitrogen mustards is via the N-7 position of guanine, phosphoramide mustard
reacts much more slowly by this pathway than does either chlorambucil or
nitrogen mustard (Hemminki & Kallama, 1986).

Table 2. Carcinogenicity of Antineoplastic Drugs in Humans: Leukemia in Cancer Survivors

Drug	Number of cases of leukemia observed	Time period (years) for incidence	Cumulative incidence (%)	Mean (or median) total dose (g)	Potency index (10-year incidence per gram total dose)	Reference
Busulfan	4	8	3.3	3.2	1.3	Stott et al., 1977
Chlorambucil						
(1)	16	8	25	7.5	4.2	Berk et al., 1981
(2)	2	7	5.7	4.4[a]	1.8	Greene et al., 1982
Cyclophosphamide	3	10	5.4	19.5	0.28	Greene et al., 1986
Melphalan						
(1)	21	10	11.2	0.60	18.7	Greene et al., 1986
(2)	34	10	1.7	0.52	3.3	Fisher et al., 1985
Treosulphan	8	5	7.6	140	0.11	Pedersen-Bjerregaard et al., 1982
Semustine	14	6	4.0	1.6[a]	4.2	Boice et al., 1983
Actinomycin D	0	9+	0.0	0.008	–	Trapido, personal communication
Methotrexate	0	10+	0.0	0.56	–	Trapido, personal communication

[a] protocol dose

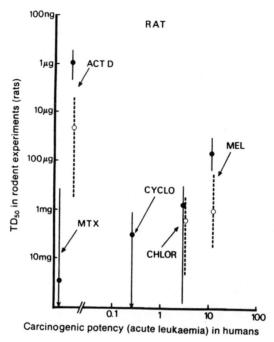

Figure 1. TD_{50}s with 99% confidence intervals for carcinogenic potency in rats (y-axis) plotted against leukemogenic potency in humans (x-axis).

_____ All tumours; – – – – hematopoietic system tumours.

Abbreviations: ACT D = actinomycin D; CHLOR = chlorambucil; CYCLO = cyclophosphamide; MEL = melphalan; MTX = methotrexate

The alkylation at N-7 of guanine is probably only one pathway by which DNA is alkylated by anticancer drugs. Alkylation at other sites in nucleic acid bases may in fact give rise to mutagenic lesions which contribute nothing or very little to the cytotoxic activity of drugs but lead to transformation and development of a second cancer. It is likely, for example, that alkylation at O^6 position of deoxyguanosine would be favoured by highly reactive, positively charged, alkylating species such as the N-2-chloroethylaziridinium intermediates common to the nitrogen mustard drugs. Such reactions may contribute less to the overall alkylation of cellular DNA, but may be more mutagenic, than the major reaction at the N-7 position, which is likely to lead to cytotoxic cross-linking.

A fundamental chemical property which may distinguish the leukemogenicity of anticancer drugs is the intrinsic reactivity of the alkylating intermediates. This property is usually characterized by the degree of "S_N1" or "S_N2" character of the intermediate. These terms refer to types of chemical reactions known respectively as unimolecular and bimolecular nucleophilic substitutions. The relevance of this concept to drug carcinogenicity is exemplified by the data shown in Table 3.

Drugs which, like methylmethanesulfonate (MMS), are almost certainly exclusively S_N2 alkylating agents (e.g. busulfan and treosulphan) are among the less potent leukemogens and this is consistent with current hypotheses suggesting that S_N2 activity is associated with weak carcinogenicity. In contrast S_N1 reagents, such as methylnitrosourea (MNU), are highly reactive and are likely to form potentially mutagenic adducts. Thus, not surprisingly, the nitrosourea semustine (MeCCNU, Tables 2 and 3), which has been used in cancer therapy, is quite potent as a leukemogen.

Recent studies have also shown that the non-alkylating moiety attached to the chloroethylaziridinium group derived from different nitrogen mustard containing drugs can strongly influence sequence selectivity of alkylation at N-7 of guanine (Kohn et al., 1987).

DISCUSSION

This review has focussed almost entirely on the chemical differences between alkylating anticancer drugs, and possible explanations for their difference in leukemogenic potency. It is clear that differences in absorption, distribution and cell membrane transport as well as metabolic effects must also play a role in the ability of a drug to exert cytotoxic and carcinogenic activity. However, since cellular DNA is the presumed target of these drugs, a knowledge of the nature of the different DNA reactions is fundamental to a better understanding of their mechanism of action.

Much more work is needed both on the DNA adducts formed by alkylating agents, and the pharmacokinetic and metabolic parameters of these drugs. Of particular importance is the amount of active metabolites which is distributed to the bone marrow, presumably the target of leukemogenesis. With full information of this kind, it should be possible to build up a model which relates administered dose to leukemia risk, at least for agents of simular structure such as the nitrogen mustards, and possibly for all alkylating anticancer agents.

Table 3. Examples and characteristics of S_N1 and S_N2 type alkylating agents.

Type of alkylating activity	S_N1	S_N2
Representative model carcinogen	$\overset{O}{\overset{\|}{H_2NCNCH_3}}$ with NO on N (NMU)	$CH_3O\overset{O}{\underset{O}{\overset{\|}{\underset{\|}{S}}}}CH_3$ (MMS)
Major sites of alkylation by model carcinogen[a]	Putative mutagenic lesion: O^6dG Other lesions: N^7dG, N^3dA	N^7dG, N^3dA
Leukemogenic drug of similar structure	$CH_3\langle\rangle{-}\overset{O}{\overset{\|}{NCNCH_2CH_2Cl}}$ with $\overset{H}{\underset{NO}{\|}}$ (MeCCNU)	$OH_3\overset{O}{\underset{O}{\overset{\|}{\underset{\|}{S}}}}O(CH_2)_4O\overset{O}{\underset{O}{\overset{\|}{\underset{\|}{S}}}}CH_3$ (Busulphan)

[a]From Margison and O'Connor, 1979

The anticancer drugs also provide the opportunity to quantify other aspects of carcinogenesis, such as variation in individual susceptibility. For example, by measuring DNA adducts following therapy in a large group of patients, and carrying out a long-term follow-up of the group, it should be possible to determine both whether there are inter-individual differences in the extent of adduct formation, and secondly, whether these differences are predictions of leukemia risk.

This review has emphasized the value of studying anticancer drug carcinogenicity as a model for quantitative risk estimation. However, it must always be kept in mind that the ultimate goal in quantifying risk is its reduction. For cancer patients, this means reducing the long-term hazards of chemotherapy as far as possible while maintaining therapeutic efficacy.

REFERENCES

BEIR, 1980, "The Effects on Populations of Exposure to Low Levels of
    Ionizing Radiation", Committee on the Biological Effects of Ionizing
    Radiation (BEIR III), National Academy of Sciences, Washington, D.C.
Berk, P. D., Goldberg, J. D., Silverstein, M. N., Weinfeld, A., Donovan,
    P. B., Ellis, J. T., Landaw, S. A., Laszlo, J., Najean, Y., Pisciotta,
    A. V., and Wasserman, L. R., 1981, Increased incidence of acute
    leukemia in polycythemia vera associated with chlorambucil therapy.
    New Engl. J. Med.. 304:441.
Boice, J. D., Greene, M. H., Killen, J. Y., Ellenberg, S. S., Keehn, R. J.,
    McFadden, E., Chen, T., and Fraumeni, J. F., 1983, Leukemia and
    preleukemia after adjuvant treatment of gastrointestinal cancer with
    semustine (methyl-CCNU). New Engl. J. Med., 309:1079.
Connors, T. A., 1987, Antitumor alkylating agents: cytotoxic actin and
    organ toxicity, in: Carcinogenicity of alkylating cytostatic drugs,
    (IARC Scientific Publications No 78)", D. Schmähl, and J. M. Kaldor,
    eds., International Agency for Research on Cancer, Lyon.
Doll, R., 1971, The age distribution of cancer: implications for models of
    carcinogenesis (with Discussion), J. Roy. Stat. Soc., 134:133.
Fisher, B., Rockette, H., Fisher, E. R., Wickerham, L., Redmond, C., and
    Brown, A., 1985, Leukemia in breast cancer patients following adjuvant
    chemotherapy or postoperative radiation: the NSAPB experience. J.
    clin. Oncol., 3:1640.
Gold, L. S., Sawyer, C. B., Magaw, R., Backman, G. M., de Veciana, M.,
    Levinson, R., Hooper, N. K., Havender, W. R., Bernstein, L., Peto, R.,
    Pike, M.C., and Ames, B. N., 1984, A carcinogenic potency database of
    the standardized results of animal bioassay. Environ Health Perspect.,
    58:9.
Greene, M. H., Boice, J. D., Greer, B. E., Blessin, J. A., and Dembo, A.
    J., 1982, Acute nonlymphocytic leukemia after therapy with alkylating
    agents for ovarian cancer – a study of five randomized trials. New
    Engl. J. Med., 307:1416.
Greene, M. H., Harris, E. L., Gershenson, D. M., Malkasian, G. D., Melton,
    L. J., Dembo, A. J., Bennett, J. M., Moloney, W. R., and Boice, J. D.,
    1986, Melphalan may be a more potent leukemogen than is cyclophospha-
    mide. Ann. intern. Med., 105:360.
Hemminki, K., Kallama, S., and Falck, K., 1983, Correlations of alkylating
    activity and mutagenicity in bacteria of cytostatic drugs, Acta
    Pharmacol. Toxicol., 53:421.
Hemminki, K., and Kallama, S., 1986, Reactions on nitrogen mustards with
    DNA, in: "Carcinogenicty of Alkylating Cytostatic Drugs (IARC
    Scientific Publications No 78)", D. Schmähl, and J. M. Kaldor, eds,
    International Agency for Research on Cancer, Lyon
IARC, 1986, "Monographs on the Evaluation of the Carcinogenic Risk of
    Chemicals to Humans, Vol. 38, Tobacco smoking", International Agency
    for Research on Cancer, Lyon
IARC, 1988, "Monographs on the Evaluation of the Carcinogenic Risk of
    Chemicals to Humans, Supplement No 7, Overall evaluations of
    carcinogenicity: An update of IARC Monographs Volumes 1-42",
    International Agency for Research on Cancer, Lyon.
Jick, H., Watkins, R. N., Hunter, J. R., Dinan, B. J., Madsen, S., Rothman,
    K. J., and Walker, A. M., 1979, Replacement estrogens and endometrial
    cancer. New Engl. J. Med., 300:218.

Kaldor, J. M., Day, N. E., and Hemminki, K., 1988, Quantifying the carcinogenicity of antineoplastic drugs. Eur. J. Cancer Clin. Oncol., 24:703.

Kinlen, L. J., Sheil, A. G. R., Peto, J., and Doll, R., 1979, Collaborative United Kingdom-Australasian study of cancer in patients treated with immunosuppressive drugs. Br. Med. J., 2:1461.

Kohn, K. W., Hartley, J. A., and Mattes, W. B., 1987, Mechanisms of DNA sequence selective alkylation of guanine-N7 positions by nitrogen mustards. Nucl. Acids Res., 15:10531.

Margison, G. P., and O'Connor, P. J., 1979, Nucleic acid modification by N-nitroso compounds, in: "Chemical carcinogens and DNA, Vol. I", P. L. Grover, ed., CRC Press, Boca Raton, Florida

Pedersen-Bjergaard, J., Nissen, N. I., Sørensen, H. M., Hou-Jensen, K., Larson, M. S., Ernst, P., Ersbøl, J., Knudtzon, S., and Rose, C., 1982, Acute non-lymphocytic leukemia in patients with ovarian carcinoma following long-term treatment with treosulfan (=dihydroxybusulfan). Cancer, 45:19.

Penn, I., 1987, Malignancies induced by drugs therapy: a review, in: Carcinogenicity of alkylating cytostatic drugs, (IARC Scientific Publications No 78)", D. Schmähl, and J. M. Kaldor, eds., International Agency for Research on Cancer, Lyon.

Peto, J., 1979, Dose response relationships for asbestos related disease: Implications for hygiene standards. II. Mortality. Ann. NY Acad. Sci., 330:195

Peto, R., Pike, M. C., Bernstein, L., Gold, L. S., and Ames, B. N., 1984, The TD_{50}: a proposed general convention for the numerical description of the carcinogenic potency of chemicals in chronic exposure animal experiments. Environ. Health Perspect., 58:1.

Stott, H., Fox, W., Girling, D. J., Stephens, R.J., and Galton, D. A. G, 1977, Acute leukaemia after busulphan. Br. med. J., 2:1513.

Tucker, M. A., Coleman, C. N., Cox, R.S., Varghese, A., Rosenberg, S. A., 1987, Risk of second cancers after treatment for Hodgkin's disease. New Engl. J. Med., 318:76.

Tuyns, A.J., Pequignot, G., Jensen, O.M., 1977, Le cancer de l'esophage en Ille-et-Vilaine en fonction des niveaux de consommation d'alcool et de tabac. Bull. Cancer, 64:45.

CONTRIBUTORS

M. E. Anderson - Harry G. Armstrong Aerospace Medical Research
     Laboratory, Wright-Patterson AFB, OH 45433-6573

M. Asamoto - First Dept. of Pathology, Nagoya City University
     Medical School, Mizuho-cho, Mizuho-ku, Nagoya 467, Japan

K. Athanasiou - Dept. of Pharmacology, Medical School, University
     of Ioannina, GR 451 10 Ioannina, Greece

P. Bannasch - Institut fur Experimentelle Pathologie, Deutsches
     Krebsforschungszentrum, 6900 Heidelberg, (F.R.G.)

J. Bax - Department of Biological Toxicology, TN)-CIVO Toxicology
     and Nutrition Institute, 3700 AJ Zeist, The Netherlands

H. M. Bolt - Institut fur Argeitsphysiologie an der Universitat
     Dortmund, Ardeystrasse 67, D-4600 Dortmund 1, (F.R.G.)

A. Buchmann - Institut of Biochemistry, German Cancer Research
     Center, Im Neuenheimer Feld 280, 6900 heidelberg (F.R.G.)

W. Bursch -   Institute of Tumorbiology-Cancer Research,
     University of Vienna, Borschkegasse 8a, A-1090 Vienna

M. Castagna - Institut de Recherches Scientifiques sur le Cancer,
     7, rue Guy Mocquet, 94802 Villejuif Cedex, France

C. C. Chang - Michigan State University, East Lansing, MI, 48824

H. J. Clewell, III. - Harry G. Armstrong Aerospace Medical
     Research Laboratory, Wright-Patterson AFB, OH 45433-6573

S. M. Cohen - University of Nebraska Medical Center, Dept. of
     Pathology and Microbiology, Omaha, NE, 68105

B. Colombo - Division of Experimental Oncology A, Istituto
     Nazionale, Tumori, Milan, Italy

R. B. Conolly - NSI Technology Services, Corp., Dayton, OH 45431-
     1482

B. Denk - GSF, Institut fur Toxikologie, Ingolstadter Landstr. 1,
     D-8042 Neuherberg, (F.R.G.)

T. A. Dragani - Division of Experimental Oncology A, Istituto
     Nazionale Tumori, Milan, Italy

L. O. Dragsted - National Food Agency of Denmark, Institute of Toxicology, Dept. of Biochemical and Molecular Toxicology, 19 Morkhoj Bygade, Dk-2860 Soborg, Denmark

L. B. Ellwein - University of Nebraska Medical Center, Dept. of Pathology and Microbiology, Omaha, NE, 68105

M. Emura - Institut fur Experimentelle Pathologie, Medizinische Hochschule Hannover, D-3000 Hannover 61, (F.R.G.)

J. G. Filser - GSF, Institut fur Toxikologie, Ingolstadter Landstr. 1, D-8042 Neuherberg, (F.R.G.)

T. Green - ICI Central toxicology Laboratory, Alderley Park, Macclesfield, Cheshire, U.K.

G. Grimmer - Biochemisches Institut fur Umweltcarcinogen, D-2070 Grosshansdorf, (F.R.G.)

R. Hasegawa - First Dept. of Pathology, Nagoya City University Medical School, Mizuho-cho, Mizuho-ku, Nagoya 467, Japan

M. Hollstein - International Agency for Research on Cancer, 69372 Lyon cedex 08, France

K. Imaida - First Dept. of Pathology, Nagoya City University Medical School, Mizuho-cho, Mizuho-ku, Nagoya 467, Japan

N. Ito - First Dept. of Pathology, Nagoya City University Medical School Mizuho-cho, Mizuho-ku, Nagoya 467, Japan

J. Jacob - Biochemisches Institut fur Umweltcarcinogene, D-2070 Grosshansdorf, (F.R.G.)

J. M. Kaldor - International Agency for Research on Cancer, Lyon, France

W. Kessler - GSF, Institut fur Toxikologie, Ingolstadter Landstr. 1, D-8042 Neuherberg, (F.R.G.)

W. Kunz - Institut of Biochemistry, German Cancer Research Center, Im Neuenheimer Feld 280, 6900 Heidelberg (F.R.G.)

R. J. Laib - Institut fur Arbeitsphysiologie an der, Universitat Dortmund, Ardeystrasse 67, D-4600 Dortmund 1, (F.R.G.)

M. Lechner - Laboratory of Biochemistry, Instituto Gulbenkian de Ciencia, Oeiras, Portugal

G. Manenti - Division of Experimental Oncology A, Istituto Nazionale Tumori, Milan, Italy

M. Marselos - Dept. of Pharmacology, Medical School, University of Ioannina, GR 451 10 Ioannina, Greece

I. Martelly - Institut de Recherches Scientifiques sur le Cancer, 7, rue Guy Mocquet, 94802 Villejuif Cedex, France

U. Mohr - Institut fur Experimentelle Pathologie, Medizinische Hochschule Hannover, D-3000 Hannover 61, (F.R.G.)

S. Moolgavkar - Fred Hutchinson Cancer Research Center, Seattle, WA, 98104

W. Parzefall - Institute of Tumorbiology-Cancer Research, University of Vienna, Borschkegasse 8a, A-1090 Vienna

D. Pearson - Institut of Biochemistry, German Cancer Research Center, Im Neuenheimer Feld 280, 6900 Heidelberg (F.R.G.)

G. D. Porta - Division of Experimental Oncology A, Istituto Nazionale Tumori, Milan, Italy

R. H. Reitz - Mammalian and Environmental Toxicology, Dow Chemical Company, Midland, MI 48674-1803

M. Riebe -Institute fur Experimentelle Pathologie, Medizinische Hochschule Hannover, D-3000 Hannover 61, (F.R.G.)

M. R. M. Sacchi - Division of Experimental Oncology A, Istituto Nazionale Tumori, Milan, Italy

E. Scherer - Division of Chemical Carcinogenesis, The Netherlands Cancer Institute, 121 Plesmanlaan, 1066 CX Amsterdam, The Netherlands

M. Schwarz - Institut of Biochemistry, German Cancer Research Center, Im Neuenheimer Feld 280, 6900 Heidelberg (R.R.G.)

R. Schulte-Herman - Institute of Tumorbiology-Cancer Research, University of Vienna, Borschkegasse 8a, A-1090 Vienna

D. E. G. Shuker - International Agency for Research on Cancer, Lyon, France

M. Straub - Institut fur Experimentelle Pathologie, Medizinische Hochschule Hannover, D-3000 61, (F.R.G.)

M. Tatematsu - First Dept. of Pathology, Nagoya City University Medical School, Mizuho-cho, Mizuho-ku, Nagoya 467, Japan

P. Tautu - German Cancer Research Centre, Institute of Epidemiology and Biometry, Dept. of Mathematical Models, D-6900 Heidelberg, INF 280

C. C. Travis - Office of Risk Analysis, Oak Ridge National Laboratory, Oak Ridge, TN 37831-6109

I. Timmermann-Trosiener - Institute of Tumorbiology-Cancer Research, University of Vienna, Borschkegasse 8a, A-1090 Vienna

J. E. Trosko - Michigan State University, East Lansing, MI 48824

H. Tsuda - First Dept. of Pathology, Nagoya City Unviersity Medical School, Mizuho-cho, Mizuho-ku, Nagoya 467, Japan

V. Vasiliou - Dept. of Pharmacology, Medical School, University of Ioannina, GR 451 10 - Ioannina, Greece

J. Wen - Institut fur Experimentelle Pathologie, Medizinische Hochschule Hannover, D-3000 Hannover 61, (F.R.G.)

J. Wilson - Monsanto Company, St. Louis, MO

R. A. Woutersen - Department of Biological Toxicology, TNO-CIVO Toxicology and Nutrition Institute, 3700 AJ Zeist, The Netherlands

H. Yamaskai - International Agency for Research on Cancer, 69372 Lyon cedex 08, France

INDEX